The twelve who survive

The twelve who survive

Strengthening programmes of early childhood development in the Third World

Robert Myers
Second edition

HIGH/SCOPE PRESS
Ypsilanti, Michigan

Published by
HIGH/SCOPE PRESS

A division of
High/Scope Educational Research Foundation
600 North River Street
Ypsilanti, Michigan 48198-2898
313/485-2000, FAX 313/485-0704

First published in 1992 in the USA and Canada
by Routledge
11 New Fetter Lane, London EC4P 4EE

A division of Routledge, Chapman and Hall Inc.
29 West 35th Street, New York, NY 10001

Library of Congress Cataloging-in-Publication Data
Myers, Robert G.
    The twelve who survive: strengthening programmes of early childhood
development in the Third World/Robert Myers.—2nd ed.
        p. cm.
    Includes bibliographical references (p.   ) and index.
    ISBN 0-929816-99-4
    1. Child welfare—Developing countries. 2. Child development—
Developing countries. 3. Children—Health and hygiene—Developing
countries. I. Title.
    HV804.M94 1995
362.7' 09172'4—dc20   95-31582
                                                            CIP

Printed in the United States of America

To Mother

My first and best teacher

Her subject:

the art of giving
and of living
simply,
with people
and nature
and books,

in harmony
and with faith
in a better world

Contents

Tables, figures and illustrations

TABLES

FIGURES

ILLUSTRATIONS

Note: All photographs were taken by the author, with the exception of 'Katie's world' which was taken by Melanie Matero.

Foreword

Urie Bronfenbrenner

This is a remarkable book. It takes the reader to the great, unknown continents of childhood, where most of the world's children live, and die before their time – Africa, Asia, and Latin America. Yet the story is not one of despair, but rather of the resilience of children themselves, and of the healing and revitalizing power of what, surely, given their ever-so-modest resources, are among the most powerful and cost-effective human service programmes now in existence.

Nor does the volume speak only to what we somewhat speciously refer to as the 'developing' world (thus conveniently dismissing it from both our consciousness and our conscience). For the same forces that diminish and distort the development of millions of children in the Third World are today undermining the future competence and character of increasing thousands of children in the so-called 'developed' nations, especially in the United States, where today one-quarter of all children are living below the poverty line (a standard based primarily on nutritional requirements). Moreover, the most effective strategies for counteracting this developmentally destructive downward trend are based on the same principles and practices that have been incorporated in the programmes so vividly described in this volume.

How does it happen that the same strategies should be optimally applicable in such diverse domains of geography and culture? The answer is to be found in a communality of cause and cure. Today we acknowledge that the massive alteration of the natural environment produced by modern technology and industrialization can destroy the ecosystem essential to life itself. We are now only beginning to recognize that this same awesome process has its analogue in the social realm as well, that the disruptive and immobilizing onslaughts of unemployment, urbanization, bureaucratization, and the frequent dislocations and growing chaos of everyday life are undermining the basic institutions that create and sustain the development of human competence and character from childhood onward. Those institutions, of course, are the family, the school, and the community.

It is precisely these three structures that form the pillars of the 'programmes that work' which come to life in this book. The programmes in turn rest on a firm foundation wrought by an ingenious fusion of scientific concepts and findings with practical experience from the field in dozens of countries across the developing world. At the foundation's centre are the results of contemporary research revealing the key processes and conditions underlying children's development.

The first of these discoveries is that the processes are *interactive*; development occurs primarily not as the result of stimulation from the outside but through the active engagement of a growing organism with its immediate environment in two domains: with other people, and – initially through them but then on its own – with objects and symbols that invite exploration, manipulation, elaboration, imagination. Characteristic of the author's masterful blend of theory with practice, the text provides a 'cognitive kit' of a rich array of developmentally instigative activities that mothers, relatives, caregivers, older children, and other members of the community can, and as documented in this volume, actually *do* carry out with young children in a wide range of quite different cultures.

And herein we encounter a second key principle that explains both how such activities are best discovered and which ones are most effective. Moreover, the principle goes far beyond these specific domains to permeate the programmes in their entirety; namely, the programme elements build on, or are adapted to, the *values and customs* of the culture in which the children and their families live or have their roots.

In a third principle, the research findings challenge the prevailing fashion in science itself, for most of today's developmental researchers are organized into separate camps, each specializing in a different aspect of human functioning – physiological, cognitive, emotional, and social. Yet, as Myers emphasizes over and over, once the findings from these domains are related to each other, they reveal that development is quintessentially *multidimensional* – that processes in each of these spheres are interrelated and reinforce each other. And, as he once again moves briskly from theory to practice, Myers points to the same paradox in the design and operation of many programmes that seek to serve what he refers to as a 'piecemeal child'. He then marshals that evidence, both from research and field experience, to demonstrate that the most effective programmes are those that are multifaceted in both structure and function. An example of special relevance and impact in the Third World now speaks also to our own.

There is a two-way interactive relationship between psychological well-being and health and nutritional status. That synergistic relationship is evident in the results of research cutting across a broad spectrum of scientific disciplines. Accordingly, health, nutrition, and psychological well-being should be approached together, whether the principal goal of the programme is survival or social or intellectual, or emotional development.

(p. 198)

Yet another principle that, in our contemporary world, has crossed earlier borders of culture and class, stresses *the necessity of stability and predictability* in the lives of children and those committed to their care. The interactive processes that produce and sustain development take time to become 'revved up' and they remain effective only if they are conducted on a regular basis, in similar circumstances, over an extended period in the child's life.

Having made these points, Myers then thoughtfully provides, for those who may have need of a 'users' handbook', descriptions of an astounding variety of settings across the world that meet these specifications and could be selected and adapted for other locations.

But such expansion of the child's world must not wait upon the emergence of new capacities. In the domain of policy and programmes, perhaps the most distinctive principle that Myers exposes and applies is the essentiality of *linkages*, the creation and strengthening of ties not only between the settings in which the child lives – such as home, child care, neighbourhood, and school – but also in the world of his parents. Particularly important in this regard is the parents' workplace as defined by space, time, and the activities in which they engage. All of these must be, and are, integrated into the programmes that are most effective.

The ultimate link in this dynamic system, and the one from which the programmes derive their greatest stability and thrust, is the community as a whole. Operationally this means that, to be effective, programmes require and achieve participation from all segments of the community across the often divided – and even divisive – domains of age, gender, class, and caste. A worthy goal, you will say, but seldom attainable. Yet the many examples in this book turn 'seldom' into 'often' and illustrate dozens of strategies through which the transformation is accomplished. The reality, and drama, of this phenomenon give the volume an appeal and importance to a wide circle of readers well beyond those most directly concerned in the helping professions.

There is yet a final principle that pervades all the rest, a primary *focus on strengths*, as opposed to deficiencies and defects, the strengths that are still to be found, even under the most horrible conditions, within the children themselves, but also within their families, neighbourhoods, and – perhaps above all – within their cultures. These are the vantage points from which it becomes possible to counteract, and even to reverse, the processes of developmental disruption and disarray.

To be sure, one question remains that is not fully confronted. Where is one to find the resources and resolve to set all these constructive processes in motion, and to sustain them after the initial period of enthusiasm and typically more generous funding has passed? Up until now, such efforts in the Third World have been supported primarily by contributions, both in money and personnel, from public and private sources in the developed countries, with the principal appeal and motivation grounded in humanitarian concerns. It is with such an appeal that Myers ends the volume in his 'call to action'.

But today there are new actors, driven by different motives, who are coming on the scene. The new element in the picture is the increasing recognition and concern on the part of national leaders worldwide – both in the public and, especially, in the private sector – with respect to two rapidly escalating economic problems. The first is the enormous cost of providing for or, alternatively and more frequently, neglecting the growing segments in national populations of so-called 'uneducables' and 'unemployables'. The second relates to the quality and dependability of the available work force in an age of increasing economic competition not only among developed but also developing nations.

The new mounting concern and watchword among those who occupy the seats of power is the preservation and rebuilding of what is now being called *human capital.* But can such 'extrinsic' motivations produce policies and programmes that still have a human face? Between the lines of this multifaceted work there lies an unspoken yet eloquent answer to this crucial question. In a key section, Myers outlines three models for bringing about community development. The first is 'imposed development', in which the initiative, expertise, and leadership are brought in from the outside. The result?

> In this, a specific problem may be solved, but without participation, except in the most superficial sense. And nothing will have been done to build a sense of 'community' in the process.
>
> (p. 319)

In a second model, which Myers calls 'self-actualized development', the community takes initiative on its own, using its own resources. On the basis of the available evidence, Myers offers the following evaluation.

> This second approach to identifying and acting upon problems is easier to talk about than to realize. It tends towards the romantic. If a sense of community does not already exist ... it may be necessary to look to outsiders as participants in at least the initial stages of discovery and community building. Moreover, very few communities are able to find within themselves all the human and material resources they need.
>
> (p. 319)

Myers' third model, and strategy of choice, which he calls 'partnership', is described as one in which communities work together 'with' institutions from the larger society to solve common problems.... Partnership implies mutual respect and equality and a sharing of responsibility for both successes and failures.

(p. 319)

It is in this partnership model that the answer to the critical question lies. The model appears again and again in the programme biographies documented in the pages that follow, and what one learns is that partnership is not something that is there at the beginning. The process starts with hope, but also with many doubts and divisions, and it is through participation that partnership is gradually achieved. And with each step comes new hope, new commitment, new accomplishment, and no small measure of human joy. Especially noteworthy is the fact that, in a number of the programmes, the sponsoring agencies get caught up in the momentum and begin to act as committed partners in the enterprise. As this happens, their own original priorities become reordered and redefined.

To be sure, such phenomena are still to be systematically documented and assessed, but there can be little doubt that they occur. To paraphrase Lord Acton, it would appear that not only power, but also virtue can corrupt to its own ends, albeit perhaps not 'absolutely'. It would be a fitting paradox if the pragmatic effort to protect and increase human capital were to pay its dividends not only in economic growth but also in the achievement of a more humane community for children and families both abroad and at home.

This fine volume takes us on that path, but we still have many miles to go.

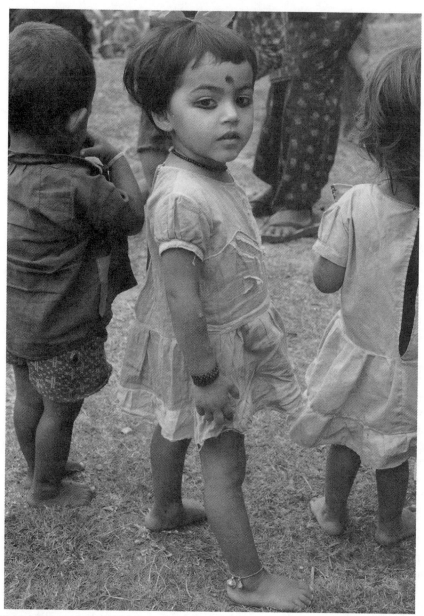

'Pride', Hill country, Nepal

Author's note

Child care and the social, intellectual, and physical development of infants and young children, especially in the so-called 'Third World', are the main concerns of this book. At issue is the well-being and development of children in Nepal and Nigeria and Nicaragua and elsewhere who are managing to survive in spite of being born into poverty, and living in life-threatening conditions. These young survivors are increasing in number. They are found in all parts of the globe. In their survival they are at the same time a delight, a hope for the future, and a daily problem for poor families struggling at the margin to survive.

At least 12 of every 13 children born (92 per cent) in 1991 will live to see their first birthday. When that survival statistic is compared with the 1960 figure of 5 for every 6 children born (83 per cent), it is clear that an important advance has been made in child survival over the three decades. Projections for the year 2000 show that 19 of 20 children born (95 per cent) are expected to survive to age one. Still, many international organizations and some governments continue to place almost exclusive emphasis in their programming for children on further reducing mortality, with little attention to the healthy development and general welfare of the survivors.

What will happen to 'the twelve who survive'? Many of the same conditions of poverty and stress that previously put children at risk to die now put them at risk of impaired physical, mental, social and emotional development in their earliest months and years. Delayed or debilitated development in the early years can affect all of later life. It can also be prevented. And, because children are amazingly resilient, it can be overcome. But overcoming early difficulties is not only inefficient, it requires greater commitment than most people in privileged positions have been willing to give, up to now. As a result, millions of children will be deprived of their right to healthy and normal development. They will fail to live up to their potential and will be further thwarted in their attempt to escape from the persistent cycle of poverty. Many of the survivors will lead lethargic, unproductive, unrewarding, and dependent lives.

As more infants survive, and as social change accelerates, a moral and social imperative grows. We must respond to the question, 'survival for what?' The obligation mounts to anticipate which children are likely to be debilitated and delayed in their social and intellectual development, and to do all in our power to prevent that from happening. In so doing, we will also be increasing the chance of survival to age five and beyond, for these disadvantaged survivors to age one are also the children who will be more likely to die before age five. Who is caring for these children? How is that care given? What is their early life like? What can be done to enhance their growth and development and to help them not only to survive, but also to realize their individual and social potential?

This book is a call to re-examine policies and approaches to enhancing early childhood care and development. It is a call for increased support to programmes that will improve the care and development of young children living in poverty. In making that call, my purpose is not to argue against trying to save lives. That would be foolish as well as inhumane. *To the contrary, I will argue that increased attention to a child's creative and coping potential and to social and emotional well-being can help to increase the survival rate, even as it enhances the quality of life.* That is so because a child's development, growth, and the struggle to survive are simultaneous, inseparable, and mutually reinforcing processes. We must, therefore, support combined programmes of child survival *and* child development.

Why is it that child survival seems to attract so much more attention than child development? One reason is certainly that starvation and death attract attention, provoking an immediate, almost visceral humanitarian response. Skeletal children whose hollow unfocused eyes peer from the cover of *Time* magazine prick the conscience of the privileged who not only live, but live reasonably well. Death and third-degree malnutrition are good fundraisers, at least in the short run, as famine in Ethiopia and elsewhere has shown. And well they should be. But how can the problems of delayed development, and their widespread social consequences, be made equally vivid?

Less dramatic, but still capable of attracting attention, are poster images of a dirty and unkempt but pretty girl, aged four, who pleads silently with mournful penetrating gaze for fostering support through one or another international organization. Those eyes symbolize the daily struggle for a better life by children who have managed to survive.

In writing this book about child development programmes there is a temptation to seek attention by using as a central image the picture of a young girl with mournful eyes. But this is not, first and foremost, a photo essay, and my approach must be different. My task is to convince with words, with facts, and examples, incorporated into a reasoned, and reasonable, argument. My audience is not 'the public' but is, rather, the group of individuals who can have a more immediate influence on policy and programming for early childhood care and development. That audience includes people in national governments as well as in non-governmental and international organizations concerned with the growth and development of young children. It includes researchers, academicians and practitioners. It includes medical doctors, nutritionists, and preschool teachers. It includes staff of women's ministries and organizations which, while focusing on the productive role of women, must also be concerned with child care and development.

Moreover, my approach is not mournful. Indeed, I would like readers to keep before them another image. Next to the picture of a child who is sad and depressed and inactive, imagine another picture – of the same child, now with a smile. This is a child who can dream, who comes from a rich cultural heritage, and who is capable of helping herself, if only given a chance, despite the ravages of poverty and accompanying health and nutritional problems. Unfortunately, this image of a smiling child comes and goes and is not as sharp as it should be. It needs to be brought into focus.

The image of a smiling child helps avoid writing or thinking about programmes only, or primarily, as social welfare efforts directed towards 'the unfortunate poor'. Instead, we are reminded that there are strengths that can serve as positive starting points in almost all environments – strengths which can be reinforced, even as new elements are added. The image symbolizes also the view that children can be active partners in a constructive and enduring endeavour, not just passive recipients of beneficent gestures. This approach – of collaboration in constructing a meaningful future, based on valid and valued current practices – contrasts with a compensatory view of programming beginning with the identification of deficits (often defined in terms of a standard brought from outside) and then focusing on ways to overcome those deficits. My emphasis on thinking 'constructively' should not, however, be confused with a romanticized view eulogizing 'the happy poor'.

A call to support programmes of early childhood care and development that features a smile instead of beginning with a profound lament, and that is built on facts and real examples, runs the risk of being ignored. Smiles rarely suggest emergency or a need for action. And, after all, few of us are really driven by logic. Facts are a secondary concern because few, if any, political decisions are made on strictly reasoned grounds. Recognizing these risks, I will be content if this book is used to justify and advance humanitarian actions based on general decisions already made by enlightened individuals or governments or other organizations concerned with the future of children. To that end, the following pages will provide a rationale and guidelines for investing in early childhood. If, along the way, some key individuals are convinced of a need they did not previously recognize, and if they act upon that recognition, the book will have more than served its purpose.

As decreasing mortality figures suggest, the need to look beyond mere survival to programmes of early childhood care and development has become increasingly apparent. Not only are more children living, but the rapid pace of social change creates conditions which require new ways of thinking about child care and development. More women are entering the labour force. Family structures are changing. Urbanization requires some different skills from those that were imparted in the past. These trends are likely to continue and to demand action. And there is increasing evidence that early investments in development of 'the whole child' can bring improvements in the life of the child and benefits to the larger society.

Once the need to look beyond survival is accepted, the question becomes, 'what can we do?' This book makes some suggestions about what can be done to promote the physical, social, intellectual, and emotional development and well-being of those who survive. In responding to the question, I will draw heavily on reviews of programme experience as well as on the growing scientific literature providing insight into child development.

Throughout this book, several emphases and points of view will be evident:

An emphasis on policy and programming

Those readers expecting a detailed academic treatment of child survival, growth and development in this book will be disappointed. A systematic attempt will be made, however, to review literature and to weave together threads from several different disciplinary approaches to the subject and to draw guidelines for policy and programming from that exercise. In so doing, my intent is to bolster the rationale for action, placing emphasis on the many actions that can be taken *now*, given the present substantial, if somewhat dispersed, knowledge base.

In addition, emphasis will be placed on the broader lines of policy and programme implementation strategy, with much less consideration given to the programme details. This book is not a practitioners' training guide or a child development curriculum manual. Setting the details of programmes is obviously an important task which requires crucial decisions about content and organization. That is better carried out once general lines are clear. And, because the specifics of implementation will vary widely from programme to programme according to the circumstances, such details must fall outside the scope of this book.

Attending to children and families living in 'at risk' conditions

An emphasis on children who live in conditions placing them at risk of delayed or debilitated development and its attendant consequences carries with it two implications. First, the emphasis in this book is on children who are living in poverty. I am not concerned with problems of the middle or upper classes, whether they be found in India or Sweden, even though some of these children may be at risk of a distorted and unhealthy development resulting from over-indulgence or from other conditions increasingly present among 'favoured' social groups. Second, the emphasis is on prevention and on anticipating problems, rather than on waiting until they occur and trying to cure them.

Interrelatedness

Throughout the book, I will be concerned with interrelated needs, and with mutually reinforcing programming responses and outcomes. The interrelationship of programming for child survival and for child development will be stressed. Unity and interaction among the physical, mental, social, and emotional dimensions of development lie at the core of the discussion. Implications of the synergistic (interactive) relationship that exists among actions directed towards these various dimensions have not yet been fully recognized nor appreciated by programmers despite the frequent call for 'integrated' programming. Within this unitary, integral view, I will emphasize the social and intellectual and emotional dimensions of development because these seem to be the least well attended to in programmes, particularly in the very early years of childhood.

The importance of home and community

The first responsibility for care and development remains in the home, with reinforcement from the local community. For that reason, empowering caregivers and communities with the knowledge, self-confidence, and organization to provide for survival and development needs of their children receives priority among a group of complementary approaches.

Complementary rather than 'alternative' approaches

While stressing the importance of programmes focused on home and community, these two approaches will be seen as part of an overall strategy that involves also direct attention to children in centres of child care, work to strengthen institutions responsible for promoting care and development, and advocacy efforts with policymakers, programmers, professionals and others who need to be convinced of the value of integrated attention to the young child. These five approaches are seen not as alternatives, but rather as complementary options.

Considering where people are

A basic principle of this book is 'building on strengths'. Rather than advocate a 'compensatory' approach, the transfer of ready-made foreign ideas about care and development, or a single 'blueprint', for success, I will stress the importance of discovering what practices are valued and in use in particular settings, giving special attention to those local, time-tested practices that are known to bring good results. With this information, one can reinforce the positive, and avoid undermining basic values, while adding other elements, rather than simply compensate for presumed deficits – the difference between taking one's cue from a vision of a smiling face rather than a mournful one.

Participation

My emphasis on participation goes beyond that of 'community participation'. I am concerned also about the participation of the child in its own development, and about learning by doing at all levels. Behind this bias are two principles. First, active involvement with others in the process of change is good in and of itself. Second, learning through experience is a sound practice.

The chapters that follow are grouped into seven parts. The first two chapters set the stage by providing a rationale, looking at the evolution of child-care and development programmes, and describing the current configuration of care and development programmes. Special attention is given to changes occurring since 1979 when the International Year of the Child (IYC) was celebrated. A second part, consisting of three chapters, seeks to clarify key concepts, and to draw implications for programming from the literature on early childhood development. A comprehensive programming strategy is suggested combining stages of development with five complementary approaches (direct attention, education of caregivers, community development, strengthening institutions, and strengthening awareness and demand) and with several programme guidelines (emphasize children at risk, be comprehensive and participatory, adjust to varying cultural contexts, reinforce and complement local ways, and seek cost-effective solutions with the potential for reaching the largest possible number of children in need).

Part III presents a 'state of the practice', providing a range of programme options available for carrying out each of the five complementary programming approaches. Some advantages and disadvantages of each approach are given and specific examples of programmes are described briefly.

Part IV focuses on the need for, and the problems associated with, trying to combine programme elements. After a look at what it means to 'integrate' programming and programmes in the first chapter of this part, individual chapters deal with: combining programming for physical, psychological and social well-being; combining programmes of early childhood development with educational programming at the primary school level; and combining programmes of child care with actions to improve women's work and welfare.

The fifth and sixth parts treat community involvement, the importance of identifying and respecting traditional wisdom in childrearing, and issues of scale and costs. A final part sets out conclusions and recommendations.

Since I began writing this book, more than two years ago, important changes have occurred, creating a much more supportive climate for increased investment in programmes favouring early childhood care and development. Dramatic political changes at a global level, an apparent end to the cold war, talk of a reduction in military expenditures, and new proposals for relieving heavy debt burdens seem to be releasing people to think and hope about social problems and solutions in new ways. We have entered a new decade, the last of the century. Both the decade marker and the nearness of the twenty-first century have stimulated reflection and creative thought about the shape of things to come, including visions of childhood in the twenty-first century.

Three specific international events have given new visibility to the child. In November 1989, a Convention of the Rights of the Child was approved by the General Assembly of the United Nations. This Convention urges signatories to, '... insure to the maximum extent possible child survival and development' (Article 6). It also indicates that, while placing primary responsibility for a child's upbringing with parents and families, states must help parents and must 'insure the development of institutions, facilities and services for the care of children' (Article 18.2). The Convention has provided the occasion for discussions at the highest government levels around the world and the number of signatories is increasing steadily.

In March of 1990, a World Conference on Education for All, organized by UNICEF, UNESCO, the World Bank and UNDP, brought together governmental representatives from over 150 nations and representatives from more than 200 non-governmental organizations. The Declaration approved at the Conference included the following statement:

> Learning begins at birth. This calls for early childhood care and initial education. These can be provided through arrangements involving families, communities, or institutional programmes, as appropriate.
>
> (Article 5)

The Framework for Action also set as one of the targets to be considered in plans for the 1990s:

(1) Expansion of early childhood care and development activities, including family and community interventions, especially for poor, disadvantaged, and disabled children.

(Paragraph 8)

A World Summit for Children occurred in September 1990 that brought together seventy heads of state to discuss the plight of children and to commit themselves to improvements. The Summit has given additional impetus to activities under way and is opening the door to new efforts to strengthen child care and development.

Meanwhile, international organizations have begun, very slowly, to open themselves to new ways of thinking about the lives as well as the death of children. Phrases such as 'beyond survival' are beginning to seep into conversations and to appear in official documents.

These recent political and economic changes at the global level and the opening that seems to be present with respect to thinking about the care, education and development of children provides some hope for 'the twelve who survive'. But the opening remains to be filled with more than words and paper and new slogans. With that challenge in mind, and fortified by the hopeful image of a smiling, if somewhat bedraggled child, let us turn to the discussion of specific ideas about what can and should be done.

Robert Myers
March 1991
Mexico City

Acknowledgements

This book has been made possible by the support of various organizations which have, over the past six years, constituted the Consultative Group on Early Childhood Care and Development. These organizations have funded many of the concept papers and reviews drawn upon so heavily in the book. Their support has also allowed me to travel and to see programmes at first hand. It has given me the luxury of time for reflection and writing. The three principal participants in, and contributors to, the Consultative Group are the Ford Foundation (which included specific funding for the writing task), UNICEF and USAID. Other participating organizations in the Group have been: UNESCO, the International Development Research Centre, the Aga Khan Foundation, the Carnegie Corporation, the World Health Organization, the World Bank, the Rockefeller Foundation, Save the Children Federation, the International Child Development Centre, the Bernard van Leer Foundation, the Swedish International Development Agency, and the American Health Foundation.

Neither the Consultative Group activities nor this writing would have been possible without the support of the High/Scope Educational Research Foundation, and particularly of its president, David Weikart, who took a risk by supporting the idea of a Consultative Group during the organizational stage, and before others had begun to participate. High/ Scope has served the Consultative Group in an advisory capacity throughout, providing both technical and professional backstopping.

UNESCO deserves special thanks. Wolfgang Schwendler, who heads the inter-divisional project on the Young Child and the Family Environment, and John Bennett, editor of UNESCO's social science series, have gone beyond the call of duty in helping this book take shape and appear. I am indebted also to Urie Bronfenbrenner for contributing the book's excellent forward.

This work could not have been written without the intellectual and moral and organizational support of my colleague, Cassie Landers, who not only provided insightful comments along the way, but who also took on extra programmatic and administrative burdens so I might have time to write.

I am grateful to members of the Advisory Committee to the Consultative Group for their comments on an early version: Cigdem Kagitcibasi, Nittaya Kotchabhakdi, Vicky Colbert, Barnabas Otaala, Elizabeth Hillman, and Judith Evans.

Finally, during this process Maru Linares, my companion and occasional security blanket, has been my best critic and supporter, adding an oft-needed sense of reality, helping to correct fuzzy thinking, and through her actions providing an unobtrusive reminder that the 'bottom line' lies in human values and our relation to others.

Part I

Setting the stage

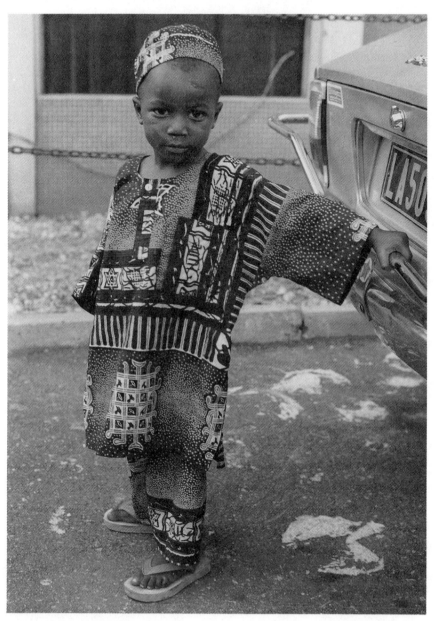

'The world in hand', Lagos, Nigeria

Chapter 1

Why invest in early childhood development?

BELIEVERS AND SCEPTICS

The world is filled with believers in the importance of good care and attention for children during their earliest months and years. That widespread
belief is embedded in many cultural traditions. The young child may be
seen as a little god – still in a state of relative perfection – or as a 'little sun'
around which the world revolves. Children are 'the butterflies of Paradise'
(Sharif, in UNICEF 1985).

Belief in the need for proper care is also grounded in the recognition
that children are the next generation; they represent the continuity of tradition as well as the hope for, and fear of, change. There is a need to believe
that the children of today can be both a rallying point for social action and
the constructors of a better world.

Personal experience creates believers in the value of early childhood
care and development. Parents, professionals, and others who are simply
close observers of how the neighbour's children grow up, recognize a
healthy effect of good care and attention to infants and young children.
They do not need an elaborate rationale or cold scientific evidence to
justify their personal feeling that rudimentary health precautions and a
good diet, combined with smiles and cuddling and talk and play, will
enhance a child's development. Such actions are not only seen as right and
just, but also as a good investment of time and money.

But if there are so many believers in the world, why is it that
programmes of early childhood care and development have received so
little support? Why do governments and other organizations not respond
more generously in their budgets to the obvious developmental needs of
'the twelve who survive' (those twelve of every thirteen children born in the
world, who manage to survive to age one, often in spite of the cruel conditions that surround them)? Why are there not more programmes designed
to improve care and enhance development?

Unfortunately for children, when it comes to investing in programmes
intended to improve early childhood development, there are sceptics as

well as believers. And, control over purse strings and planning processes often falls to sceptics whose way of viewing the world is conditioned by their job. These sceptics need more to go on than someone else's belief that investing in programmes of child care and development is a good thing to do. They want to be shown that early childhood is a better investment than roads or dams or primary schools (or bombers?). They want visible and hard evidence that the proposed programmes will work. In order to justify action, they demand a rationale – a set of convincing arguments based on something other than unsubstantiated beliefs, combining both scientific and political arguments.

In setting out a rationale, it is important to respond to sceptics' concerns. These sources of scepticism are as varied (and sometimes irrational) as are the arguments used in favour of investing in early childhood development. For instance, a typical sceptic might say:

'*But I don't understand.*'   One source of scepticism lies in simple mis-understandings about what child development is. For the uninitiated, child development sometimes appears to be either too vague and simple, or too complicated and mysterious to be dealt with in programmes of any scale and significance. 'Who wants to programme hugs for a child?' 'What do you mean by inadequate interaction adversely affecting the maturation of neural pathways?' Lack of understanding arises also from the fact that 'early childhood development' crosses disciplinary lines and seems to mean different things to different people, blurring the basis for action. The same imprecision attaches to 'child care'.

Moreover, an investment in early childhood development is not like an investment in a road or a dam. Roads and dams can be seen once they are completed and their function is relatively easy to understand. Sceptics would like a similarly visible result and a clear set of concrete guidelines and examples of various kinds of programmes that have been shown to work for early childhood development.

We will take on the challenge in this book of trying to present child care and development in straightforward language. We will begin, for instance, with a simple definition of child development as 'a process of change in which a child learns to handle ever more difficult levels of moving, thinking, speaking, feeling, and relating to others'. We will suggest guide-lines and a variety of programme approaches that can help that process of. change to occur as it can and should in order to improve physical, social, and emotional well-being. We will bring together some seemingly disparate views, extracting from them common elements that provide a basis for action.

'*It's already taken care of.*'   Ironically, many individuals who view programmes of early childhood care and development with a sceptical eye have grown up in advantaged conditions – in a loving home, with food on the table and good health care, and with parents who provide a stimulating environment for growing and learning. As a result of their own experience, they feel that families can and do provide the attention needed for healthy growth and development. They may agree that the early years of a child's life are important but they see no need for special programmes to assist children and families during that period. Sometimes, they see child development primarily as a matter of loving a child and they argue, with good reason, that love is not something to be programmed.

In brief, some sceptics believe that families are doing a good job, for the most part, of bringing up their children. And sometimes they are right. So why interfere? Their experience does little to help them to understand why it is hard for a young and harried mother, struggling alone to survive in an unsupportive urban environment, to provide the love, health care, and attention to her child that she would like to provide.

'*It's a mother's job.*' In some cases, the above view about what families should be and do is related closely to another source of scepticism – the belief that a mother's place is in the home. Early childhood programmes, particularly if they are outside the home, are sometimes seen as eroding the traditional role of the mother. Scepticism rooted in this view of the maternal role persists even though programmes to enhance early care and development can reach into the home and can respect the primary role of mothers and families in the process. It persists even though mothers, traditionally, have seldom been the only person providing care to their young children (see Chapter 11). It persists in spite of the fact that many women must work outside the home, and that studies show provision of alternate care in these cases can be good for both mother and child.

'*Give me evidence.*' Some sceptics are open to the idea that early development is important and should be fostered, but they lack hard evidence that early interventions produce results, particularly over the longer term. Sometimes, this scepticism simply reflects a lack of information, combined with the fact that the chain of causality is long. Indeed, it is difficult to imagine (and even harder to prove) effects extending into adult life from actions taken in the early years. Sometimes, evidence is cited to show that programme results do *not* occur – or, if they occur, do not last. Sceptics may, for instance, point to findings of studies carried out in the early 1970s, suggesting that the effects of early childhood programmes 'wash out' when children reach age seven or eight. They are not aware, however, that over the last ten to fifteen years, these findings have been superseded by new research information.

'*What is the rate of return?*' Still other sceptics seek, and do not find, an economic justification for investment in child care or early childhood programmes. They would like to be able to compare an economic rate of return to programmes of early childhood development with other possible investments in order to choose that one carrying the highest rate. At a minimum, they would like to know that proposed programmes will effect-ively produce results justifying the cost of the programme. Reasonably, they would like to feel that money is not being wasted.

Any rationale for investment in programmes of early childhood care and development should include responses to the different sources of scepticism sketched above. Doing so should, at a minimum, bolster the position of those who would like to support programmes of care and devel-opment but are under pressure to support other programmes instead.

LINES OF ARGUMENT

The rationale that follows draws upon eight complementary lines of argu-ment for increased support to programmes of early child care and devel-opment. These are:

1 *A human rights argument.*   Children have a right to live and to develop to their full potential.

2 *A moral and social values argument.*   Through children humanity transmits its values. That transmission begins with infants. To preserve desirable moral and social values in the future, one must begin with children.

3 *An economic argument.*   Society benefits economically from investing in child development, through increased production and cost savings.

4 *A programme efficacy argument.*   The efficacy of other programmes (e.g., health, nutrition, education, women's programmes) can be improved through their combination with programmes of child development.

5 *A social equity argument.*   By providing a 'fair start', it is possible to modify distressing socioeconomic and gender-related inequities.

6 *A social mobilization argument.*   Children provide a rallying point for social and political actions that build consensus and solidarity.

7 *A scientific argument.*   Research evidence demonstrates forcefully that the early years are critical in the development of intelligence, personality, and social behaviour, and that there are long-term effects associated with a variety of early intervention programmes.

8 *Changing social and demographic circumstances.*   The increasing survival of vulnerable children, changing family structures, urban–rural migration, women in the labour force, and other changes require increased attention to early care and development.

Some of these lines of argument will be more relevant to one situation than to another. Different individuals will find appeal in different arguments, reflecting their particular concerns about the rights of children, about economic benefits, about social equity, about adjusting to changing circum-stances affecting families and work.

We turn now to a brief elaboration of each argument.

Children have a human right to develop to their full potential

For many people, the obligation to protect a child's human rights is the most fundamental and convincing reason to invest in programmes to enhance early childhood development. The Declaration of the Rights of the Child, adopted unanimously in 1959 by the United Nations General Assembly, recognized among its ten principles:

> Principle 2: 'The child will enjoy special protection and will have at its disposal opportunities and services, dispensed under the law and through other means, *allowing physical, mental, moral, spiritual, and social development in a healthy and normal way*, with liberty and dignity.' (Italics added)

Thirty years after approval of the 1959 Declaration, a Convention on the Rights of the Child has been ratified, in 1989, by the United Nations Assembly that urges signatories to:

> ... ensure to the maximum extent possible child survival *and development.*'
>
> (Article 6)

> ... render appropriate assistance to parents and legal guardians *in the performance of their child-rearing responsibilities and shall insure the development of institutions, facilities and services for the care of children.*
>
> (Article 18.2)

Further:

> ... children of working parents have the right to benefit from child care services and facilities for which they are eligible.
>
> (Article 18.3)

Allowing disability and arrested development to occur each year in millions of young children, when it could be prevented, is, then, a violation of a basic human right. The fact that children are dependent on others for satisfaction of their rights creates an even greater obligation to help and protect them, and in this process families may require help.

The Declaration of Children's Rights and the Convention suggest that the right for children to develop to their full potential is widely accepted internationally, providing the cornerstone for an early childhood programme rationale. However, the human rights rhetoric needs to be translated into actions.

Humanity transmits its values through children

We are continually reminded that 'children are our future'. The transmission of social and moral values that will guide that future begins in the earliest months and years of life.

In societies where there is a concern that crucial values are being eroded, there is a strong incentive to find ways in which those values can be strengthened. Early childhood programmes can assist in that effort, both by strengthening the resolve of parents and by providing environments for children to play and learn that include specific attention to desired values. Attending to the development of basic values in children must be a high priority in a world racked by violence, but seeking peace, in a world facing environmental degradation but seeking cooperative and sane solutions, and in a world where consumerism, competition, and individualism seem to be winning out over altruism, cooperation, and solidarity as core values.

If children are our future, they are the agents of change as well as the custodians of continuity. For many, that is frightening. But for many revolutionary governments early childhood has represented an opportunity. They have consistently recognized the importance of inculcating values at an early age. The idea that the 'New Man' begins with the 'New Child' has provided a basic and adequate rationale for massive early childhood programmes following revolutions. Although the centralized, proselytizing nature of many such programmes is not always palatable to outsiders (any more than the proselytizing of missionaries is to many revolutionaries), what the post-revolutionary spread of child-care centres and preschools shows clearly is that the decision whether or not to invest in early childhood programmes is fundamentally a political decision.

Society benefits through increased productivity and cost savings associated with enhanced early childhood development

Without referring to a scientific literature, common sense suggests that a person who is well developed physically, mentally, socially, and emotionally will be in a better position to contribute economically to family, community, and country than a person who is not. And in most countries of the world, that economic contribution begins at a very early age.

Increased productivity   Early childhood programmes have the potential to improve both physical and mental capacity. They can also affect enrolment, progress and performance of children in schooling which is associated with important changes in skills and outlooks affecting adult behaviour. Schooling helps build such skills as the ability to organize knowledge into meaningful categories, to transfer knowledge from one situation to another, and to be more selective in the use of information (Rogoff 1980; Triandis 1980). Schooling facilitates greater technological adaptiveness (Grawe 1979). It relates directly to both increased farmer productivity (Lockheed, Lau and Jamison 1980) and productivity in the informal market sector (Colclough 1980). This complicated chain of relationships will be traced in more detail in Chapter 10, and evidence will be presented from longitudinal studies to help substantiate the effects, over time, of early support for developmental programmes.

Income generation Economic benefits from early childhood programmes may also occur through effects on the employment and earnings of care-givers. Child-care and development programmes offer the possibility of increased labour force participation by women and they can free older siblings to learn and earn as well. They can provide employment for individuals as paid caregivers and can bring new sources of income to local suppliers of materials and services needed to make the programme function.

Cost savings Another way in which investments in health, nutrition, and psychosocial development during the early years can bring an economic return is through cost savings – by reducing work losses, by cutting the later need for social welfare programmes, by improving the efficiency of educational systems through reductions in dropout, repetition, and remedial programmes, and by reducing health costs.

One often-quoted example of an economic pay-off to an investment in early development comes from the United States where a longitudinal study of the effects of participation by children from low-income families in a preschool programme produced benefits estimated at seven times the original cost of the programme (Berruta-Clement *et al.* 1984). Most of these benefits occurred as a result of cost savings. Another example comes from Brazil where an evaluation shows that it is possible for a programme of integrated attention to preschool children to pay for itself (see Chapter 15) by reducing the extra primary school costs associated with repetition (Ministerio da Saude 1983).

A rate of return? It is difficult to calculate a ratio of programme costs to programme benefits or an economic 'rate of return' for social investments of any kind, including programmes of early childhood care and develop-ment. But when such estimates have been made, they suggest a high return on an investment in early childhood is possible. For instance, Selowsky, using Latin American data, concluded that:

> Yearly investments per child in programmes that can induce a change in ability equal to one standard deviation can be 'justified' if they cost between 0.37 and 0.51 the yearly wage of an illiterate worker.
>
> (Selowsky 1981, p. 342)

Both the hoped-for increase in what Selowsky calls 'ability' and the costs cited are well within the realm of possibility to achieve (see Chapter 15).

In brief, increased productivity, income generation possibilities, and potential cost savings provide compelling reasons why economic benefits can be expected from investment in programmes of early childhood care and development.

The efficacy of other programmes can be improved through joint investment in early childhood development

Early childhood development programmes can affect cost savings in programmes of health, nutrition, and education, as suggested above. But at least as important, integrated attention to child development can increase the effectiveness of health and nutrition programmes. Combining programmes takes advantage of the interactive effect among health, nutrition and early stimulation (see Chapter 9). In addition, child-care and development programmes are potentially useful as vehicles for extending primary health care.

If children arrive at primary school better prepared, they can make better use of the school. Not only will dropout and repetition decrease, affecting costs, but the quality of education will rise because one of the most important 'inputs' into the school system is the child. When children are better prepared, teachers can be more effective, facilities and materials can be used better, and children can learn more from each other.

In a different vein, income-generating programmes for women that respond to child-care and development needs are likely to be more successful than programmes that do not. If proper care for their children is assured, women will lose less work time as a result of child-related concerns (Galinsky 1986). They will also be able to seek steadier and better-paying employment (see Chapter 11).

Because investments in early childhood care and development can help to make other programmes more efficient and effective, it is not appropriate to look at them as a direct 'trade-off' against, for instance, primary schooling or primary health care. They should be considered as part of the same package, bringing increased benefits at marginal, or even no additional, cost.

Programmes can help to modify distressing inequalities

Investments in early childhood development can help to modify inequalities rooted in poverty and discrimination (social, religious, gender) by giving children from so-called 'disadvantaged' backgrounds a 'fair start'. Poverty and/or discrimination produce stressful conditions and unequal treatment that can inhibit healthy and comprehensive development in the early years. For instance, children from poor families often fall quickly and progressively behind their more advantaged peers in their readiness for school, and that gap is never closed.

Boys, traditionally, have been better prepared for schooling than girls and have had more opportunities to enter and continue in school. The differences begin with gender-linked disparities in the patterns and practices of early development that need to be changed if the discrimination is to be overcome. These are often deeply rooted in culture, but there is evidence that integrated attention to early development can produce changes in the way families perceive the abilities and the future of a girl child.

By not intervening to foster early childhood development where assistance is most needed, governments have tacitly endorsed and strengthened inequalities. Ironically, one argument used against early education programmes is that they are discriminatory – favouring the upper class. That is certainly true if no special effort is made to assist the poor and if programmes of early education are left to the rich who can pay for them. But evidence to be provided in Chapter 10 shows that early childhood programmes can moderate rather than reinforce these social differences. As an example, one evaluation of the huge Integrated Child Development Service of India shows clearly that benefits are greatest for lower castes and for girls (Lal and Wati 1986).

Children provide a rallying point for social and political actions that build consensus and solidarity

Mozambique, Lebanon, Peru, Sri Lanka, El Salvador, Ethiopia, Iraq and a significant number of other countries are victims of violent actions that place the problem of living together in peace high on the list of social goals. In many locations, lesser political and social tensions make it extremely difficult to mobilise people for actions that will be to their own benefit. In such circumstances, it has been shown that placing 'Children First' can be an effective political strategy.

Perhaps the most dramatic, but short-lived, examples of mobilisation around programmes to benefit young children are those in which cease-fires have been obtained between warring groups, as in El Salvador, in order to carry out national immunization campaigns. Less spectacular are the many community-based programmes that take children as an 'entry point' for common action. Examples of such programmes will be scattered throughout the book, and the topic will be treated in more detail when discussing community participation in Chapter 12.

Scientific evidence demonstrates lasting effects of early attention to child development

Evidence from the fields of physiology, nutrition and psychology continues to accumulate to indicate that the early years are critical in the formation of intelligence, personality, and social behaviour. This evidence begins with the not-so-new discovery that brain cells are formed during the first two years of life. But recent research has strengthened the argument for early attention by showing that sensory stimulation from the environment affects the structure and organization of the neural pathways in the brain during the formative period. Thus, opportunities for complex perceptual and motor experiences at an early age favourably affect various learning abilities in later life and are able to compensate, at least partly, for the deficit associated with early malnutrition. Recent research also demonstrates that children whose mothers interact with them in consistent, caring ways will be better nourished and less apt to be sick than children not so attended. Chapter 9 will present some of this information.

In the 1970s, evaluations of some early intervention programmes in the United States indicated that the effect of these programmes on the intelligence quotient of children seemed to 'wash out' by the time they were in the second or third grade of primary school. More recently, longitudinal data clearly demonstrate major long-term effects associated with a variety of early intervention programmes. These results, which will be presented in Chapter 10, include improved school attendance and performance, increased employment and reduced delinquency during the teenage years, and reduced teenage pregnancy.

Changing social and economic conditions require new responses

Over the last decade, the effects of a world recession have been felt increasingly – by individual families and by governments seeking to adjust their behaviours and programmes to the new realities (Cornia *et al.*, 1987). But even prior to the recession and, in some settings, independently of it, major social changes have been occurring that call out for new approaches to early childhood care and development.

Increasing labour force participation by women   The increased pressure for women to work for wages and the need to take over men's farming chores as they have migrated to cities or sought work in mines has brought additional burdens affecting child care and creating a need for alternative forms of care. The trend towards increasing labour force participation pre-dates, but has been strengthened by, the world recession of the 1980s. These trends are likely to continue, and even to increase in the coming years.

The mother in these or other settings who works so that she and her family can survive may love her child and believe that she should devote time and energy to her baby, but she may not be able to do so; she needs help.

Modification of traditional family patterns   Extended families are no longer as common as they once were. As migration and progressive urbanization occurs, members of an extended family are not as available for child care as in the past. Grandmothers are no longer as easily available, either because they remain in rural areas or because they too are working outside the home in wage-earning jobs. The number of women-headed households has increased. In some developing countries the percentage is high (over 40 per cent in rural Kenya, Botswana, Ghana, Sierra Leone, and Lesotho, according to Youssef and Hertler 1984). In these households, women must work, creating a major need for complementary child care. If care is available, the earnings of these women are more likely than would be the earnings of men to go towards improving the welfare of the children in the household (see Chapter 11).

Associated with these changes in families (and in economic conditions) are increases in the numbers of abused children and of street children. These growing problems are often dealt with after the fact rather than seeking solutions in the earliest years by helping distressed families with very young children.

Increased primary school attendance has decreased the availability of older siblings to act as supplementary caretakers. Or, siblings have been forced to drop out of school to provide such care, in which case there is a strong argument for child-care initiatives that will help siblings continue their education, at least to the point of literacy.

Changes in mortality and survival rates   Over the last 30 years, the infant mortality rate has been more than cut in half. More children are surviving who in the past would have died an early death. As survival to age one has increased from 5 of 6 in 1960 to 12 of 13 in 1988, the pressure increases to mount programmes for those who survive.

IN SUMMARY

The rationale developed here brings together several lines of argument supporting the value of investing in early childhood development. Each argument stands on its own, but when combined they are particularly compelling. Whatever the differences in individual predilections and local circumstances, it is clear that the set of arguments provides a strong base from which to argue for investment in programmes of early childhood care and development – by individuals and families, by communities, by governments, by non-governmental organizations, and by international funders.

When early childhood is made a priority, the financial support is forthcoming, even in situations of relative poverty. Financing for early childhood programmes is not the basic problem. The problem is to recognize the value of such programmes and build the personal and political resolve necessary to carry them out.

The general rationale developed here will be strengthened by the chapters that follow which seek clarification of concepts, provide evidence to substantiate the general arguments and give examples of what can be done.

REFERENCES

Berruta-Clement, J.R., L.J. Schweinhart, W.S. Barnett, A.S. Epstein and D.T. Weikart, *Changed Lives: The Effects of the Perry Preschool Program on Youths Through Age 19*. Ypsilanti, Mich: High/Scope Educational Research Foundation, Monograph No. 8, 1984.

Colclough, C. 'Primary Schooling and Economic Development: A Review of the Evidence', Washington D.C: World Bank Staff Working Paper No. 399, 1980.

Cornia, A., R. Jolly and F. Stewart, *Adjustment with a Human Face: Protecting the Vulnerable and Promoting Growth*. New York: Oxford University Press, 1988.

Galinsky, E. *Investing in Quality Child Care: A Report for AT & T*. New York: Bank Street College of Education, 1986.

Grawe, R. 'Ability in Preschoolers, Earnings, and Home Environment', Washington DC: World Bank Staff Working Paper No. 319, 1979.

Lal, S. and R. Wati. 'Non-Formal Preschool Education – An Effort to Enhance School Enrolment', a paper presented to the National Conference on Research on ICDS, February 25–29, 1986. New Delhi: National Institute for Public Cooperation in Child Development (NIPCCD). Mimeo.

Lockheed, M.D., D. Jamison, and L. Lau. 'Farmer Education and Farm Efficiency: A Survey', *Economic Development and Cultural Change*, 29 (October 1980), pp. 37–76.

Ministerio de Saude, y Instituto Nacional de Alimentação e Nutrição, 'Analição do PROAPE/Alagoas com Enfoque na Area Econômica', Brasilia, MS/INAN, 1983. Mimeo.

Rogoff, B. 'Schooling and the Development of Cognitive Skills', in H. Triandis & A. Heron (eds), *Handbook of Cross-cultural Psychology, Vol. 4*. Boston: Allyn-Bacon, 1980.

Selowsky, Marcelo. 'Nutrition, Health, and Education: The Economic Significance of Complementarities at Early Age', *Journal of Development Economics*, Vol. 9 (1981), pp. 331–46.

Sharif, Hadith, in *Child Care in Islam*. Cairo: UNICEF, 1985. This volume collects sayings from the Holy Koran and from major Muslim writers regarding attention to children.

Triandis, H. 'Reflections on Trends in Cross-Cultural Research', *Journal of Cross-Cultural Psychology*, Vol. 11, No. 1 (1980), pp. 35–58.

United Nations Secretariat. 'The Draft Convention on the Rights of the Child, Third Version', New York: the United Nations, May 1989.

Youssef, N. and C.B. Hertler. 'Rural Households Headed by Women: A Priority Concern for Development', Rural Employment Programme Research Working Paper, Geneva: International Labour Organisation, 1984.

Chapter 2

Where we are and how we got there

Before attempting to describe in as systematic a way as possible the current state of programming for early childhood care and development, a brief note about the evolution of such programmes will help put the present in perspective. After all, neither child development nor child care is new. But as societies and circumstances have changed over the years, forms of care and development have also changed. Among those changes of form has been the growth of institutionalized programmes of care and development. Recalling origins of these child-care and development programmes not only reminds us that things have changed, but also suggests how slow we are to adapt in some cases while we go overboard in others.

CHANGING CONTEXTS, CHANGING NEEDS

In the Western world, one origin of child-care and development programmes as we know them today lies in changes accompanying the Industrial Revolution in the eighteenth century. In the predominantly agricultural and rural society that preceded industrialization, children were usually found within an intact, extended family. These children of the field were socialized to a relatively limited and unchanging world in which community values were generally agreed upon. The rural setting provided space to explore and a stimulating environment. The responsibility for child care lay clearly with women whose work usually permitted them to breast-feed and to attend directly to the child in the early years. Families were often large and older children were expected to help with the child-care tasks. Indeed, children quickly entered an adult world and, in a sense, did not have a separate 'childhood' as is the case today (Aries 1962).

The rural conditions of the eighteenth and nineteenth centuries should not be romanticized; life was demanding and survival was continually threatened by disease, and occasionally by lack of food. But for those children who managed to survive their early months, 'development' was less problematic than it would be for many of their peers in new urban environments. The child-care practices evolved over the years were suited

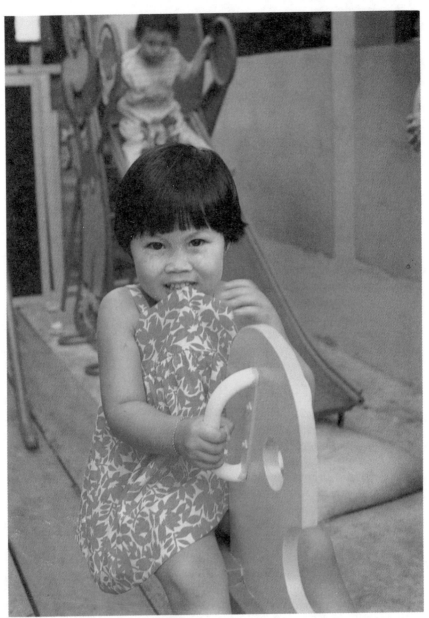

'Becoming shy', Bangkok, Thailand

to socialization in the rural environment; they were not so suited to cities.

With industrialization and moves to the city came changes in values, in living conditions, in family arrangements, and in working patterns. The new conditions brought with them a need to care for children of working mothers. They led to a need for ways to foster exploration and provide adequate stimulation for children within a more restricted physical environment. They called for new parenting skills and a different kind of socialization. With these changes, the older forms of child care and development were not adequate guides.

In response to the changing circumstances, two kinds of programmes began to appear. One set of programmes was established principally to care for foundling or indigent children. These social welfare programmes, often run by upper class women, were protective and custodial, putting some food in the stomach and a roof over the head, but little more.

Another strain of programmes also evolved that often catered to the growing urban middle class and/or to children of working mothers (van der Eyken 1969). These programmes emphasized enrichment and stimulation more than protection and custodial care and they were, in a sense, designed to substitute for the rich possibilities offered by rural environments. They brought toys and play activities into a restricted classroom in order to give children the stimulation and practice that rural children came by more naturally. (As these centre-based models are carried from Western capitals to rural areas of the Third World today, it is well to remember this origin to avoid the introduction of unnecessary and foreign elements.)

The parallel between the changes in values, living patterns, family structure, and work associated with the Industrial Revolution and changes occurring today in the rapidly urbanizing and sometimes industrializing nations of the Third World is marked. And many countries have turned to a similarly bifurcated structure in responding to the changes: a welfare approach for the poor, providing at best protective care, and an enrichment approach for the middle classes, with more of a developmental focus.

During the twentieth century, and particularly since 1945, other changes have been at work that did not figure strongly at the time of the Industrial Revolution. A communications revolution has helped to create the 'global village' (the African historian, Ki-Zerbo, would characterize it as a 'global supermarket' (Ki-Zerbo et al. 1990). Transistor radios now reach into most corners of the world, and even television is reaching rural areas to a degree not thought possible 25 years ago.

Another twentieth century revolution has occurred in education, or perhaps more accurately in schooling. A premium is now placed on literacy, and literacy rates have expanded dramatically. Almost as dramatic is the growth of primary schooling. Much greater emphasis is being placed today on the acquisition of cognitive skills related to abstract reasoning. The arrival (intrusion?) of schools in rural areas has brought competition with indigenous educational forms. It has carried with it a new kind of certification that is increasingly required by rural as well as urban children.

Transportation and organizational revolutions have occurred as well. Buses not only help rural people visit cities and migrate to them; they also aid periodic or permanent return to villages where new ideas and new clothes can be displayed. Communication and transportation revolutions have facilitated the outreach of business and governmental organization, such that reaching the villages is no longer unusual. These organizational representatives hawk their commercial or social wares, backed by large cadres of city-based individuals creating new products for sale and looking for new ways to get them sold.

There is, then, not only a shift to the city with accompanying changes, but also reach of the city into rural areas, with accompanying changes. With that spread come bottle-feeding, Pepsi-Cola, blue jeans and plastics. The changes also bring uncertainty about old values and ways of doing things, including rearing children. There is a changing sense of 'community', and new confusion about loyalties. The implication of all this is that even children who remain in rural areas increasingly live simultaneously in multiple, and sometimes conflicting, environments. They are affected by national and global cultures, but are rooted in a local culture sometimes unsure about its own roots and directions.

In general, ideas about early childhood development have been slow to change, despite increasing access to information that might help that happen. That is so for rural residents who are asked to assimilate new ways but resist changes that may indeed be necessary for their children to function in the transitional world, or multiple worlds, that surround them. It is true for migrants to cities who need to make adjustments to a new environment. And it is true for urban-based professionals and bureaucrats looking to rural areas. Having been reared and trained in a Western (and probably urban) tradition, they hold fast to Western-influenced forms and content as they venture into rural areas, failing to recognize and build upon the rich cultural base and the time-honoured practices that are known to work well. If individuals are slow to adjust, cultures are even slower.

Consider, for instance, another revolution that is in progress: the emancipation of women and associated changes in family structures (Tilly and Scott 1978). The effect of this revolution is yet to be felt in many parts of the world, but it is arriving. Again, there is need to adjust ways of thinking about child care and development, as they are being influenced by this revolution. But we have been slow to react. And, ironically, when reactions come, they may be too fast or too drastic, failing to take into consideration the need and desire to maintain basic values reinforced by the previous socialization process.

A more complete recounting of changes influencing our ways of thinking about early childhood care and development would discuss also the effects of increasing affluence, changing distributions of wealth and economic swings requiring difficult adjustments, the major shifts in geo-politics of the 1950s and 1960s that brought independence to many nations, and the growth of international organizations with their trend-setting and loan-making powers. But the purpose of this chapter is not to attempt an extensive historical analysis of social and economic changes as they affect childhood (see Wall 1975 and Levine and White 1986); it is, rather, to suggest to the reader that models and ways of thinking about early childhood development require considerable modification in the face of the major changes that have occurred and in light of the dual worlds in which so many 'at risk' children live. Another purpose is to point to the challenge of supporting cultural heritages and values while working out those modifications.

Let us turn, then, to the recent past to see how we are adjusting. With the declaration of 1979 as the International Year of the Child (IYC), an opportunity was provided for new child-care and development thinking and initiatives. What was the result?

THE INTERNATIONAL YEAR OF THE CHILD: A TURNING POINT?

Without doubt, the IYC generated a new enthusiasm and interest in the child. Many descriptive and analytical exercises were undertaken at the national level, intended to identify needs, to create awareness, and to mobilize people around the idea of attention to 'the whole child.' A plethora of small-scale pilot or demonstration projects were begun that marked a significant opening towards 'non-formal' programmes set within a context of community development. Parental education programmes were also begun, as were programmes directed towards the care of younger children by older brothers and sisters. At the same time, considerable energy was devoted to promoting more formal preschools.

What happened as a result of the IYC? One retrospective look has concluded that '... awareness of the rights and needs of children has increased a hundredfold over the past ten years' (Smyke 1989, p. 53). That awareness is reflected in the Convention of the Rights of the Child, ratified by the United Nations ten years later.

But what about changes in policies and programmes since 1979? At a general level, it is clear that increased awareness has helped lead to new laws and national policies. There has been significant progress in the level of programming intended to improve child survival, and more modest advances with respect to child care and development. Various organi-zations formed at the time of the IYC continue to be productive and active. Undoubtedly, providing a more detailed response than this regarding effects of the IYC is difficult because there has been no systematic mechanism to trace most of the efforts begun in 1979. That is especially so for projects and programmes that began from a child development, as contrasted with a child survival, viewpoint. (These views will be described in the next chapter.)

Meanwhile, it is clear that although the IYC generated a high level of enthusiasm and activity, much of the momentum gained in 1979 with respect to programming for child care and development was lost. National governments and international organizations often did not follow up the new initiatives with special funding. There was considerable dabbling but no concerted and sustained campaign to expand child development. Internationally, children did not win a 'decade' as had women and water. No specific institution in the United Nations family was charged with, or took on, follow-up responsibility. Without the needed leadership and continuity, information and advocacy exercises and pilot initiatives related to child development were soon swallowed up in a stronger international current, focusing on primary health care. That movement had already begun to gain force in 1978 at the Alma Ata Conference dealing with 'Health for All'.

As the 1980s began, increasing emphasis was being placed in international circles on primary health care and on infant and child survival, as the Alma Ata recommendations began to be implemented. UNICEF, with the World Health Organisation, launched a Child Survival and Development Revolution (CSDR) which, while containing 'development' in the title, focused narrowly on survival. The CSDR initiative was first captured in the acronym GOBI-FFF (Growth monitoring, Oral rehydration, Breast-feeding, and Immunization, together with Food supplementation, Family spacing and Female education as tag-along themes). As the crusade evolved, however, more and more emphasis began to be placed on immunization and oral rehydration, as the 'twin engines' of CSDR. Only now are other elements being given greater attention, still within a posture emphasizing survival and growth. Other international and bilateral organizations collaborated in this worldwide survival crusade. Governments responded, cognizant both of their still-high infant mortality rates and of the international climate favouring assistance to reduce those rates.

At the same time, mounting economic problems in most Third World countries during the 1980s left little room for programme expansion of any kind. In general, the economic adjustments that became necessary worked against the social sectors of health and education. And, with emphasis given to health-related programmes directed towards improving survival, large-scale support of programmes stressing, or even including, attention to psychosocial development in early childhood years did not materialize as it should have if the IYC recommendations and initiatives had been followed.

In spite of these handicaps, growth has occurred in child-care programmes and in the preschool sector in selected countries. Whether the IYC provided already dedicated individuals with enough additional strength to carry on against considerable odds, or whether the expansion of efforts occurred independently of the IYC because local pressures required a response, is not clear. But the situation in 1989 was considerably better than that of 1979. And, because child development is a multidimensional and interactive process, the child survival programmes did have an effect on child development as well.

But how far have we come?

CHILD CARE AND DEVELOPMENT IN 1989: A PANORAMA

The general picture that emerges from an attempt to describe programmes of early childhood care and development in 1989 is more than a bit blurry and contains apparent contradictions. On one hand, it seems that immense strides have been made in the last 20 years, and particularly in the last 5 or 10 years. As will be evident from the statistics to be presented later in this chapter and from the 'state of the practice' to be presented in Chapters 5 and 6, some countries have made dramatic advances and there are innumerable examples of innovative and sometimes widespread programmes. But another general impression appears as well – that the situation is far from adequate. Based on the evidence we can marshall, it seems that:

1 In most countries, coverage in identifiable, organized programmes is still relatively low. That is particularly true for Sub-Saharan countries.
2 Many projects and programmes continue to be pilot or demonstration activities that are innovative, effective, and feasible to replicate, but have not been extended in a significant way.
3 The distribution of programmes, particularly the more institutionalized programmes, while improving, usually continues to favour the cities.
4 Reaching children before the age of three, and particularly between the ages of one and three, continues to be a challenge. Day care that takes into account both the needs of children and of their working mothers remains at a very low level, both in extension and in quality.
5 Programmes of support and education for parents have grown dramatically in some countries but are virtually non-existent in others, particularly with respect to the psychosocial components of early development. And there is a tendency in these programmes to impose, rather than to reconstruct and expand knowledge.
6 Many 'volunteer' programmes have now passed the point of initial enthusiasm and the volunteer spirit that was so critical in getting programmes under way is growing thin. And yet these programmes have not been recognized as bona fide claims on the public purse; they are in danger of fading.

7 Often, the quality of the programmes is poor, so that the effects on children are minimal. The combining of elements in programmes of integrated attention to the child remains a challenge, despite some successes and an increasing awareness.

These points may help to explain a conclusion that the field is growing significantly but is still very fragile and in need of increased attention, both to maintain gains and to fill in major gaps.

An impossible task?

At present, a detailed and comprehensive description of child care and development in the Third World is impossible. There are at least two basic reasons why that is so. First, a great deal of child care is so informal that it is not included within any set of statistics. It not only escapes the attention of national and international organizations concerned with care and development, but it also fails to appear in national systems of economic accounting as a productive activity.

Even among the more organized programmes, the diversity is so great that no one set of statistics can do a proper job. To cover the field properly, one should include information not only about the number of centres in operation, but also about home visiting, parental education programmes, child care related to women's income-generating projects, programmes of care and development within broader community efforts, and disability programmes that include young children. Moreover, if one takes a truly holistic view of development, all programmes of health and nutrition and early education and care should be included. When one considers that different organizations, public and private, and operating at the level of the community, the region, and the nation, are in charge of programmes emphasizing different aspects of development, the task becomes overwhelming.

We will be more modest in defining our task, focusing on organized programmes of child care and development, and leaving aside mono-focal programmes of health and nutrition (even though these will have an effect on development). We will concentrate on programmes that are labelled as child care, child development, or preschool programmes, or that have one of these as a major component. This reflects our own desire to highlight the psychosocial dimension of child development. Even so, the task is complex, and rarely does one find information about the different programmes together in one place.

An example from São Paulo, Brazil, illustrates the complexity of describing early childhood programmes. In their thorough study, Campos and Rosemberg (1988) found that in the Greater Metropolitan Area of São Paulo, four major programmes were run by Federal (national) agencies, six by state agencies, and three by municipal agencies. Each of these 13 different public organizations operated with a somewhat different model. The most basic variants were a 'complete creche', (attending to children ages 0 to 6), a 'complete preschool' (ages 2 to 6), preschool classes (for children ages 5 and 6), 'emergency' preschools (less formal versions of a complete preschool, also for ages 2 to 6), and emergency creches (ages 0 to 6). In most sets of statistics, these so-called emergency programmes would not be included. In addition to the above models there were also 'infant parks' (a holdover from the 1930s, attending children from ages 3 to 12) and child-care centres organized in private businesses (ages 0 to 6). Moreover, a wide range of private programmes existed, accounting for approximately 38 per cent of the total coverage.

Another example: the International Year of the Child provided the stimulus in India for a mammoth project, undertaken by the Ministry of Welfare, to provide a statistical profile of 'The Child in India'. Finally published in 1985, the 1500-page work included extensive information about nutrition programmes, including infant feeding, 'child welfare services', and 'welfare of the handicapped, ages 0 to 6'. The welfare services included central- and state-sponsored Integrated Child Development Service projects, central and state homes for destitute children, central and state foster care schemes, creches run by central and state and municipal governments, and private sector agencies, and services offered by such unusual organizations as the Tea/Coffee, and other 'Boards'. By the time the report was published in 1985, the compendium was out of date in some major respects. The ICDS system had grown rapidly in the period from 1980 to 1985 and there had been some improvements in the health and nutritional status of the Indian child in this period. Nevertheless, the exercise provided an excellent framework for continued monitoring of programmes to improve the condition of the Indian child.

Statistics and impressions

Although no source can give us a full picture, there are several from which one might expect to obtain a general idea of the current state of programming for early childhood care and development. We will examine figures contained in documents from UNESCO and UNICEF, the two main United Nations agencies concerned with child development.

UNESCO

Educational Statistics   Included in the periodic publication of educational statistics by UNESCO is information about 'Education preceding the first level'. The 1988 edition includes (Table 3.3) enrolment figures for most countries, covering the period from 1980 to 1985 (or 1986 in some cases).

The UNESCO data refer to 'kindergarten, nursery schools, as well as infant classes attached to schools at higher levels. Nursery play centres, etc. have been excluded whenever possible'. Although the UNESCO figures cover various kinds of programmes, they do not always pick up non-formal programmes and most of those that have been included refer to organized programmes for children in the 3 to 6 age range. Accordingly, UNESCO figures provide a floor, or minimum idea of coverage of early childhood programmes.

Because the programmes included in UNESCO statistics vary so much from country to country (e.g. Quranic preschools in Morocco, community-based schools in Kenya, formal preschools for an elite in Niger), it is impossible to make much sense of inter-country comparisons. However, it is possible to look at the growth of this part of early childhood programming within each country over the five or six years following the IYC. An analysis of data from that perspective yields the following:

– With very few exceptions, coverage grew during the period, despite difficult economic circumstances. The few countries in which growth did not occur are the war-torn countries of Angola, Mozambique, Iran, and Lebanon. A fifth country that reported slightly lower coverage was Cuba. All other developing countries (the approximately 100 others for which data were included) showed at least some expansion.

– In some cases, expansion was dramatic, but that expansion occurred with reference to a very small base. For example:
    Burkina Faso grew five-fold (but from a total enrolment of only 732 children in 1980 to 3751 in 1986).
    Oman grew six-fold (from 396 to 2,542).
    Somewhat higher, the Dominican Republic grew five-fold (from 27,278 to 125,780).

– Some countries with relatively large numbers of children participating nevertheless grew relatively fast:
    Brazil reports doubled coverage, from 1980 to 1986 (from 1,335,000 to 2,699,000).
    Thailand jumped almost three-fold (from 367,313 to 1,009,131) in the same period.

– Among the largest countries:
    China is listed as having expanded from approximately 11,507,000 in 1980 to 16,289,800 in 1986 (still a relatively low percentage coverage overall).
    India reported an increase in participation from 918,238 in 1980 to 1,033,315 in 1984. (It is clear from this statistic that children participating in the non-formal preschool component of the huge Integrated Child Development Service are not included in the statistics for India. Coverage in the preschool centres of that programme

was estimated to be approximately 3,000,000 children in 1985: UNICEF 1988.)

Indonesia: 'Enrolment' increased from 1,005,226 in 1980 to 1,258,468 in 1985.

Brazil: see above.

Data were not provided for Bangladesh, Pakistan or Nigeria.

The UNESCO statistics also provide a figure for the percentage of enrolled children who are girls. In all but three countries (Morocco, Oman, and Nepal), the percentage of girls in 'education preceding the first level' is 45 per cent or above. This suggests a potential levelling effect for early education programmes.

Without knowing the size of the corresponding age group, it is difficult to get a good idea of what the numbers reported in the UNESCO document mean. When a population adjustment is introduced, the Dominican Republic, for instance, with a population of 6.4 million people and a preschool enrolment of 126,000, makes a slightly better showing than China with an enrolment of over 16,000,000 but a population of 1.2 billion.

Latin American preschool enrolments   A better idea of coverage, relative to the number of children below the age of 6 can be obtained from statistics compiled by the Latin American Regional Office of UNESCO (Calvo 1988). Table 2.1 in this chapter shows the 'rate of enrolment' for the years 1981 and 1985, for selected countries. The statistics suggest that:

- A relatively high percentage of children, ages 4 to 6, enrolled in unspecified forms of preschool education.
- A relatively low percentage of children under 4 are in pre-school programmes.
- A general trend of expansion, in percentage terms, occurred over the four-year period. (Note that in these statistics, Cuba shows growth, whereas in the earlier set, Cuba showed a slight decline.)

For the Latin American region as a whole, it is estimated by UNESCO that 'initial education' (pre-primaria for children 0 to 5 years of age) grew from coverage of 7.9 per cent in 1980 to 15 per cent in 1986 – a growth rate of 19 per cent per year during that period (Tedesco 1989, p. 11).

A world survey   In 1988, UNESCO carried out a special survey of early childhood care and education (ECCE) in its Member States (Fisher 1990). Respondents were asked to include both formal and non-formal types of ECCE programmes (not just formal preschools). But the response rate to the questionnaire was only 54 per cent, and some of the world's most populous countries (including Brazil, Pakistan, Bangladesh and Nigeria)

Table 2.1 Rate of *escolarización* at the preschool level, selected Latin American
countries[*]

Country	Age range	Rate of escolarización[†] 1981	1985
Bolivia	4–5	31.5%	34.1%
Brazil	0–6	9.8	13.9
Chile (1982/4)	0–5	11.9	13.9
	0–3	2.4	2.3
	4–5	32.2	38.3
Colombia	0–4	10.5	14.3
	5	31.9	36.0
Cuba (1980/4)	4–5	36.9	43.8
Ecuador	5	19.7	29.6
El Salvador	4–6	15.0	20.1
Honduras	4–6	9.5	11.2
Dominican Rep.	6		29.2

[*] *Source*: UNESCO-CREALC, 1987, as quoted in Gilberto Calvo, 'El proceso de transición
entre los programas de atención a la niñez y los de educación primaria en América Latina',
a discussion paper prepared for the workshop on the articulation of initial and primary
school education, March 14–18, 1988. UNICEF, Bogota and UNESCO-CREALC, Santiago
1988.
[†]The rate of *escolarización* refers to the indicated percentage of the age group that is
enrolled in preschool programmes.

did not reply. Moreover, the results are heavily biased by replies from
industrialized countries and from the Arab States. In addition, the level of
details of the replies varied enormously, as did the kinds of programmes
included. Although the survey provides some interesting national descriptions, it is difficult to try to use the data to paint a general picture of ECCE.

The world survey does confirm the general, and sometimes dramatic,
growth of ECCE institutions and enrolments in the 1980–88 period. It also
confirms the still relatively low coverage in most Third World countries and
an urban bias in a significant number of places. In addition, the Survey
suggests that more than half of the programmes reported were 'fee
charging' programmes.

UNICEF

Another source of information from which one might expect to obtain an
overview of the state of early childhood care and development
programming is the yearly production by UNICEF of annual reports and,
for many of the countries in which UNICEF works, situation analyses
covering the condition of women and children.

To explore the potential of this source, we undertook a review of all UNICEF's annual reports for 1988, and of 46 situation analyses produced between 1986 and 1988. The first, and principal, conclusion of that review is that the statistics are spotty and unsystematically presented. Indeed, UNICEF field offices are not requested to provide information on programmes of child care or of child development. What emerged from the review, therefore, were interesting bits and pieces that help to form an impression but cannot be added together in a coherent whole. By way of example, the following items are presented for Asia and Africa, gleaned from the reports.

Asia

- China, with its 16.3 million in preschools, covers 24 per cent of its 3 to 6 year olds. Over a three-year period from 1986–88, a programme of parental education had grown from virtually nothing to 130,000 parent schools.
- Sri Lanka covers 15 per cent of its children, ages 0 to 5, in early childhood care and development programmes of several types.
- By the end of 1988, it was estimated that the Philippines would be reaching 24 per cent of the 11.5 million preschool aged children (0 to 5) in that country.
- In Vietnam, 30 per cent of all children aged 0 to 3, and 35 per cent of all 3 to 6 year olds are in formal day-care centres.
- Approximately 35 per cent of India's 5144 development blocks are covered by the Integrated Child Development Service.
- In Laos, 4 per cent of all children ages 4 to 6 are in early childhood centre-based programmes.

Africa

- Programmes in Kenya cover 11 per cent of its children aged 3 to 5. (This seems to be an understatement. Another source indicates coverage of over 20 per cent for 1987: Riak *et al.* 1989.)
- In Benin, only 1 per cent of preschool aged children were in any kind of organized programme of day care or child development.
- Botswana covers 2.6 per cent of its children aged 2½ to 6 in preschools.

The UNICEF reports yielded fascinating information about particular programmes in which UNICEF was collaborating. But they seldom included the kind of information that would let one describe the larger programme picture for one country in a systematic way. A clear idea did not emerge of the strength of various actors – government, non-governmental organizations, and international organizations – in helping to organize and support care and development initiatives. Rarely was there information about parent or adult education programmes. Occasionally a community development programme or an integrated survival and development programme would be described that included a child-care and development component. Training programmes were mentioned in which UNICEF was involved, but there was no overview. Attention was given to advocacy efforts, but in only a very few instances was the child development component of such programmes discussed explicitly.

Some general conclusions

1   The review of UNESCO and UNICEF documents provides support for the contention that the field has grown significantly since 1979, and it is possible that the figures are underestimated.
2   The statistics also illustrate vividly the uneven nature of the growth. Not surprisingly, they verify that Latin American and Asian countries have made much greater progress in terms of organized programmes than have African countries.
3   Another conclusion emerges from the review of available information: a country does not have to be rich or boast an expanding economy in order to give early childhood care and development sufficient priority to mount a significant programme or set of programmes. India and Kenya are particularly good examples of countries with relatively low per capita incomes but fairly extensive programmes of attention to pre-school children. In Latin America, generally, a radical decline has occurred in the standard of living during the 1980s, but 'initial education' in the region has grown rapidly. In Mexico, where the problem of the international debt is among the most serious in the world, preschool coverage grew by 9 per cent each year during the period from 1982 to 1988.

Beyond guestimates

From the review, we have drawn some very general conclusions. But for the most part, the interpretations have to be hedged for lack of consistent information. Emerging from the analysis is a clear need for a more systematic way to follow the progress of early childhood care and development programmes. A method is also needed to help record the coverage and quality of various kinds of initiatives that, when taken together, adequately describe the effort being put into providing organized care and into enhancing early development.

As a first very rough step, a general set of categories should be set up that would cover the range of early childhood programmes, serving different age groups and implemented by different governmental and non-governmental organizations. That accounting should include non-formal programmes, such as home day care or parent-to-parent education programmes that operate on a volunteer or quasi-volunteer basis, with the caregivers functioning outside any formal bureaucratic system. The particular set of categories for a country would have to be evolved locally in order to reflect the organizational profile of that country. The examples from São Paulo, Brazil and from India presented on pages 22 and 23 provide examples of the kind of approach that might be taken.

There is a need also to have a more systematic idea of who the main actors are in the field. Programmes of non-governmental organizations can easily go unrecorded, even though the work of church groups and other non-governmental organizations may be extremely important in a particular context.

It may be that the most accurate and complete way of describing child care and development in a particular country will be through a household sample survey, rather than by polling institutions. Many countries are already in a position to do this, with sampling frames set and a solid survey research capacity in place. The utility of this method is being tested in a multi-country study now under way, organized by the International Association for the Study of School Achievement (see Olmsted 1989).

Once a general description of types of programmes and coverage and actors has been organized, it would be possible to begin looking at the quality of programmes in a more systematic way. Again, a sampling basis might be required, this time, of institutions. Institutional inputs and programme content criteria, determined locally, could be monitored. (In the UNESCO survey, questions were asked about staffing and specialists, the training of teachers, the objectives of ECCE, the content of ECCE classes, and about equipment and buildings. These were, however, at a general level and did not necessarily represent what actually goes on in the early childhood institutions.)

Attention to quality seems particularly important when considering how values are being imparted in the early socialization process. If one had to guess, the guess would be that early childhood programmes more often than not are taking their cues from imported models that reinforce value shifts towards the individualistic, production-oriented cultures of the West. Is that where we want to be?

Beyond these organizational and programmatic descriptions, concerned mainly with inputs and coverage, there is a need also for measures of programme impact. In other fields it is possible not only to provide a panorama of institutions and programmes, but also to monitor progress in the field in terms of an indicator such as the reduction of the infant mortality rate or of third degree malnutrition. The field of child development does not yet have agreement on such a measure of 'where we are'. We will return to that issue later in the book, recommending creation of a 'Child Readiness Profile'.

In Part I, we have presented a rationale for investing in programmes of early childhood care and development. We have provided a general impression of the changing contexts and needs associated with the growth of organized care and development programmes, and have presented data suggesting that programme coverage has been increasing significantly, and differentially, but remains relatively low in most Third World countries. The need for a more systematic approach to monitoring these programmes and the general state of child development has been emphasized. We now turn, in Part II, to a more thorough examination of what it means to invest in early childhood care and development and of how that can be done.

REFERENCES

Aries, P. *Centuries of Childhood: A Social History of Family Life.* New York: Vintage Books, 1962.

Calvo, G. 'El proceso de transición entre los programas de atención a la niñez y los de educación primaria en América Latina', a discussion paper prepared for the workshop on the articulation of initial and primary school education, 14–18 March, 1988, Bogotá, UNICEF, and Santiago, UNESCO-CREALC, March, 1988.

Campos, M. and F. Rosemberg. *Diagnostico da Situação da Educação Pre-Escolar na Região Metropolitana de São Paulo.* São Paulo, Brasil: Fundação Carlos Chagas, julho de 1988.

Fisher, E.A. 'Statistical Analysis of Questionnaires on Early Childhood Care and Education (ECCE)', Paris: UNESCO, January 1990. (Draft)

Government of India, Ministry of Welfare. *Child in India: A Statistical Profile.* New Delhi, 1985.

Ki-Zerbo, J. *Educate or Perish.* Dakar: UNESCO Regional Office, 1990.

Levine, R. and M. White. *The Human Condition: The Cultural Basis of Educational Development.* London: Routledge and Kegan Paul, 1986.

Olmsted, P. and D. Weikart (eds). *How Nations Serve Young Children: Profiles of Child Care and Education in 14 Countries.* Ypsilanti, Michigan: The High/Scope Press, 1989.

Riak, P., R. Rono, F. Kiragu and M. Nyukuri, 'Early Childhood Care and Education in Kenya', in Olmsted, P. and D. Weikart (eds), ibid., pp. 203–18.

Smyke, Patricia. 'Caught in the Cross Currents (What's Happened to Children and People Who Work for Children in the Ten Years since the International Year of the Child)', a review of NGO/UN action for children 1979–1989. New York: the Non-Governmental Organizations Committee on UNICEF, 1989.

Tedesco, J.C., 'La Situación Educativa y las Estrategias en Marcha Frente a la Conferencia Mundial, "Educación para Todos", Notas para la Exposición, a paper presented to the Regional Consultation on Education for All in Quito, Ecuador, November 28, 1989. Santiago, Chile, UNESCO, November, 1989.

Tilly, L. and J.W. Scott. *Women, Work, and Family.* New York: Holt, Rinehart and Winston, 1978.

UNESCO, *Educational Statistics, 1988.* Paris: UNESCO, 1988.

UNESCO. '1988 World Survey on Early Childhood Care and Education (ECCE): Summary of Findings', Paris: UNESCO, September, 1989. Doc ED-89/617.ECCE/3. Mimeo.

UNICEF/India. Annual Report. New Delhi: UNICEF, 1988.

van der Eyken, Willem. *The Pre-school Years.* Harmondsworth, England: Penguin Books, 1969.

Wall, W.D. *Constructive Education for Children.* London: George G. Harrap and Co. Ltd and Paris: The UNESCO Press, 1975.

Part II

In search of conceptual clarity

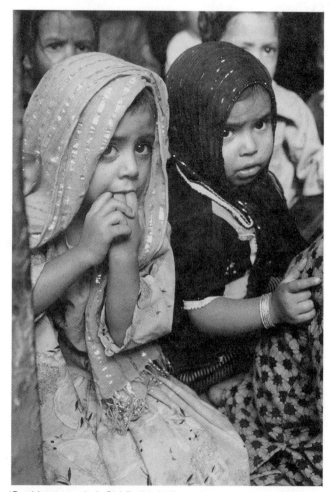

'Seeking security', Old Delhi, India

Chapter 3

What do they mean and what do we know?

A programme officer in an international organization recently asserted, 'Obviously, a child has to survive before it develops'. We will argue that is a misconception – that survival, growth, and development are simultaneous (not sequential) processes. Actions promoting survival or growth enhance development and vice versa.

A pregnant woman expresses her surprise to a community worker: 'You mean that when my baby is born it will be able to see me? I didn't know that'. Yes, that is so if you are close to her – and she can hear and feel your touch and communicate with you and do lots of other things that will help you to help her develop.

A director of a child-care centre explains with pride to a visitor that, 'The children in our nursery get good care. They get fed on time – and good food too. See how clean the place is. We keep them warm. The doctor comes in to see them once a month'. That is all to the good, but her concept of child care is limited. It does not seem to include responding to social and intellectual needs.

A government official, asked about support given to programmes of child development, seeks clarification from the questioner: 'A child development programme? Oh, you mean like the preschools where the children play a lot with coloured blocks?' No, not exactly; child development can be fostered in many kinds of programmes, including nutrition, health, and education programmes, and by working with parents and community members as well as with children.

Each of the introductory comments or questions provides an example of a fundamental misconception or lack of knowledge about child development and care. This lack of understanding and clarity can have a major and negative effect on the actions of parents, professionals, planners, politicians, and funders, and through them on developing children. But the concepts of child survival, growth, development and care are not always clear and the evolving terms mean different things to different people, sometimes creating confusion. And, although we know a great deal about how the child develops, that knowledge is not always available to those who care for children or who make decisions about programmes of care and development.

It is important, therefore, to be clear about how child survival, growth, development and care are defined and employed in this book. It is equally important to demonstrate that a substantial knowledge base exists that can be drawn upon now to foster and improve child care and development. Accordingly, this chapter has two purposes:

1 To clarify what we mean by child survival, growth, development and care.
2 To suggest that we know more than we think we know about child care and development, using examples to show that the state of the art provides us with a more-than-adequate base to begin our programming.

WHAT DO THEY MEAN?

Child survival

A negative definition   Somewhat ironically, 'survival' is usually defined negatively: to survive is *not to die*. Infant survival is not dying before age one; child survival is not dying before age five. Consistent with this view of survival, programmes of child survival place emphasis on avoiding death, usually measured by reduction of the infant mortality rate (IMR) or the mortality rate of children under five years of age (U5MR). That emphasis is made easier by the fact that death is a dramatic and final event and can be counted with relative ease and accuracy, even allowing for failures to report infant and child deaths.

A positive definition   But child survival can be thought of as something more than simply avoiding death. Death seldom occurs instantly. Most deaths follow a period of illness and deterioration that can be painfully prolonged or relatively short. Dying is a process, the end of which is death (Mosley and Chen 1984). Living is a process, the end of which is not only survival, but physical, mental, and social health and welfare.

Surviving children fall along a continuum running from near death through sickness to a healthy state. The further a child is along that continuum towards a healthy state, the better the chances are of continued survival. The process of surviving, then, can be thought of as actively seeking a healthy state – of moving towards the healthy end of the death–sickness–health spectrum – rather than simply preventing or arresting the process of dying.

Accepting this positive reconceptualization of child survival – as a process of seeking a healthy state at birth and in the early months and years of life – requires looking beyond the analysis of causes of mortality and beyond programmes that reduce mortality. It means examining where children are along a health–growth–development continuum. It means searching for programmes that will improve their health. This requires clarity about what, in a positive sense, constitutes moving towards a 'healthy state'. That must include seeking mental and social health as well as physical well-being for young children.

An infant survival ratio (ISR)   If survival is to be defined positively rather than as 'not dying', it should be indexed by an infant (or child) *survival* ratio (ISR or CSR) rather than by infant and child mortality ratios. The success of programmes should be measured by increases in a survival ratio rather than by decreases in a mortality ratio.

An ISR simply turns the IMR upside down. For instance, in 1988, the IMR was approximately 77 deaths for every 1000 children born; i.e. 1 of every 13 children born was expected to die before the age of one year (Grant 1988). The ISR would be 923 per 1000, emphasizing that 12 of 13 children live to age one. Using the ISR, we can say that the rate of survival has increased from 5 of 6 children born in 1960 to 12 of 13 children born in 1988.

Suggesting an ISR[1] in contrast to an IMR is more than just an alphabet or numbers game. To emphasize living, as represented by an ISR, provokes a different way of thinking than emphasizing the avoidance of death, as represented in the IMR. It dramatizes the fact that many children somehow manage to live in spite of being 'at risk'. It provokes questions about the condition of those who live and about what is being done for the welfare of the increasing number of poor and 'at risk' children who are surviving.

Growth

To grow is to increase in size. Growth occurs as cells are added to the body or as cells increase in size. The measures of growth most commonly used are weight or height or both. These measures are relatively easy to obtain (compared with measures of social or psychological development), and norms have been developed against which the measures can be compared. This relative ease of measurement and the availability of standards has given rise to the use of growth charts, based on height and/or weight for age, as a convenient means of monitoring a child's growth.

Growth, for children, can be thought of as having attained a certain 'growth norm' or it can be seen as a process of steadily increasing in size. There has been a slow shift in recent years from the normative emphasis towards viewing growth as a process. Steady growth indicates progress. Failure to grow (as indicated by failure to gain weight, for instance) points to a need for remedial action. Thus, the particular point where a child falls on a growth chart is less important than the pattern of change – i.e.

whether there has been an increase or decrease since the previous measurement.

The shift towards viewing growth as a process parallels the shifting conceptualization of survival sketched above, and, as we shall see, is consistent also with changing ideas about child development.

Obviously, growth depends on the amount and kind of food a child eats. The relationship between food intake and growth has been a main concern of nutritionists. However, there is a strong tendency among nutritionists to overlook the fact that intake is not only a matter of whether or not food is available; it is also affected by the fact that feeding, particularly in the early years, is a social process. Feeding involves an interaction between the mother, or another caregiver, and the young child. This point will be elaborated in Chapter 9.

Growth not only depends on the quantity and quality of the food a child takes in, but also depends on how well that food is assimilated and used by the body. How well food is used depends in part on the health of a child. A child with diarrhoea certainly will not use its food well. Although it was not always the case, the combined effect of food intake and health status on growth is now widely recognized. However, we shall argue (see Chapter 9) that physical growth (and survival) can be influenced also by how well a child is developing socially and psychologically, and by how free a child and the child's caregiver are from stress. In most discussions of growth and nutrition, the social and psychological health of caregiver and child is not included. The effect on nutrition and health of developmentally sensitive interactions is not understood to be important and is not given its due.

Child development

Child development and child growth   Development is not the same as growth, although, as suggested in the preceding discussion, the two are interrelated and the terms are often used interchangeably. Whereas growth is described by a change in *size*, development is characterized by changes in *complexity* and *function*. A child who learns to coordinate eye and hand movements in order to grasp an object shows a sign of developing a more complex way of thinking, independently of the size of the child. The ability to grasp signifies greater control over one's environment. These changes are very different from an increase in height from 70 to 75 centimetres or in weight from 10 to 12 kilograms.

A working definition of child development   Although it is difficult to arrive at a consensus about some aspects of child development, the following definition, presented in intentionally simple language and extended below through the discussion of characteristics, provides an appropriate starting point for discussion and action:

Child development is a process of change in which the child learns to handle ever more complex levels of moving, thinking, feeling, and relating to others.

As with survival and growth, development can be conceptualized as attaining a certain state (as measured, for instance, by a developmental or intellectual quotient or by whether a child has achieved the coordination that allows walking by a certain age). Or, child development can be viewed, as we prefer to do, as a process with several characteristics.

1 *Development is multidimensional.* As suggested by our definition, development includes improving:

- A physical (or motor) dimension – the ability to move, coordinate;
- A mental (or, more broadly, cognitive) dimension – the ability to think and reason;
- An emotional dimension – the ability to feel; and
- A social dimension – the ability to relate to others.

To describe adequately a child's development, therefore, requires more than measuring how well a child is developing its ability to think or to walk; it requires looking at all of the developmental dimensions.[2]

In this book, emphasis will be placed on the mental, social, and emotional dimensions of development. Accordingly, reference will be made periodically to 'psychosocial' development, a term that encompasses these three dimensions.

2 *Development is integral.* By describing development as integral we mean that the several dimensions of child development are interrelated and must be considered together; changes along one dimension both influence and are influenced by development along the others. Emotional development, for instance, affects physical and cognitive development. If a child is under emotional stress and has not developed an ability to cope with that stress, the ability to develop physically and to learn will both be affected. This interaction among conceptually distinct but organically interrelated dimensions requires attention to 'the whole child' and emphasis on a 'total' or 'integrated' approach to programming for child development.

Because child development is integral, our emphasis on 'psychosocial development' cannot be exclusive and must be seen within the broader view of development that includes physical development.

3 *Development occurs continually.* The process of development begins prenatally and continues throughout life. In its time dimension as well as its content, then, child development must be seen as part of human development occurring over the entire life span. We are concerned here with the child from conception to age five or six when a child moves beyond the home. But that concern requires also attention to the effects of early

development on later development and on behaviours and attainments in all of later life.

Viewing development as a continuing process means that a child is always developing; whatever happens at a given moment helps to prepare the way for what happens in the future. However, the idea of continuity, as used here, does not imply that attainments at one point will continue indefinitely or that the path of development is always positive. Changing conditions can undercut or support what has been attained. Nor does the notion of continuity imply that a child with delays and problems in early life will necessarily remain forever behind others. On the contrary, children are very resilient, particularly in their earliest years. Changed circumstances can open the way to improvement. If the environment does not change, however, deficits can accumulate, leading to developmental delays. Conversely, appropriate interventions can have a recuperative effect, as will be shown later on.

4 *Development occurs in interaction.* Development happens as a child responds to, learns from, and seeks to affect his or her biophysical and social environments. It occurs in interaction with people and things. For this reason, fostering development requires more than providing a child with 'stimulation'. It requires also responses to initiatives taken by the child. A child helps to construct its own environment. A child takes initiatives and influences its surroundings. This fact is central to an understanding of how health and nutrition are affected by a child's psychological and social development, and vice versa.

There is a strong tendency to think that a child first survives, then grows and develops. But survival, growth, and development occur simultaneously, not sequentially. Moreover, by attending to developmental needs it is possible to have a positive effect on survival and growth. Put another way, improved development, including psychosocial development, will have a positive effect on nutrition and health (disease and infection) and on the chance of survival.

5 *Development is patterned, but unique.* All children develop and there is a general sequence[3] or outline to that development. But the rate and character and quality of development will vary from child to child. Individual variation is the product of a child's special biological makeup and the particular environment in which it struggles to survive and develop. The rate of development will vary from culture to culture as well as from child to child.

The main goal of a child's development.   A developing child adapts to and seeks some mastery over his or her surroundings. Because surroundings can be very limiting, some analysts include in the goal of child development the ability to transform one's surroundings. In the short run, adaptation and mastery is to immediate conditions. Over a lifetime, however, mastery and adaptation can include adjustment to a variety of surroundings with very different requirements for survival and development. Consistent with this goal, we may view development as '... a lasting change in the way in which a person perceives and deals with his environment' (Bronfenbrenner, 1979).

The developmental goal of adaptation to and mastery (and transformation) of one's surroundings differs radically from a goal of survival, or of being healthy, or of attaining a certain level of coordination or of achieving a higher intelligence quotient. It takes into account that different cultural and ecological surroundings place different demands on the child. It requires a disaggregated and decentralized view of early childhood development.

Child care

Child care falls in a somewhat different category from the three previous key concepts. Care consists of the actions necessary to promote survival, growth, and development. Caring for a child means responding to basic needs. The basic needs of development go beyond protection, food, and health care to include the need for affection, interaction and stimulation, security provided through consistency and predictability, and play allowing exploration and discovery. These needs appear together. A supportive environment will respond to all a child's needs which will, however, be defined somewhat differently and given different priorities by different cultures.

At a minimum, the following child-care activities can be specified:

providing security
sheltering
clothing
feeding
bathing
supervising a child's toilet
preventing and attending to sickness
nurturing and showing affection
interacting with and stimulating a child
playing
socializing the child to its culture

Defining child care in this way means that *programmes of child care and of integrated child development should be the same.* In this book, child care is used in the broad sense described above, including health and other elements of custodial care, but looking beyond them to include also care directed to the psychological, social, and emotional welfare of children.

But child care is commonly used in a much narrower way. Moreover, the meaning attached to 'care' is different for different groups attending to young children. In the health community, for instance, care is fundamentally health care defined in terms of preventing or attending to infection and disease. Appropriately, child care is linked to care for the mother in maternal and child health (MCH) programmes.

When associated with programmes designed to improve the 'productive' role of women, child care refers to the arrangements made to look after a child while the mother works. Often, that arrangement is 'custodial', assigning to another person or institution the temporary responsibility for assuring that a child has shelter, clothing, food, and attention to health needs. This association with custodial care means that child-care programmes are usually put in a different category from child development programmes. Child-care programmes have not, for the most part, placed much emphasis on stimulation and education components intended to foster the mental and social development of the children being cared for.[4]

If child care is approached from a social welfare perspective, it is usually associated with institutionalized care, and often with programmes for abused or abandoned or indigent children. These programmes also have a strong custodial tradition.

When discussing programmes of child care, we shall look beyond centre-based or institutional care and include also direct care by a mother, and delegation of responsibility for care to extended family members or to others on a personal social network.

The foregoing discussion of terms may seem rather laboured to some readers; others will find it horribly over-simplified. However, existing misconceptions and the general lack of clarity that marks many discussions seem to demand both the attempt to clarify and to present these central concepts in straightforward language. At a minimum, the reader should now understand how the concepts of child survival, growth, development, and care are used in this book, and we can turn now to examples of the knowledge base that is (or should be) available to parents, planners and others.

WE KNOW MORE THAN WE THINK WE KNOW

Somewhere between the obvious and the uncertain, we know more than we think we know about early childhood development and about programming to facilitate and foster that development. The field has grown rapidly in the last two decades, bringing new knowledge and some changes in orientation. At the same time, experience has been accumulating at a rapid rate. Undoubtedly, the field will continue to develop and we shall continue to improve our knowledge on the basis of concrete experiences. However, a more-than-reasonable base of knowledge and experience already exists that is sufficient to guide programming, even while we are filling in gaps in our knowledge.

Consider the following affirmations, derived from the literature on child development, each with an important implication for programming. The statements illustrate scientifically derived knowledge that is useful for programming. Some of the statements are obvious, but bear repeating because they provide a basis for programme actions. The less obvious statements could be the subject of some debate, but even these would be accepted as reasonable working hypotheses by most experts in the field of early childhood development.

1 A child can see and hear at birth and is also born with predispositions that prepare it to perceive, learn from, and make demands upon the external world. An infant can communicate from birth – by crying and through its facial expressions and movements.

Implication: From birth, an infant can interact with and learn from its environment. Therefore, programmes designed to enhance development can include the newborn, helping parents to be responsive to and promote communication through their interaction with the newborn.

2 As a child interacts with its surroundings, it is both influenced by and influences them. For example, a child that is alert and/or a child that cries is more likely to obtain a response and to be fed than a child that is listless.

Implication: Activities that help a child to develop socially and psychologically will make the child more alert and will, therefore, also help to improve the nutritional status and health of a child and its chances for survival. There is a two-way relationship between psychosocial development and the physical aspects of growth and development.

3 Infants differ from birth in their disposition to activity, irritability, and fearfulness, among other characteristics, and therefore differ in what they require from their environment and in their reaction to what caregivers do.

Implication: The same actions by caregivers can produce different effects in different children. Therefore, parents need to be alert to how each particular child responds to the conditions around it. They need to be flexible. And, they need to have a range of skills and expectations to match the temperament of a given child.

4 Cognitive and social development are affected by the growth of brain cells and the development of neural connections.

Implication: Health and nutrition conditions that damage the brain, even prenatally, when the most growth is occurring, will influence development.

5 Stimulation that provides the brain with exercise will help to improve the connections made and will set a stronger base for later development.

Implication: Environments should provide appropriate stimulation, particularly during the early years when connections are being formed in the brain.

6 The cognitive development of infants living in environments with little variety is generally lower than that of infants living in environments that contain variety.

Implication: Attention should be given to determining the degree of variety present in different environments and to either reinforcing or adding to that variety, according to the needs of the particular child. (Most environments offer variation and there is not a need to import things or people to provide needed variation. Also, in exceptional cases, environments are too varied and stimulating, creating confusion.)

7 Children are amazingly resilient, particularly in the earliest years, when they seem to have a series of built-in mechanisms to help them develop. A child's development may be delayed, or damage may occur, as a result of problems at birth or because the environment after birth is cruel. However, unless early, prolonged, and severe difficulties (e.g. an extended period of severe malnutrition) occur, a child has the potential to recover and develop normally.

Implication: The fact that a child has suffered from poor health or has been moderately malnourished does not automatically mean the child's development will be delayed. Recuperation is possible. However, preventive programmes beginning with prenatal care of the mother are preferable.

8 In addition to needs for food, shelter, health care and protection, young children have basic psychological and social developmental needs. These include:

- A need for love and affection;
- A need for interaction (both providing stimulation and reacting to the child);
- A need for consistency and predictability in their caregiving environment; and
- A need to explore and discover.

Implication: Programmes of integrated attention to the child should respond to these basic needs as well as to the needs for food, shelter, health care, and protection.

9 Although all children have certain basic needs, each child will have a set of individual needs, determined by its own genetic makeup, by the immediate conditions in the family that satisfy (or do not satisfy) some of the basic needs, and by conditions in the community and larger society, both of which set goals and impose limits on the child affecting its development.

Implication: Programming must take into account these differences in individual needs and in the conditions at the level of family, community, and society that affect development. A programme formula, to be applied to all children and circumstances, is therefore inappropriate.

10 There is a synergistic relationship among the various facets of development – the physical, social, intellectual, and emotional facets are part of a

whole so that affecting one area brings effects in the others as well. For example, in infants as well as in adults, cognitive processes are related to emotional states because they are related to the onset, control, and reduction of anxiety.

Implication: Multifaceted approaches to programming are needed.

11 The social experience of a child will usually have a much stronger influence on future achievement, IQ score, and socially deviant behaviour than condition at birth.

Implication: A benevolent environment is critical. It is possible for recuperation to occur, even in relatively high 'at risk' circumstances related to conditions at birth.

12 All children develop, but some children develop faster than others and their development is qualitatively different (applying whatever criterion seems appropriate).

Implication: Although developmental norms may be useful for judging a large population of children, they should be applied with caution to individuals.

The above are given as examples. Throughout the book we shall add to the examples of the knowledge base that can be drawn upon in the design and implementation of programmes for early childhood care and development.

There is another source of knowledge that needs to be taken into account: that source is 'traditional wisdom'. Failure to recognize and draw upon traditional wisdom with respect to childrearing practices is common. Until recently, a similar failure was present with respect to health practices, but the last ten to twenty years have begun to break down resistance to considering traditional medicine in any way other than as quackery. The same needs to occur for childrearing practices related to child development. This source of knowledge will be examined as childrearing practices and beliefs are discussed in Chapter 13. As traditional wisdom is given its proper place, and when the currently applicable wisdom is separated from that which no longer applies, the conclusion is reinforced that we know more than we think we know.

In view of the above, it seems appropriate to observe that the state of the art is ahead of the state of the practice. Consider the following:

State of the art	*State of the practice*
1 Development is a continuing process beginning during the prenatal period	1 Programmes emphasize children ages 3 to 6
2 Development is an interactive process	2 Emphasis is placed on one-way 'stimulation'

| 3 There is a synergism between health, nutrition, and psychosocial development | 3 Programmes continue to be mono-focal and to lack integration |
| 4 Indigenous childrearing practices are often helpful | 4 Solutions are often imported |

It is time to act on these differences, even while new ideas accumulate to inform programming.

NOTES

1   In UNICEF's publication, *The State of the World's Children, 1989*, in a special section titled 'Measuring Real Development' (pp. 73–90), a table is presented grouping countries according to a child survival ratio (p. 80). In the text, however, discussion continues in terms of a U5MR.

2   Sometimes included as separate dimensions are moral and spiritual dimensions of development. Kohlberg (1976), for instance, has set out stages of moral development. An inner sense of contentment and peace resulting from self-control over greed or anger or envy defines a spiritual goal in some cultures that is central to personal development and that begins in early childhood. While recognizing the need for moral and spiritual development, we have not included these dimensions specifically, preferring to approach them as culturally determined goals guiding social and emotional and cognitive development.

3   As a general guide to understanding where a child is in the process of continuous change, the process is often described theoretically in terms of 'stages'. Theorists differ with respect to: whether it is really possible to identify distinct traits distinguishing one stage or period or step from another; the particular aspects of development used to define stages (e.g. physical or social or sexual); the relationship of stages to chronological age, how small and limited in time each stage is (vs. broad definitions encompassing long periods); the universality of stages (must they be the same in all cultures?); whether or not a child must pass sequentially through stages; whether regression is possible; and how problems at one stage will affect actions at another (Thomas 1985, Chapter 2). For all these differences, the notion of stages can still be useful practically as well as theoretically if the proper cautions are exercised.

4   When 'care' is translated into French, the corresponding word is 'protection', leaving little room for a broader definition of care that includes attention to a child's development. In the following chapter, that is illustrated dramatically as child care enters one of the models through 'injury', consistent with the idea of protection.

REFERENCES

Bronfenbrenner, U. *The Ecology of Human Development.* Cambridge, Mass: Harvard University Press, 1979.

Grant, James. *The State of the World's Children, 1988.* New York: UNICEF, 1988. Ibid., 1989.

Kohlberg, L. 'Moral Stages and Moralization: The Cognitive-Developmental Approach', in T. Likona (ed.), *Moral Development and Behavior: Theory,*

Research, and Social Issues. New York: Holt, Rinehart and Winston, 1976, pp. 12–60.

Mosley, H. and L. Chen. 'An Analytical Framework for the Study of Child Survival in Developing Countries', *Population and Development Review*, supplement to Vol. 10 (1984), pp. 25–45.

Thomas, R.M. *Comparing Theories of Child Development* (2nd ed.). Belmont, Calif: Wadsworth Publishing Company, Inc., 1985.

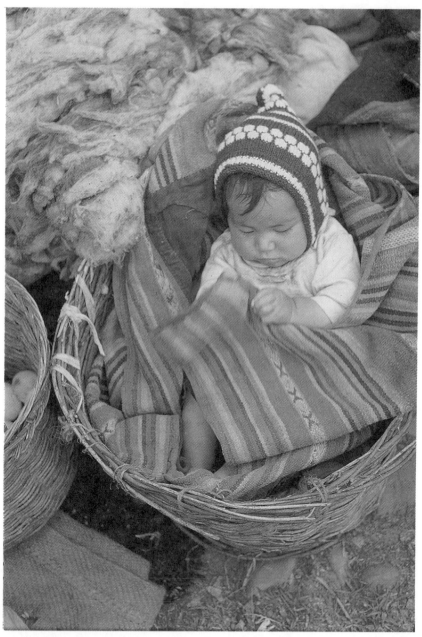

'Exploration', Huancayo, Peru

Chapter 4

Trends, frameworks and relationships: collecting the pieces

The search for clarity requires more than specification of terms. Because child survival, growth, development, and care cut across many fields and can be approached from many perspectives, diverse models and analyses exist, side by side, that can confuse as well as enlighten. In addition, the field of child development has been changing. Scientific thinking is running well ahead of its translation into programme actions based on that thinking. There is, then, a pressing need to sort through, and try to make sense of, the multitude of models and frameworks that guide analyses of child survival, growth, development, and care. And there is a need to identify changing interpretations, with policy and programme implications in mind.

This chapter has two purposes:

1 To examine a set of frameworks that look in diverse ways at survival, growth and development, in order to understand better the variables affecting these processes.
2 To identify trends in thinking about survival, growth and development.
The review provides a basis for moving beyond programming focused on child survival and growth, to combined programming for child survival and development, viewed broadly. The analysis leads to identification of five complementary programming approaches, to be presented in the following chapter.

THE PIECEMEAL CHILD

Unfortunately, when it comes to studying child development and care, or to formulating policy and implementing programmes, we are victims of the age of specialization in which we live. Academic and bureaucratic divisions of labour cut the child into small pieces. The 'whole child', so often present in the rhetoric of child development, is slowly dissected in a series of unconnected, narrowly conceived analyses. Doctors, psychologists, nutritionists, sociologists, educators, anthropologists, economists and others each approach the topic from a distinct point of view. Narrow analyses are reinforced by equally narrow sectoral approaches to planning and programming. How to overcome these divisions is a major challenge.

With such a wide spread of interests related to child development and with such different treatments of the topic it is not surprising that sceptics often shake their heads, wondering which version of child development is the real one. The academic discipline or professional posture that gives rise to each framework influences the statement of the problem and the particular set of assumptions, variables, and relationships incorporated into the framework. The language used varies widely, sometimes requiring translation. For instance, 'child development' may be treated as growth or socialization or acculturation, depending on the discipline.

Collecting the pieces

One way to try to bring the pieces back together is to look for commonalities and complementarities among approaches to child survival, growth, care and development that are rooted in different disciplines. To that end, we have selected for discussion seven overlapping frameworks from the vast array.

The seven have been chosen because:

1 Each makes an attempt at conceptual integration by bridging disciplines, combining, for instance, a medical viewpoint with a social science one, or linking anthropology and psychology.
2 Taken together, the complementary and overlapping perspectives introduce a wide range of variables, operating at different levels of specificity and at different points in a child's progress to survive and develop.
3 The frameworks illustrate a process of redefinition that has been occurring over approximately the last 15 years.

Each of the seven frameworks is useful in attempting to understand some part of the larger picture of intertwined influences and relationships affecting child survival, growth, development, and care. Inevitably, each is incomplete. Bringing together the different approaches is intended to help reintegrate thinking, with the hope that overcoming piecemeal thinking will help to overcome piecemeal programming and action.

The frameworks selected are summarized briefly in Table 4.1. The table shows how the seven differ with respect to their disciplinary origin and the dependent variable or focus of analytical attention. The list includes frameworks based in the fields of epidemiology, nutrition, psychology (particularly that part of psychology concerned with child development), anthropology, sociology, and economics. The frameworks focus variously on survival, child welfare, the ability to thrive nutritionally and to grow, the ability to function well in one's particular environment, and the combined

Table 4.1 Frameworks for the analysis of child survival, growth, development and care

Authors and sources	Fields	Main dependent variable
1 W. Henry Mosley and Lincoln Chen, 'An Analytical Framework for the Study of Child Survival in Developing Countries', *Population and Development Review*, A Supplement, Vol. 10 (1984), pp. 25–45.	Epidemiology Demography	Child survival
2 A. Cornia, R. Jolly, and F. Stewart, *Adjustment with a Human Face: Protecting the Vulnerable and Promoting Growth*. New York: Oxford University Press, 1988, Chapter 2.	Economics Epidemiology	Child welfare
3 M. Zeitlin, H. Ghassemi, and M. Mansour, *Positive Deviance in Child Nutrition*. Tokyo: The United Nations University, 1990.	Nutrition Sociology	Growth
4 Urie Bronfenbrenner, *The Ecology of Human Development*. Cambridge, Mass: Harvard University Press, 1979.	Psychology Sociology	Interactive model
5 Charles Super and Sara Harkness, 'The Developmental Niche: A Conceptualization at the Interface of Child and Culture', *International Journal of Behavioral Development*, Vol. 9 (1987), pp. 1–25.	Anthropology Psychology	Interactive model
6 Barry Lester and T. Berry Brazelton, 'Cross-Cultural Assessment of Neonatal Behaviour', in D. Wagner and H. Stevenson (eds), *Cultural Perspectives on Child Development*. San Francisco: W.H. Freeman and Co., 1982, Chapter 2.	Biology Psychology	Interactive model
7 Lynn Bennett, 'The Role of Women in Income Production and Intra-Household Allocation of Resources as a Determinant of Child Health and Nutrition', *Food and Nutrition Bulletin*, Vol. 10, No. 3 (1988), pp. 16–26.	Anthropology Economics	Family welfare

welfare of family members. They vary greatly in their complexity and their breadth of vision.

The brief description and discussion of each framework that follows is intended to provide the interested reader with a feel for the information used to draw conclusions about changes in the field and about implications of these changes for policy and programmes.

SEVEN FRAMEWORKS

The first two models presented below are somewhat different from the remaining five. They illustrate how analyses based on a medical model, focusing on child survival, lead to neglect of child development variables that both affect the probability of dying and should be considered as part of the process of healthy survival.

Framework 1: Mosley and Chen

The purpose of the model presented by Mosley and Chen (see Figure 4.1) is to aid the study of social, economic, biological, and environmental factors affecting the probability of survival. This epidemiological model is the work of two medical doctors with field experience in developing countries and with a strong public health bias. The model is particularly important for several reasons:

1 It represents a conscious, prudent, and influential effort to overcome communication barriers between medical and social science communities by seeking common ground, combining variables from the social science with medical variables in one operational model.

2 The model looks at survival (and death) as process(es) occurring in time and defined in terms of a health/sickness continuum. In so doing, the model redefines 'cause of death' as the cumulative consequence of multiple disease processes (including their biosocial interactions). Growth faltering is taken as an indicator of a child's general condition, with death incorporated as the end point of growth faltering.

3 Within the medical community, this is a revisionist model. By giving an important place to socioeconomic determinants of survival, it shifts analysis and action from extending and improving the supply of health technologies and services to working on the demand for technologies and services while strengthening the 'home production' of health.

4 By grouping 14 variables into a set of 5 'proximate' (intermediate) variables, Mosley and Chen arrive at a relatively parsimonious model in which socioeconomic determinants are seen to act through biological mechanisms to insert an influence on mortality.

In brief, this is an integrative and broad, yet relatively tidy, analytical

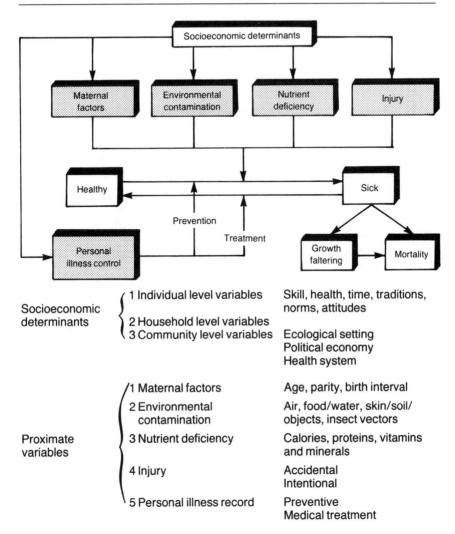

Figure 4.1 Operation of the five groups of proximate determinants on the health dynamics of a population
Source: Mosley and Chen (1984), p. 27.

scheme marking an advance in thinking about child health and survival.

Featured in the Mosley/Chen model are five 'proximate variables', labelled by Mosley and Chen as: maternal factors, environmental contamination, nutrient deficiency, injury, and personal illness control (see Figure 4.1). The operation of the model is described in the following terms:

The socioeconomic determinants must operate through more 'proximate variables' (intermediate variables) that in turn influence the risk of disease and the outcome of disease processes. The specific diseases and nutrient deficiencies observed in a surviving population may be viewed as biological indicators of the operations of the proximate determinants.

(Mosley and Chen, p. 27)

All proximate determinants in the first four groups influence the rate of shift of healthy individuals towards sickness. The personal illness control factor influences both the rate of illness (through prevention) and the rate of recovery (through treatment). Specific states of sickness (infection or nutrient deficiency) are basically transitory: ultimately there is either complete recovery or irreversible consequences manifested by increasing degrees of permanent growth faltering (or other disability among the survivors) and/or death. A novel aspect of this conceptual model is its definition of a specific disease state in an individual as an indicator of the operation of the proximate determinants rather than as a 'cause' of illness and death.

(Mosley and Chen, p. 28)

Adapting the model

How can these ideas of child health and survival be applied to shed light on our concern with child development and care for children who are surviving? How might the model be used, adapted, built upon? The following observations seem relevant:

Incorporating 'development' into the survival model

The child survival model of Mosley and Chen makes no specific reference to child development. However, making a developmental component explicit in the model is a relatively easy task and can be done from a health standpoint by including psychological health and social adjustment as components of 'a healthy state'. Indeed, it is common for the medical community to include these in the definition of a healthy state. Affecting that part of the healthy state as well as the probability of death are conditions that can be incorporated into a sixth 'proximate determinant' we have labelled 'psychosocial stress'. Along with nutrients and cleanliness, etc. a child needs loving, stimulating, reciprocal attention. Failure to receive such attention creates stress and can reduce activity, affecting where an individual is on the health–sickness–death continuum.

'Development faltering' can be introduced into the model as an outcome parallel to 'growth faltering', making explicit the developmental dimension of being healthy or sick. Growth faltering and developmental faltering are interrelated, and both are interrelated with health. The Mosley/Chen model is presented again in Figure 4.2, with these additions made.

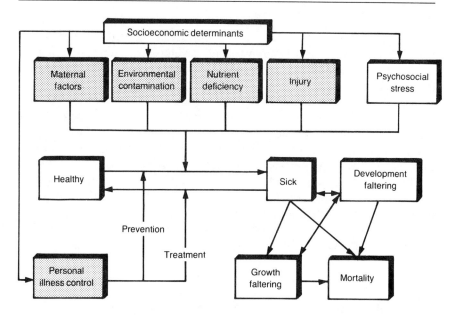

Figure 4.2 An adaptation of the Mosley/Chen model

Attending to the mother–child dyad

Missing from the Mosley/Chen model and from their discussion of the operation of the model is reference to the mother–child dyad. Individual characteristics of the mother and father are included among the socioeconomic determinants. But healthiness and development are very much a product of how a mother (or other caregivers) interacts with a child. More than time and education are required. In the list of traditions, norms, and attitudes presented by Mosley and Chen should be included childrearing practices and beliefs influencing the mother–child interaction. (These were not included in their explanation of the model.) What do parents believe about the ability of their newborn to see and hear? What are the feeding practices (not just the food preferences)? Does a caregiver talk to a child?

Community organization and support systems

Mosley and Chen describe socioeconomic variables at three levels: individual, household, and 'community'. In their treatment of 'community-level' variables the authors move directly to discussion of larger system variables operating at a national level. Missing is reference to community participation and organization in which 'community' refers to an immediate social grouping, larger than the household, of which children and families are a part. Although an immense literature has been devoted to ways in which social organization and participation might be strengthened at the grass roots in support of survival and development, this dimension is missing from the model. It could be incorporated into the socioeconomic determinants with relative ease.

Also appearing as important in the literature dealing with growth and development are 'personal support networks'. How a mother can use her time depends in part on her social support system. Her self-esteem and confidence, also important in improving care for a young child, can be influenced heavily by her social support system. Although 'the family' is the first level of social support, it is not the only, or always the best, support mechanism. Consider, for instance, the case of the single mother without access to extended family members. The Mosley/Chen model does not incorporate this social dimension which is, however, picked up in other models to be discussed below.

A linear view

The social science model that Mosley and Chen build upon is essentially a demographic model seeking 'main effects', describing the presumed effect of a set of independent variables on intermediate variables which, in turn, affect dependent variables. This linear flow does not allow for possible interactions among variables. The model differs fundamentally from an interactive or transactional or ecological or anthropological treatment of the same topic.

A Western view

In their discussion of the model, Mosley and Chen emphasize interventions that have their origin in concepts and practices of Western medicine. The question, for them, is whether or not the Western methods and technologies used are effective and have an impact. They state:

> Anthropological literature is replete with examples of how a society's beliefs about disease causation shape behavior that has an impact on the proximate determinants of child survival. These range from ritualistic practices, to choice of therapies and practitioners for sickness care, to sexual taboos and abstinence to prevent illness in the suckling child. One manifestation of this phenomenon is the commonly reported 'under-utilization' of modern (Western) health facilities when they are introduced into traditional societies. Probably one of the most powerful influences of formal education is the transmission of concepts of modern scientific medicine. When the mother is exposed to such information, it can transform her preferences for health care practices so as to signi-

ficantly improve child survival, often without investment of additional economic resources.

(Mosley and Chen, p. 36)

Another way of approaching the problem might be to ask what methods and technologies work. By phrasing the question in that way, one opens the door to effective traditional wisdom – to the possibility that local methods can be identified and supported that are different from, but as effective as, the Western methods.

Throughout this book, we shall insist that an effort be made to see what healthful practices the household carries out, then build on and around those. This approach differs from (and can be complementary to) a programming approach which centres exclusively on the introduction of new practices. Again, an anthropological perspective provides a useful and necessary counterpart to the demographic and epidemiological approach taken by Mosley and Chen.

Framework 2: Cornia/UNICEF

The Mosley/Chen model has provided a starting point for various analysts who have gone on to create their own adaptation of the model (e.g. van Norren and van Vianen 1986). One of these (see Figure 4.3) is the work of Andrea Cornia and colleagues at UNICEF in their examination of causes underlying losses in child welfare in times of economic recession and in their search for ways to prevent or overcome such losses. The model evolved by Cornia/UNICEF reinterprets and extends the Mosley/Chen framework.

The variables, relationships, and language of the Cornia/UNICEF model reflect its creation by economists and its origin in a set of questions related to national policies of economic adjustment. The model focuses on 'resources' affecting the 'production' of 'child welfare'.

Although the Cornia/UNICEF model appears complicated at first glance, its logical flow and grouping of variables into four major sets makes it easy to follow. An important feature of the model is its specification of macroeconomic variables (variable set 1) and relations that begin with changes in the world economy, national policies of economic adjustment, and macro-economic trends at the national level. These changes influence the availability of (variable set 2) six classes of resources, each susceptible to influence, directly or indirectly, by decisions made about adjustment to declining economic conditions. The six classes of resources are:

–   The level of subsistence production;
–   Family income and its distribution;
–   The price of food, as affected particularly by inflation;

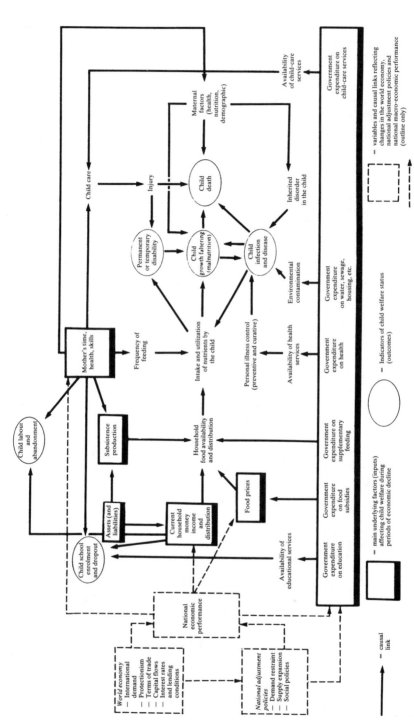

Figure 4.3 An analytical framework linking changes in selected economic determinants and changes in selected indicators of child welfare

Source: Cornia et al. (1987), p. 36.

- Public expenditures (health, education, food subsidies, water, housing, child care, and others);
- Time, health, and instruction of mothers;
- Assets and liabilities.

These first two sets of variables pick up and recast the socioeconomic conditions specified by Mosley and Chen. They include individual, family, and national-level variables.

The effects of the resource variables (variable set 2), which are designated as 'underlying causes', are traced in a linear causal way through a large set of intermediate health- and nutrition-related variables (variable set 3) that are similar to, but expand upon, the five proximate variables of Mosley and Chen.

A set of outcomes (variable set 4) describe child welfare in different ways. By taking 'child welfare' as the outcome, rather than 'child survival', Cornia and colleagues broaden the analysis. In addition to survival (mortality) and to the health (infection/sickness) and nutrition (growth faltering) indicators found in the Mosley/Chen model, Cornia includes as indicators of child welfare: temporary or permanent disability, child abandonment and child labour, and school enrolment and dropout. These additional variables place greater attention on those children who are managing to survive, and they incorporate effects on children beyond the age of five.

Incorporating child care and 'development' into the model

1 *Child care* is explicitly incorporated, linked both to the availability of services and to the time, health, and education (instruction) of the mother. However, child care is pictured as having a direct causal relationship only through 'injury'. This placement of care in the model reflects a very narrow view of care – even narrower than the normal definition of custodial care – focusing on protecting a child from bodily harm.

2 *Child care and women's work.* The model appropriately reflects the fact that child care may be carried out by the mother or by a 'service'. However, the mother is assigned full responsibility for 'feeding'; the model relates the frequency of feeding directly (and only) to mother's time, health, and instruction even though feeding may occur in an institutional setting or be done by other family members or caretakers.

The availability of child-care arrangements will influence the time use and health of a mother (of all family members) and therefore her (their) ability to participate in 'productive' as well as 'reproductive' activities such as feeding. This important relationship – of alternative care to time and of time to productive activities – is not picked up in the model. Rather, women appear to be assigned a predominantly reproductive role, extended somewhat by recognizing their participation in subsistence activities. Any potential contribution women might make to family income is not considered. (In Chapter 11, we shall discuss a more general tendency of economic models to adopt questionable assumptions about the productive and reproductive roles of women as they affect care, survival, growth, and development. The Bennett framework – see below – will pick up this topic from a different perspective.)

3 *Development and disability.*   Psychosocial development is not explicitly included in the framework. Perhaps the closest the model comes to incorporating child development is the inclusion of a disability outcome variable. This outcome was not included by Mosley and Chen. Disability is pictured in the model as a product of faulty child care leading to injuries and/or as a result of malnutrition. Although it is possible to interpret temporary disability as including a psychosocial dimension, disability is more commonly associated with physical disabilities, including blindness, lack of hearing, or loss of a limb. The model lends itself to this physical interpretation, particularly through the association with injury.

In brief, the Cornia/UNICEF model, like the Mosley/Chen model, does not include explicitly a psychosocial dimension of early childhood development. To do so would have further complicated an already complicated model. The omissions, however, indicate a failure to put child care and development in proper perspective as they affect growth and survival.

Linearity

With one exception, the Cornia/UNICEF model is linear. The exception depicts an interaction between nutrition (or growth faltering) and health (infection and disease). The linear nature of the model facilitates analysis but is also misleading because it misses important interactions among variables. For instance, 'frequency of feeding' is affected by the ability of the child to demand food which is affected by its nutritional and health status. This interaction is not presented in the model.

Missing variables

Cornia and colleagues consciously omit from their analysis attention to social and cultural values, arguing that during periods of pronounced economic fluctuations the variation in values will be minor. But it may be that this very lack of variation may create a problem. One response to economic adversity is to migrate. As families move to cities, the values that served them well in the rural areas may no longer serve as well.

The Cornia model does not incorporate community organization or participation.

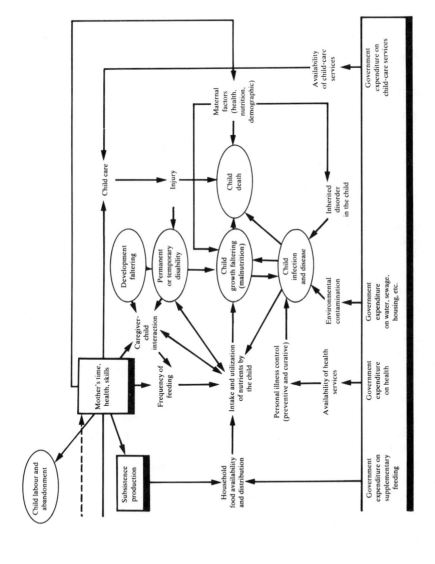

Figure 4.4 An adaptation of the Cornia/UNICEF framework

Recasting the model

At the risk of further complicating an already complicated model, it is possible to indicate how child development might be incorporated into the Cornia/UNICEF model and how a different view of child care and women's work might be captured in the model. Figure 4.4 displays a recasting of the portion of the model focusing on the intermediate and outcome variables. The reader will note the attempt to incorporate interactions among variables, rather than staying with the linear configuration of the original model.

Framework 3: Zeitlin and Mansour

The previous two frameworks were formulated, respectively, by epidemiologists and economists. This third framework (see Figure 4.5) is the work of nutritionists. The conceptual framework is directed towards discovering why some children thrive nutritionally in conditions that put them at risk whereas other children become undernourished while living in essentially the same conditions. The emphasis is on understanding what has been termed 'positive deviance' – on identifying the mechanisms of social and behavioural adaptability to conditions of nutritional stress that allow children to grow and develop well. This viewpoint and the findings associated with application of the framework have provided invaluable support to the position taken in this book.

Whereas the Mosley/Chen and Cornia/UNICEF frameworks were created primarily for analyses at a high level of aggregation – at a national level in order to formulate national policies – the Zeitlin/Mansour framework is more concerned with what happens in the immediate environment in which a child grows and develops. As shown in Figure 4.5, the child–caregiver interaction is central to the Zeitlin/Mansour model. That interaction is influenced by characteristics of the child and the caregiver and by the social support system for the dyad. Implications for policy are drawn from microlevel analyses of the growth and development process. 'Potential interventions' are included in the framework, but the authors do not treat them as variables.

The Zeitlin/Mansour framework, while focusing on growth, incorporates a psychosocial dimension. Growth is shown in the model as affected by stress, as well as by food intake and health, and these three are shown as related in a synergistic way. Indeed, in their review and analysis applying the model, the authors place emphasis on psychological factors rather than on physiological factors, saying that,

> In fact, we have no evidence that the purely physiological components of positive deviance are strong enough to predominate over or to seriously confound the interpretation of psychosocial components.

> (Zeitlin and Mansour, p. 53)

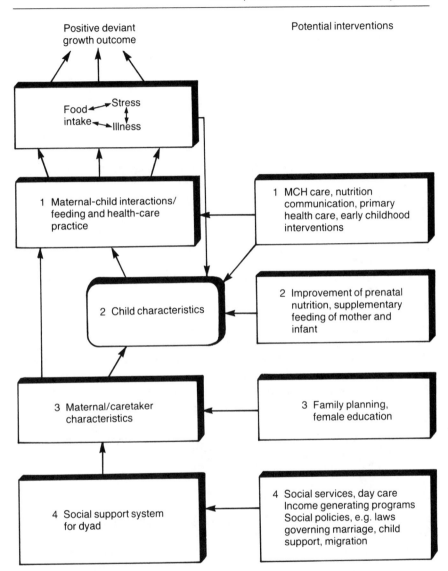

Figure 4.5 A conceptual framework of factors influencing positive deviance
Source: Zeitlin *et al.* (1990), p. 46

The negative effect of psychological stress on the use of nutrients and resistance to infection has been documented. We shall return to these results later on.

By specifically including stress and stipulating the three-way synergistic relationship, this model goes beyond that of the earlier formulations. Although Mosley and Chen would certainly accept the synergistic relationship between health and nutrition, it is not made clear in their model. The Cornia/UNICEF model does recognize the synergism with a double arrow between health and nutrition. However, these authors do not incorporate stress into their models.

Figure 4.5 also pictures an interaction between the combined health–nutrition–stress trio and a child's characteristics (e.g. its ability to elicit responses). By making that interaction explicit, the model further deviates from strict linear causality. What the formulation suggests is a kind of spiral effect in which a child that is better fed, healthier, and under less stress contributes more effectively to the mother–child interaction which, in turn, leads to its being better fed, healthier, and less stressed.

In an elaboration by Zeitlin and Mansour of the more general model of Figure 4.5, Figure 4.6 traces the effects of maternal characteristics on positive deviant growth and development. In their conceptualization, attention is given to both the 'ability' and the 'motivation' of mothers (one might substitute 'caregivers'). Affecting these traits are many of the same socio-economic factors included in the first two models.

In dealing with maternal characteristics, greater emphasis is placed by Zeitlin and Mansour on values and attitudes than was done in previous models. The framework also gives a prominent place to the social support caregivers receive (or lack). As in the Cornia model, organized care (called 'day care' in this model) is included. Interestingly, however, as in both of the earlier formulations, community organization and social networks are left out, although these can affect access to services and can make a major difference in caregiver stress which, in turn, affects the mother–child interaction.

We turn now to a set of three frameworks that are directed more specifically to questions of infant and early childhood care and development.

Framework 4: Bronfenbrenner

In general, the field of human (and child) development has been dominated by the field of psychology, focusing on the evolution of cognitive, emotional, and social processes within individuals and over their lifetimes (and in the case of child development, in their earliest months and years). However, in the 1970s, a much broader approach to the study of development took shape and began to gain prominence. This approach views development as progressive mutual accommodation between a growing human being and the changing nature of the immediate environment in which the person lives (Sameroff and Chandler 1975; Bronfenbrenner 1979). The mutual accommodation is mediated by the nature of the larger and more complicated settings in which the accommodation is taking place.

A primary exponent of this view has been Urie Bronfenbrenner. His

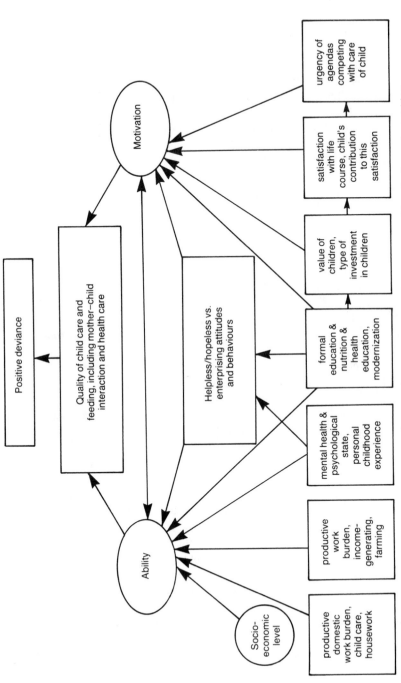

Figure 4.6 A conceptual framework illustrating maternal characteristics that influence positive deviance in nutrition
Source: Zeitlin et al. (1990), p. 63

major work, *The Ecology of Human Development*, concentrates on describing and analyzing the environmental part of the accommodation process, and in so doing draws heavily on social psychology, sociology, and anthropology – more so than on psychology. Bronfenbrenner's framework describes four environmental systems which are visualized as 'nesting structures', or concentric circles.

1   *The micro-system.*   The immediate setting within which a child acts and interacts with others is called a micro-system by Bronfenbrenner. For the child, 0 to 5, the main setting is the home. A child may also spend time in other child-care environments outside the home – a child-care centre or preschool, for instance. At this innermost level of the ecological scheme is the 'dyad', or two-person system of the caregiver and child, whose interaction is influenced by the presence and participation of other family members, friends and neighbours who form an informal social support network.

2   *The meso-system.*   As a child grows and develops, it becomes part of more than one immediate setting (e.g. the home and a day-care centre), and moves among them. The interrelations of these different settings constitute a second level of analysis labelled a meso-system. A child's development is influenced at this level by the number of different settings, by whether or not the settings are similar or different, whether the child's participation in the different settings is accompanied by supportive links (e.g. parental participation, levels of communication and knowledge, etc.). Without stretching too much, this set of immediate settings might be equated with the immediate 'community' within which a child moves.

3   *The exo-system.*   Both immediate settings and the interaction among them are related to broader societal organizations and practices. Thus, settings in which a child does not participate influence the activities and interactions occurring in immediate settings (level 1) as well as the relationships among those settings (level 2). The conditions and organization of the workplace provide one example. Governing organizations, social services, mass media, and other legally established structures form part of this third-order system, labelled by Bronfenbrenner as the exo-system.

4   *The macro-system.*   At a still higher level of generality in the framework is a macro-system that gives continuity to the form and content of all three previous levels and consists of overarching patterns of ideology and organization of the social institutions that are common to a particular culture or sub-culture. The macro-system sets the blueprint for broad social institutions, and for the relationships among immediate settings and within them. Bronfenbrenner argues that the blueprint can become markedly altered and produce corresponding changes in behaviour and development. The introduction of a new health practice or persistent economic recession, for example, might produce such changes.

Figure 4.7 provides one attempt to capture the framework in graphic

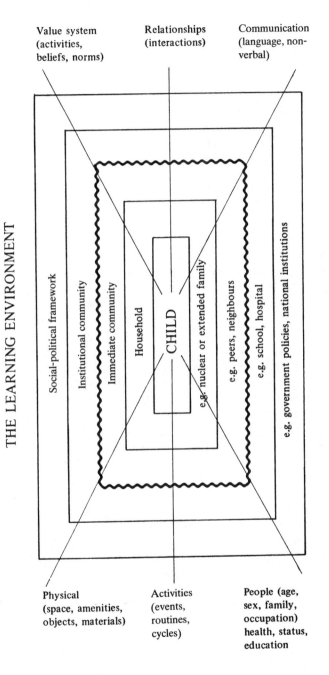

THE LEARNING ENVIRONMENT

Value system (activities, beliefs, norms)

Relationships (interactions)

Communication (language, non-verbal)

Social-political framework

Institutional community

Immediate community

Household

CHILD

e.g. nuclear or extended family

e.g. peers, neighbours

e.g. school, hospital

e.g. government policies, national institutions

Physical (space, amenities, objects, materials)

Activities (events, routines, cycles)

People (age, sex, family, occupation) health, status, education

Figure 4.7 The learning environment
Source: International Development Research Centre (1988)

form. The figure represents a slight reinterpretation at the level of the child because it puts the child in the centre rather than the dyad.

Comments on the framework

The importance of genetic and physical variables   In his discussion, Bronfenbrenner notes the crucial part played in development by biological influences but admits that his work does not give them their due. He chose, rather, to concentrate on what he felt was the less well-articulated part of the picture – on environmental influences. That seemed a necessary step prior to trying to analyse the interaction of biological and social–environmental forces.

An untidy world   The image of 'nesting systems' or concentric circles helps to visualize the Bronfenbrenner framework. However, the world in which most children live is not so tidy; they may experience different cultures and be subject to different blueprints at the same time. For example, in most rural areas of the Third World, the culture and values of the school represent a different ideological and cultural blueprint from that of the home. Entrance into school represents more than a transition from one institution to another within one overarching blueprint (as suggested at the meso-level of the framework); it creates a need for articulation between two different blueprints. At the micro- as well as the meso-level, the two blueprints that may be at work simultaneously can create a conflict in individual or family behaviour between, for instance, going to a Western doctor or to the local healer. This divergence is not captured well within the Bronfenbrenner framework, even though the framework does allow for changes in a 'blueprint'.

An ecological model is homeostatic   The ecological model which provides the foundation for Bronfenbrenner's framework is essentially a homeostatic model in which there is a search for equilibrium. But there may be a need to seek imbalance at times and to change (not just adjust) systems. This need for fundamental change is recognized by Bronfenbrenner in his discussion of the goal of development which includes as the highest form of development the 'capacity to remold reality in accordance with human requirements and aspirations' (p. 10). In general, however, an ecological model assumes adjustment over long periods and does not serve well when analysing situations in which rapid change is occurring.

Community   In contrast with the Mosley/Chen and Cornia/UNICEF models, this framework brings in a level beyond the family but below the level of national institutions. It makes a place for informal social support networks in their support of the caregiver. However, 'community' as such is not a basic concept and the discussion of community cohesion and solidarity is at best indirect.

Linearity   The Bronfenbrenner framework recognizes that the development process is not a linear process. This is not a 'main effects' model.

The Bronfenbrenner framework keeps before us, simultaneously, several levels at which programme interventions might be made, directly with the child and/or the caregiver, at the level of the immediate environment with the family, at a community level, at the level of broader social institutions, and at the level of cultural values. These levels provide the basis for a set of complementary programme approaches to be discussed in the following chapter.

Framework 5: Super and Harkness

Rooted in an anthropological tradition (e.g. LeVine 1970; Whiting and Whiting 1975; and Monroe *et al.* 1981), this treatment of child development emphasizes the effects of cultural features on childrearing. The model remains at a higher level of generality than those discussed previously.

As might be expected, emphasis is placed on interpreting differences rather than on seeking universals in values and actions. The authors reject the idea of a 'universal child' to whom universal programmes should be directed. At the same time, the model builds on the strain of psychology applied to human development represented by Bronfenbrenner and others (including the early pioneering work of Kurt Lewin 1936).

Super and Harkness provide a 'framework for studying cultural regulation of the micro-environment of the child'. They introduce the concept of a 'development niche' which is defined by three integrated components, or sub-systems, as depicted in Figure 4.8.

While focusing on the micro-environment, this framework, as the notion

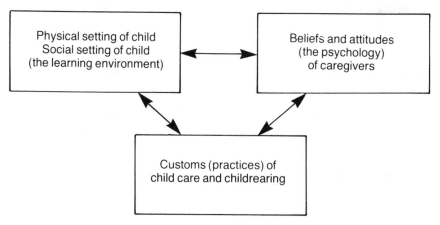

Figure 4.8 Sub-systems of the 'developmental niche'
Source: Super and Harkness (1987)

of a 'niche' implies, is set within a broader view. The three components are seen as mediating an individual's developmental experience within the larger culture.

Settings, customs of child care, and caretakers' beliefs may be in balance or diverge. In changing physical and social circumstances (for example, a move to the city), the customs of child care that served formerly may no longer be appropriate. Or, a changing set of expectations and beliefs (as introduced, for instance, by radio or television or a missionary or a technical 'expert') may lead to changes in child-care customs (e.g. bottle feeding) that are not consistent with the existing, and unchanging (or slowly changing), physical and social setting.

Super and Harkness contend that:

> Homeostatic mechanisms tend to keep the three subsystems in harmony with each other and appropriate to the developmental level and individual characteristics of the child. Nevertheless, they have different relationships to other features of the larger environment and thus constitute somewhat independent routes of disequilibrium and change. Regularities within and among the sub-systems, and thematic continuities and progressions across the niches of childhood provide material from which the child abstracts the social, affective, and cognitive rules of the culture.

(p. 545)

The above passage points to the active role of the child in constructing its view of the culture – of developing. It also gives a prominent place to homeostatic regulation, a mechanism that we have already commented may not work well in conditions of rapid social change. At the same time, by making explicit the three sub-systems, the model provides a basis for understanding disequilibrium and for insight into why some useful practices are being lost and why some new practices are not as helpful as expected by those who introduce them.

Whereas Mosley and Chen (Framework 1) emphasize ways in which people do or do not adjust to Western beliefs and practices about care and development, this model begins with what people actually believe and practise, without judging in advance whether these are good or bad beliefs and practices. This includes positive practices and beliefs that can be built upon in conditions of rapid social change, helping the homeostatic process along.

Framework 6: Lester and Brazleton

In this sixth framework, a paediatrician and psychologist have teamed to present a 'psychobiological' model for cross-cultural assessment of neonatal behaviour.

The conceptual model has the following features:

1 The framework focuses on the process of development (the *how* rather than the *what* or *why* of development). Development is a process of increasing differentiation and integration that proceeds hierarchically. Because it is a process, it can only be seen in motion, and not by looking at its component parts.

2 The framework begins prenatally. At birth, the child's psychobiological organization is a product of the synergistic interactions among:

- the obstetrical/reproductive history of the mother;
- the genetic endowment of the child; and,
- the prenatal environment.

The prenatal environment includes conditions or complications associated with pregnancy and delivery – particularly nutritional status and maternal attitude.

3 The model postulates an interaction between physical maturation, the child's temperament, and the environment in which the child is found. The neonate is described as having 'a pre-programmed response repertoire designed to maximize the survival of the individual and the species'. With this repertoire, the neonate is 'a competent organism that is skilled, selective, and socially influential, who interacts with and makes demands on the caretaking environment' (p. 52).

4 'While basic organizational processes may remain constant from culture to culture – for example, infants universally become more alert and develop increasing interactive skills in the first few weeks of postnatal life – the range and form of adaptation to a particular culture will depend upon the demands of the culture' (p. 52).

5 The model focuses on the immediate environment of the child, with allusions to broader influences (the ecological milieu, the family constellation, the physical setting, larger goals, experiences and needs of culture).

6 A great deal of emphasis is placed on the interaction of the child and its mother. In this process, the child is given an active role.

A pictorial representation of the organization of infant behaviour, as conceived by Lester and Brazleton, is presented in Figure 4.9.

Framework 7: Bennett

Yet another approach to understanding survival, growth, and development of young children begins with an examination of the household economy and works outward. This approach contrasts with one that begins with macro-level variables and traces their effect through various mediating variables to the child. It also differs from a focus on the characteristics of the child or the caregiver.

The approach taken by Bennett combines an anthropological look at the

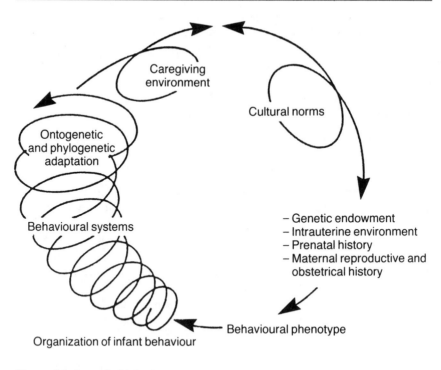

Caregiving environment

Cultural norms

Ontogenetic and phylogenetic adaptation

Behavioural systems

– Genetic endowment
– Intrauterine environment
– Prenatal history
– Maternal reproductive and
  obstetrical history

Behavioural phenotype

Organization of infant behaviour

Figure 4.9 A psychobiological model for the cross-cultural study of the organization of infant behaviour
Source: Lester and Brazleton (1982), p. 52

internal dynamics of the family with an economic viewpoint that focuses on the use of the scarce resource, time. Beginning inside the household allows exploration of the relationship between income earning and the ability to influence how household resources, including time, are used (see Figure 4.10).

Bennett's framework has several points of contact with the Mosley/ Chen and the Cornia/UNICEF models. It sets family-level influences within a broad macro-level context that includes economic, demographic, and sociocultural factors as well as biological and environmental factors. The framework includes time, knowledge, and income resources that are available to the family.

Although many of the variables are the same, Bennett's framework is in marked contrast with the Mosley/Chen and UNICEF/Cornia models in several important ways:

1 The model takes as the outcome variable the health and nutritional status of *all* household members. This recognizes that there may be some trade-offs between the condition of a young child and other family members – for example, the mother's health. Rather than take mother's

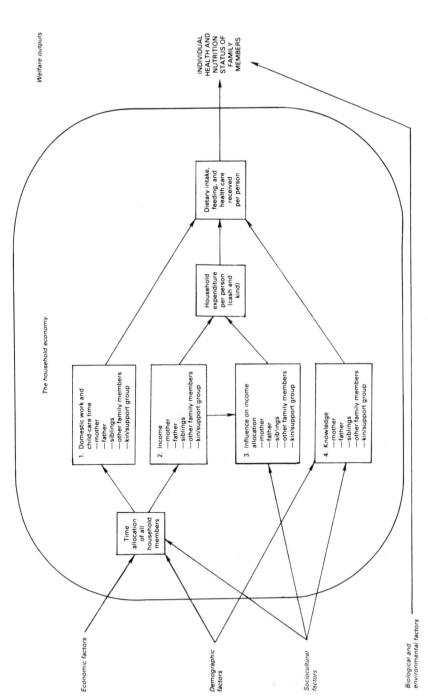

Figure 4.10 A framework for the analysis of the household economy
Source: Bennett (1988), p. 20

health simply as an input into a process directed towards survival and development of the child, it becomes an outcome variable as well.

2 Women are seen as income earners as well as mothers.

3 Income contributions by all family members are considered, but their effect is mediated partially by consideration of the way in which income is allocated and controlled within the family. This recognizes that income earned by women and children is sometimes controlled by a male head of household who does not allocate that income to improve the health and nutritional status of women and children. Bennett avoids the assumption that all members of a household give priority to the same use of resources (i.e., have a common utility function) by looking separately at the per person household earnings and expenditures.

4 The framework is cast in terms of the household rather than the family. Although these terms are often used interchangeably, families are defined by blood ties whereas households can consist of several families and do not necessarily require a consanguinal relationship.

5 Time is the key variable.

Bennett's framework, as others, incorporates major conceptual advances. By focusing on the household, it helps to fill in gaps in the previous frameworks and elaborates relationships at one of the several levels of environment affecting a child's development. The model is particularly important in reminding us that women should not be viewed only in their reproductive role and that their own health and welfare is intimately linked to the welfare of the child upon whom we are focusing. This framework provides an excellent backdrop for the discussion of child care, child development, and women's work that will be presented in Chapter 11.

As with the other frameworks, this one can be questioned on several counts. It has a linear quality to it. It does not, for instance, incorporate the probable feedback of the improved health and nutritional status of children on how time is allocated.

Maternal health (or the health of other household members) is not included as a variable affecting outcomes.

With the focus on health and nutrition outcomes, Bennett does not take a holistic view of the child, failing to attend to the psychosocial dimension of development. With this omission, the treatment of child care becomes custodial.

Interestingly, the author does not incorporate the possibility of care outside the household in centres or another arrangement, but she does allow for the possibility of multiple caretakers within the household. Discarding the extra-household care option facilitates analysis, makes it possible to look at the direct trade-offs between the time of household members spent in income earning and time spent in household production or child care. (It does not allow for overlapping care and production activities.) However, extra-familial care is increasingly common. By not including the availability of services (which are included in the Cornia/UNICEF model) the framework fails to reflect an important influence on time use within households.

It would have been possible to include many more models in this discussion. Each reader will immediately identify a favourite framework that was not included and could have been, within the criteria for selection of frameworks applied. Rather than extend the analysis, however, it seems appropriate at this point to extract some general points of agreement and some weaknesses in the models.

Weaknesses

Weaknesses of the particular frameworks have been examined along the way. There are, however, at least three weaknesses that are common to several of the models:

1 A linear treatment of relationships in three of the frameworks makes it difficult to pick up the mutual interaction (synergism) among the various components of development or the mutually adjusting process between child and environment that marks the developmental process as it moves through time.

2 Treatment of the 'community' variable or context is not strong in any of the models. This seems strange in view of the repeated calls for community participation one often hears in connection with programmes of child survival and development. In part, this weakness simply reflects the biases in both medicine and psychology towards emphasis on the individual.

3 The frameworks do not handle divergence or dissonance or conflict well. As noted when discussing the Bronfenbrenner and the Super/Harkness frameworks, many children and their families live simultaneously in at least two worlds, each governed by a different set of cultural beliefs, rituals, symbolic systems, and so forth. These are represented by the traditional healer and the doctor, the 'bush' school and the Western primary school, the national language and the local language, the secret society and the political party, etc. To some degree these separate 'blueprints' can be brought together, but often they are in conflict. The process of interaction and dynamic adjustment and coping within such circumstances will not work in the same way that is postulated in the frameworks because the adjustments required are too big; they are in fact fundamental changes requiring major leaps rather than small adjustments.

Changing interpretations

Partly because of the way in which they were chosen, the frameworks illustrate a process of redefinition that has been occurring slowly and in several fields with respect to child survival and early childhood growth and development. Several tendencies are identifiable:

1 *From a definition of survival, growth, and development as states or conditions to considering them as processes.* Our treatment of key concepts in the preceding chapter reflects this changing point of view. Survival is seen as a continuous process of seeking a healthy state (Mosley and Chen). Growth is indexed by whether or not an increase in size occurs rather than in terms of reaching a certain size at a certain time. Child development is a process of change in a child's ability to handle ever more complex levels of activity in several domains.

2 *From isolated emphasis on one or another dimension of child survival and development to a multidimensional and 'integrated' view.* In most of the frameworks, physical and psychosocial dimensions of development are included. In some the inclusion of the psychosocial is implicit, but is not made clear. The medical model of Mosley and Chen, focusing on survival, and the Bennett framework, relating women's time allocation to family welfare, are the least explicit in this respect.

3 *From a one-way relationship between health or nutrition actions affecting early childhood development to a two-way interactive relationship in which developmentally sensitive interactions affect health and nutritional status.* The work of Brazleton and Lester, and of Zeitlin and Mansour, represent this tendency. The absence of this interactive relationship is most notable in the Mosley–Chen framework. The related framework set out by Cornia includes an interaction between health and nutrition, but does not incorporate a psychosocial dimension in interaction with these two.

4 *From a view of the child as a passive recipient of 'stimulation', or of other interventions, to the child as an actor, influencing the developmental process.* This active view of the child's role is particularly present in the work of Brazleton and Lester, Bronfenbrenner, Super and Harkness, and Zeitlin and Mansour.

5 *From a 'universal' definition of the goals and outcomes of child development to a more culturally relative and sensitive view.* Super and Harkness, Bronfenbrenner, and Lester and Brazleton are explicit about the importance of cultural differences in their frameworks which, more than others, are addressed specifically to child development. The four frameworks emphasizing survival or growth or nutrition tend to be less explicit about cultural differences.

The set of frameworks also demonstrates tendencies in particular fields that have an influence on how we think about programming for child care and development. For instance, the treatment of nutrition in the Zeitlin model includes attention to feeding as a social and developmental, as well as a nutritional, process. It establishes the influence of psychosocial development variables on nutritional status as well as vice versa.

The treatment of women's roles, as shown in the Bennett framework, is beginning to move from one in which the productive and reproductive roles are treated separately and in terms of a 'trade-off', to one in which they are considered simultaneously.

Within medicine, as shown by Mosley and Chen, the shift is occurring from a curative to a preventive stance and from service delivery to 'home production' of health.

WHAT CAUSES EARLY CHILDHOOD DEVELOPMENT TO OCCUR AS IT DOES?

A look at the frameworks sheds light on several positions we have taken with respect to development that have important implications for programming:

- Both biological and environmental factors are important in the developmental process.
- Developmental outcomes result from a dynamic interaction of the child and its environment.
- Several levels of environment need to be considered when analysing the developmental process and when programming to affect it.
- Developmental problems do not have a single cause.

Nature and nurture

Although the frameworks are very different in many respects, they share a view that both biological/physiological and environmental factors are important influences on the development of the young child. The relative importance given to the two varies among frameworks. It also varies with the age of a child. The clear tendency is to give greater importance to environment as the child grows older. Consequently, the frameworks that emphasize children in the earliest months of life, including the survival frameworks, give more attention to the biological state at birth and in the early months than those looking across the age range or those oriented principally towards the immediate preschool years.

The most obvious implication of this balanced view is that programmes cannot expect to be as successful as they could be if they only intervene to change the child or to change the environment. Changes must be sought in both.

Another implication is that the risk of delayed or debilitated development, as well as the risk of an early death, is influenced by what happens prenatally as well as what happens after birth. Programmes of child survival and development must, therefore, attend to the mother during pregnancy and to practices at the time of the delivery, both for the sake of the mother and the child.

Child and environment in dynamic interaction

Several of the frameworks chosen go beyond recognizing the importance of both child and environment to recognizing a continuous and dynamic inter- action (or transactional process) between an active and changing child and the changing physical and social environment surrounding the child. Perhaps most explicit in taking this position are the frameworks of Bron- fenbrenner, Zeitlin/Mansour, Super/Harkness, and Lester/Brazleton.

In statistical terms, the idea of 'interaction' carries with it the idea that results will be greater than the sum of the parts – a multiplying of results rather than simply adding them up.

Interaction also implies influences running in both directions, not simply in one direction. A mother (part of a child's environment) not only influ- ences the actions and development of the child, but the child takes initi- atives (or does not), influencing the actions of the mother. A process of mutual adaptation takes place that is at the very centre of development.

This viewpoint has important implications for programming. For instance, it puts emphasis on the interaction between caregiver and child, going beyond interventions that seek changes only in the characteristics of the child or of the caregiver (which is one way of changing the child's environment). Mothers (or other caregivers) can be helped to recognize the importance of the way in which they interact and to be sensitive to their own reactions to the child, which may be unresponsive or unnecessarily negative or, on the other hand, too overwhelming. They can be helped to see how different forms of interaction affect the feeding process, and there- fore both the nutritional and social condition of the child.

Environmental levels

Present in all the frameworks in some form or other is the idea that a child's development is affected by influences at various levels. It is common to refer to the work of Bronfenbrenner when discussing these levels (1979), and the following paragraphs correspond, more or less, to the distinctions he makes. Some of the authors emphasize a particular level in their models while making reference to others. The terminology used for the levels differs from framework to framework and the number of levels implied or made explicit varies somewhat as well. In general, however, the set of frameworks supports the idea that we must be concerned with family, community, institutional, and cultural environments.

Family and community

In the process of developing, a child interacts directly with a caregiver and with immediate surroundings. That interaction occurs within the context of a family or household with a certain structure, set of relationships, economic and social position, practices and beliefs, and store of knowledge. The developing child is influenced by and influences these characteristics of the family in a process of mutual adjustment. Families differ widely in their ability to satisfy a child's needs for protection, food, health, love, security, stimulation, and exploration, as mediated by the child's biological inheritance, temperament, age, and physical condition. At the same time, the presence and actions of a child can change the family structure and affect the relationships, make demands on resources, and test family practices and knowledge.

One step further removed from the child–caregiver dyad is the community environment of which the child and family are a part – a community with varying degrees of cohesiveness, organization, and resources. For statistical purposes, a community is often defined in geo-political or bureaucratic terms, as a town or another administrative unit covering a particular area. But a community is more properly conceived of as a group of people who are knit together by common interests and needs and who interact with each other on a regular basis. 'Community' might be found in a social network or a tribal group or in a cooperative. These communities may or may not correspond with a particular political or geographic unit. The different frameworks reflect different definitions of community, and none treats the community level adequately, but most include at least passing reference to the importance of the community environment.

Although it is more difficult to envision an effect of a preschool-aged child on the community as part of a process of mutual adjustment, there is an influence. A child has particular and changing needs to which communities as well as families and immediate caregivers respond (or should respond but do not or cannot, as the case may be). As the develop-mental process continues beyond the preschool years, the mutual adjust-ment of a community's children and community to each other becomes more direct.

Social institutions

Communities and families are part of a larger system of social and political and economic organization, with attendant institutions, laws, policies, and norms governing activities. This social environment regulates to some degree the actions of families and communities with respect to the develop-ment of their children, both opening opportunities (e.g. the availability of primary health care or child-care centres, or a law providing for maternal leave from work) and setting limits (e.g. laws regarding child abuse).

Does interaction between the child and its environment occur at this environmental level or is the effect one-way? Most frameworks treat the social environment as a one-way influence on child development, within a generally linear model of influences. However, others suggest an interaction at this level as well. Children, primarily through the community and family, present demands on social institutions and thus constitute a pressure for institutional adjustment over time. Recognizing this possibility is important in programmes designed to empower parents and communities. Empowerment must include the possibility for parents and communities to make demands on the larger social community. As we examine the transition from home to school in Chapter 10, we will stress a process of mutual accommodation that should include adjustments by the school to the developing child as well as by the child to the social institution called a school.

Culture and ideology

A set of shared beliefs common to a culture or sub-culture guides the organization and action of social institutions, communities, families, and individuals. This 'code' (Sameroff and Fiese 1990) is evident in such actions as the form of prenatal care, the birthing process, weaning practices, when informal education begins, the values to be emphasized in the socialization process, etc. These cultural beliefs are subject to change. Changing physical and social environments (a crisis in world economic conditions, introduction of a new technology) may require adjustments in practices that are not supported by old beliefs and ideologies (the Super and Harkness framework lends itself to an analysis of converging or diverging beliefs, practices and physical and social environments). Change in the cultural ethos or ideology can also occur with a shift in the knowledge and information base. We will return to these possibilities of influencing the cultural environment when discussing programmes.

No single cause

From the foregoing it is clear that no single cause can be identified for delayed or for accelerated child development. Any programme strategy that limits itself to a single cause will, at best, be a partial solution and, at worst, a wasted effort. But we now have a basis for identifying complementary approaches and principles that will let adjustments be made to the particular conditions that will best foster survival and development in a particular place with particular children.

Let us now appropriate the results of analyses in Chapters 3 and 4 to set out a programming strategy.

REFERENCES

Bennett, L. 'The Role of Women in Income Production and Intra-Household Allocation of Resources as a Determinant of Child Health and Nutrition', *Food and Nutrition Bulletin*, Vol. 10, No. 3 (1988), pp. 16–26.

Bronfenbrenner, U. *The Ecology of Human Development*. Cambridge, Mass: Harvard University Press, 1979.

Cornia, A., R. Jolly, and F. Stewart. *Adjustment with a Human Face: Protecting the Vulnerable and Promoting Growth*. New York: Oxford University Press, 1988, Chapter 2.

International Development Research Centre, 'The Learning Environments of Early Childhood in Asia', Bangkok: UNESCO, 1988.

Lester, B. and T. Berry Brazelton. 'Cross-cultural Assessment of Neonatal Behavior', in D. Wagner and H. Stevenson (eds), *Cultural Perspectives on Child Development*. San Francisco: W.H. Freeman and Co., 1982, Chapter 2.

LeVine, R. 'Cross-cultural Study in Child Development', in P.H. Mussen (ed.), *Carmichael's Manual of Child Psychology, Vol. 2*. New York: Wiley, 1970, pp. 559–612.

Lewin, K. *Principles of Topological Psychology*. New York: McGraw-Hill, 1936.

Monroe, R.H., R.L. Monroe, and B.B. Whiting (eds). *Handbook of Cross-cultural Human Development*. New York: Garland Press, 1981.

Mosley, W.H. and L. Chen. 'An Analytical Framework for the Study of Child Survival in Developing Countries', *Population and Development Review*, a supplement to Vol. 10 (1984), pp. 25–45.

Sameroff, A.J. and B.H. Fiese. 'Transactional Regulation and Early Intervention', in S.J. Meisels and J.P. Shonkoff (eds), *Early Intervention, A Handbook of Theory, Practice, and Analysis*. New York: Cambridge University Press, 1990.

Sameroff, A.J. and M.J. Chandler. 'Reproductive Risk and the Continuum of Care-taking Casualty', in F.D. Horowitz *et al.* (eds), *Review of Child Development Research, Vol. 4*. Chicago: University of Chicago Press, 1975.

Super, C. and S. Harkness. 'The Developmental Niche: A Conceptualization at the Interface of Child and Culture', *International Journal of Behavioral Development*, Vol. 9 (1987), pp. 1–25.

van Norren, B. and H.A.W. van Vianen. 'The Malnutrition Infection Syndrome and its Demographic Outcome in Developing Countries', Publication No. 4, The Hague: Programming Committee for Demographic Research, 1986.

Whiting, B.B. and J.W.M. Whiting. *Children of Six Cultures: A Psycho-Cultural Analysis*. Cambridge, Mass: Harvard University Press, 1975.

Zeitlin, M., H. Ghassemi and M. Mansour. *Positive Deviance in Child Nutrition, with Emphasis on Psychosocial and Behavioural Aspects and Implications for Development*. Tokyo: The United Nations University, 1990.

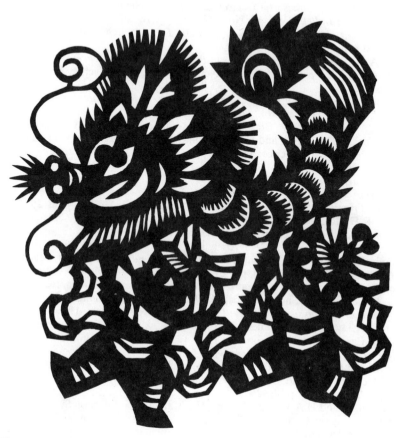

'Dragon dance'
A paper cut designed by Shen Peinong for the All-China
Women's Federation

Chapter 5

Programming approaches and guidelines[1]

For too many people, a child development project or programme immediately conjures up the image of 25 or 30 small children, ages 3 to 5, playing with blocks or fitting triangles and squares into brightly coloured puzzle boards, supervised by a professional teacher in a 'preschool' classroom. Associating child development exclusively with this 'preschool' model is unfortunate because it focuses narrowly on a child's mental development, is relatively expensive, and begins late in a child's life. It also involves a direct, 'institutional' approach, relying on creation of centres that 'compensate' for missing elements in the family and community environment while, too often, leaving parents and community members out of the programme. This image seldom provides the most appropriate guide to programming for child care and development in Third World locations.

The previous two chapters have provided us with a basis for expanding our vision of childhood development programmes beyond the preschool, or centre-based, model providing direct attention to the child beginning at age three or four. We will now try to put that broader view in a systematic form by bringing together three sets of considerations to be taken into account when planning and implementing programmes of early childhood care and development. That guide, presumptuously labelled a comprehensive programming framework, is presented in Figure 5.1.

The programming framework has three dimensions.

1 *Variations in a child's developmental status* The first dimension is defined by changes in a child's developmental needs over the first years of life. Needs will be different during the prenatal period, in infancy, in the 'toddler' and post-toddler period, as a preschooler, and as the child moves from the limited environment of the home to the school and the larger world beyond.

2 *Complementary programme approaches* A second dimension distinguishes five complementary programme approaches. Each approach is directed to a different set of environmental factors influencing the child's development, as set out in the previous chapter. In addition to centre-based programmes that attend directly to the child are complementary

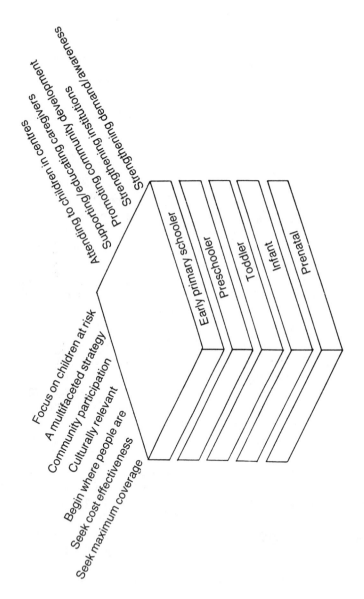

Focus on children at risk
A multifaceted strategy
Community participation
Culturally relevant
Begin where people are
Seek cost effectiveness
Seek maximum coverage

Attending to children in centres
Supporting/educating caregivers
Promoting community development
Strengthening demand/institutions/awareness

Early primary schooler
Preschooler
Toddler
Infant
Prenatal

Figure 5.1 Programming for early childhood development: a comprehensive framework

programmes that focus, respectively, on working with family, community, institutional and cultural environments.

3 *Programme characteristics/guidelines* A third dimension is derived from a set of guidelines dictating programme characteristics. In addition to serving children who are 'at risk', programmes should be comprehensive and 'integrated', participatory and community-based, flexible, based on (but not restricted to) local ways, financially feasible and cost-effective, and extended over as wide a population of at-risk children as possible.

The main reason for setting out a comprehensive programme framework is to help overcome the narrow, piecemeal thinking and actions that so dominate the early childhood development field. Rarely, if ever, will it be possible for a programme to cover all the categories set out in the framework. However, having an overall vision helps locate where specific initiatives fall and can point out the missing pieces to planners and programmers.

Let us look now at each of the three dimensions.

DEVELOPMENTAL STATUS

We have seen from the previous two chapters that early childhood development is a continuing process in which the child is changing constantly. That process begins prenatally and extends through the entire period of the child's early life. Clearly, different moments in this process will require somewhat different approaches. A child in the womb is obviously not the same as the child that is beginning to walk or talk. If a child development strategy is to be comprehensive, it should respond to changing needs throughout the development process. It is not enough to begin programming for child development when the child reaches age three. Nor is it sufficient to think only in terms of improving conditions that will lead to the birth of a healthy, well-developed child.

Because child development follows a general pattern (even though the process will vary from individual to individual and culture to culture), it is possible to establish programme activities appropriate to general stages or levels of a child's development. These stages correspond roughly to certain age periods, but they are more accurately thought of in terms of particular developmental advances that occur as a child grows older. Very roughly, it is possible to think in terms of programmes appropriate to:

- a prenatal period;
- infancy (up to about 18 months) that encompasses weaning, learning to walk, and early language development;
- a toddler and post-toddler period (about 18 to 48 months) during which a child's coordination, language, ability to think, and social skills advance by leaps and bounds;

- a preschool period (approximately ages 4 and 5) when coordination is relatively well developed, and when cognitive development and development of pre-literacy skills occurs rapidly, along with greater attention to relationships with peers; and,
- a period of accommodation to school and the world at large (roughly ages 6 to 8).

Within governments, the organizational responsibility for programmes of early childhood development tends to follow developmental stages and/or the age of children. Prior to age two or three, responsibility for these programmes often falls to the health sector and/or to organizations concerned with family welfare. From age three onward, child development is more likely to be associated with education and preschools. This division is logical in the sense that survival and the early months of development are closely tied to the biophysical condition and maturation of the child, and, during this time, most children are cared for within the family; in the later preschool years, socialization and preparation for schooling take on greater importance, and the circle of caregivers widens. However, the division also hides the need for continuous attention of a coordinated nature. It reinforces the unfortunate tendency to omit psychosocial components prior to age three and to think of child development programmes as essentially educational programmes beginning at age three.

In order to counteract the tendency to restrict programming for child development to one particular age group (for example, the preschool period as described at the outset of the chapter) and, in order to emphasize the simultaneous character of survival, growth, and development, a comprehensive framework must make explicit the need for child development programmes that cover the several periods, taking into account the variations that are occurring in the child.

COMPLEMENTARY APPROACHES

In Chapters 3 and 4, early childhood development was described as a continuous process of interaction between the child (with a maturing set of biophysical characteristics) and the people and objects in its constantly changing world. That changing world (environment) was seen to include several levels of environments influencing the child's development, including the immediate environments of the family (or household) and the community, a larger social, political and economic context (with attendant institutions, laws, policies, and norms), and a culture (providing values, rituals, and beliefs).

Although the interaction with home, community, institutions and cultural values occurs at different distances from the child, each of these environmental levels influences the process of early development, either directly, or through the actions and beliefs of the caregivers with whom the child interacts. It is evident, therefore, that a comprehensive child-care and development programming strategy, seeking real and lasting improvements in survival, growth and development, must be conceived in such a way that it works at all of these levels. It must do more than provide direct attention to the child; it must strengthen and improve the various environments within which the child is developing.

These considerations lead to a set of five complementary programme approaches:

1 *Attending to children in centres.*   The immediate goal of this direct approach, focusing on the *child* (or mother in the case of prenatal attention), is to enhance child development by attending to the immediate needs of children in centres organized outside the home.

2 *Supporting and educating caregivers.*   This approach focuses on *family* members and is intended to educate and 'empower' parents and other family members in ways that improve their care and interaction with the child and enrich the immediate environment in which child development is occurring rather than provide a substitute for it.

3 *Promoting community development.*   Here, emphasis is on working to change *community* conditions that may adversely affect child development. This strategy stresses community initiative, organization, and participation in a range of interrelated activities, to improve the physical environment, the knowledge and practices of community members, and the organizational structure, allowing common action and improving the base for political and social negotiations.

4 *Strengthening institutional resources and capacities.*   There are many *institutions* involved in carrying out the three approaches mentioned above. In order to do an adequate job, they need financial, material, and human resources with a capacity for planning, organization, implementation, and evaluation of programmes. Programmes to strengthen institutions may involve institution-building, training, provision of materials, or experimentation with innovative techniques and models (improving the 'technology' available to them). They may also involve providing the legal underpinnings for proper functioning of the institutions.

5 *Strengthening demand and awareness.*   This programme approach concentrates on the production and distribution of *knowledge* in order to create awareness and demand. It may function at the level of policymakers and planners, or be directed broadly towards changing the cultural ethos that affects child development.

Although all five approaches are intended to enhance early childhood development, each has different immediate objectives and each is directed, initially, towards a different audience or group of participants. Table 5.1

Table 5.1 Complementary approaches to programming for early childhood care and development

Programme approaches	Participants/beneficiaries	Objectives

1 Attending to children (delivering a service)	– The child
	  – 0–2
	  – 3–6
	  – 0–6
	– Pregnant women
		– Survival
		– Comprehensive development
		– Socialization
		– Rehabilitation
		– Child care
		– Reduce disparities

2 Educating or supporting caregivers	– Parents – Siblings – Other family – Parents-to-be	– Create awareness – Change attitudes – Improve/change practices – Reduce disparities

3 Promoting community development	– Community
	  – leaders
	  – promoters
	  – members
		– Create awareness
		– Mobilize for action
		– Change conditions

4 Strengthening national resources, capabilities	– Programme actors
	  – professionals
	  – paraprofessionals
		– Create awareness
		– Upgrade skills
		– Increase material resources

5 Strengthening demand and awareness	– Policymakers – The public – Professionals	– Create awareness – Build political will – Increase demand – Change attitudes

also summarizes the main objectives and audiences (or participants, or beneficiaries, or, in the unfortunate language of some programming, 'target groups') for each approach. In the following chapters, we will return to these five approaches, discussing each in somewhat more detail, suggesting advantages and disadvantages of each, examining different models that might be applied within each approach, and providing some examples of each.

Although any overall plan for enhancing child development must pay attention to all five of the approaches distinguished here, the emphasis to be given to each approach within the overall strategy will, of course, vary considerably depending on the conditions of the particular place in which the programme is being developed.

Programme guidelines

In planning and implementing programmes of child development, several principles and guidelines defining desirable programme characteristics should be kept in mind.

1 *Priority should be given to families and communities living in conditions that put their children 'at risk' of delayed or debilitated development.*

If programming is to be guided by a principle of social justice, then emphasis must be given to those most in need. Selecting those deemed to be most 'at risk' will involve some combination of information about:

- the condition of children (birth weight, infant mortality rates, nutritional and health status);
- the condition of women (educational levels, health and nutritional status, age at first pregnancy, work demands and earnings);
- family and support systems (size and composition, employment and income, the availability of adequate alternative child care);
- childrearing beliefs and practices (feeding, health habits, nurturing, communication); and
- more general socioeconomic conditions (earnings and income distribution, literacy rates, availability of potable water, access to health and other services, conditions of rapid social or economic change).

This guideline is easy to declare but not so easy to follow, regardless of what indicators are decided upon to define 'at risk' children and families. Political realities and existing economic and social inequalities make it difficult to live up to the rhetoric. However, there are sufficient examples of political will, combined with social conscience and technical competence, to think that the guideline can be followed. Moreover, the plight of children is less politically charged than many issues and can, therefore, be a leading edge in efforts to reduce inequalities.

2 *Programmes should form part of a comprehensive, multifaceted strategy.*

A programming strategy must begin with a set of objectives. Often mentioned as a starting point for child development programmes is the right of each child to be able to realize his or her potential. What it means to realize one's potential is defined somewhat differently in different cultures so the specific objectives flowing from this goal will be different for different societies. For this reason, we have taken as the main goal of child development, and hence of child development programmes, the competence of children in adjusting to, performing in, and transforming their own surroundings. In some cultures that will mean greater emphasis on independence; in others greater emphasis on group solidarity. In some cases, physical coordination will be central; in others abstract reasoning. In all, however, there will be physical, intellectual, and social dimensions of development.

We have stressed that there is unity in a child's needs. Further, we have insisted that as these needs are fulfilled together there is an interaction effect at work enhancing child development in more than just an additive way. A clear implication of this unitary, interactive view is that programmes should be multifaceted and integrative. But we have noted the tendency for a piecemeal approach to predominate, with some programmes focusing on health or nutrition without attending to the stimulation and caregiver–child interaction that fosters psychosocial development – or vice versa.

Attempting to adhere to this guideline does not mean that all components must appear in all programmes of all organizations. Nevertheless, an overall strategy that is comprehensive and multifaceted should frame all child development programme efforts. And opportunities should be sought to blend services, to encourage multisectoral collaboration, and to fit new components into ongoing programmes lacking that component.

Can this guideline be applied to each of the five complementary programme approaches? Consider the **centre-based approach**. Many child development centres do not include medical and feeding facilities and may or may not teach good health and nutrition habits to young children. A child-care centre, even with medical attention and feeding, may function with or without attention to early stimulation, organized play, and/or educational activities. However, these several dimensions of child development can be incorporated into one 'integrated' service. Or, they can be delivered separately, in pieces, through separate bureaucracies that nevertheless 'converge' on one community or one location (a community or home day-care centre, a preschool, a workplace, a health post, a community kitchen, a supplementary feeding centre, or another location).

Caregiver education, the second approach, is often focused on one component of development, say health, when it could include several – for example, health, nutrition, and education. This occurs even though it is easier to integrate the content of education programmes than it is to integrate services. **Community development** programmes sometimes emphasize one area – water and sanitation, for instance – instead of taking a multifocal view. Unfortunately, community development programmes, even though they may be justified in terms of their potential impact on children, often neglect specific attention to a child's psychosocial development needs. This neglect is based on the false assumption that if changes can be made in the physical conditions of the community, the child's mental and social development will take care of itself.

Strengthening institutions is frequently conceived in a closed and unintegrated way. For instance, efforts may be limited to the upgrading of preschool teachers by providing training in Piagetian techniques related principally to the process of cognitive development. Or paediatricians may be trained to do a better job of diagnosing early childhood diseases, but not taught about the process of early childhood development. Less often will programmes cross lines to, for instance, introduce a psychosocial development component into the training of health personnel or into the routines of health institutions.

Finally, attempts to **create a new ethos** or new cultural values can be narrowly directed towards changing people's ideas about survival or about disease, or they can take a broader view, reinforcing the natural tendency for most caregivers to consider the child as a unity.

A full section of this book will be devoted to multifocal or integrated programming. Special chapters will deal with combining health, nutrition and education, combining early interventions with primary school education, and combining child care with programmes of women's work.

3 *Programmes should be participatory and community-based.*

Community participation is sometimes encouraged for its own sake, as a basis for developing solidarity and greater control over one's own life. More often, however, participation is viewed instrumentally – as a means of making programmes more effective by engaging potential recipients actively so that usage will increase and so that the programme will respond appropriately to local needs. A growing body of experience shows that community participation increases the effectiveness of most programmes. And, community participation allows extension of services beyond what would be possible using only the budgets and resources of the public sector.

Participation in a programme can be defined in many ways. To the extent that centres are used, participation exists. Use, however, does not imply input into the content or financing or running of a programme. It may mean simply using services offered. This simple use is not the kind of participation to which the guideline refers. More common is a definition in terms of the donation of materials or labour needed to build facilities. This view of participation is still extremely limited in concept and in time. It is not the kind of participation that leads to acquisition of new knowledge and skills. It does not include the sustained involvement that will be necessary for most programmes to survive.

A more complete definition of community participation in a programme includes mobilization and direct involvement of the community in all phases of programme activity – in design, implementation, and evaluation. It implies the existence and growth of organizational mechanisms through which participation can be expressed. It means involving the community at large, not just a selected few individuals, in a process of discussion and action on a continuing basis.

Rhetoric to the contrary, most programming for child survival, growth and development is biased against participation by a significant portion of 'users' over a sustained period and in various phases of programme formulation, implementation and evaluation. This is particularly true of most centre-based initiatives providing direct attention to children; they tend to be designed, financed, and organized from outside local communities. That is more often the case if they are centralized public programmes and if broad coverage is sought. However, child-care and development centres can be, and sometimes are, set up and run with local participation even if financing comes from outside sources and general guidelines are set nationally.

A caregiver education approach can also range from an extremely participative approach based on the specific experiences and knowledge of groups of parents who learn and support each other in discussion groups, to programmes in which the caregivers are simply given information deemed appropriate to their situation, without adjustment to local circumstances and without discussion of the content. 'Teachers' may be outsiders; or they may be local individuals who are themselves successful caregivers. The difference between a participatory and a non-participatory outlook is captured in a distinction between '*transmitting* child development *messages*' and '*discussing* child development *themes*'.

Similarly, community development programmes and efforts to strengthen institutions can be highly participatory and locally controlled or can be imposed and virtually without involvement in planning, financing, or implementation.

Finally, creating awareness in the general public or among political leaders, professionals, or opinion-makers can also be approached in a more or less participatory way. Again, people can be told what they should value and believe, or they can be helped to discover these through participation.

The following two guidelines are closely related to the above discussion, emphasizing the need to be participatory and community-based.

4 *Programmes should be flexible and adjusted to different sociocultural contexts.*

Nations, communities, and cultures differ widely in the particular needs of their children. Unless programmes can identify varying needs of diverse communities and respond accordingly, programmes run the risk of being irrelevant to the prevailing conditions and needs. Moreover, achieving real participation will be difficult. Arriving with a standard package of solutions to preconceived problems does not favour participation or achieving the desired outcomes. If, however, community participation is to include consultation at all stages, programmes must be flexible enough to incorporate the results of that consultation. Nevertheless, there is a natural tendency for programmers to seek standard solutions that can be spread widely (see also Guideline 7).

5 *Programmes should support and build upon local ways that have been devised to cope effectively with problems of child care and development.*

This guideline is based on the assumption that programmes are more likely to work if they begin with solutions devised and tried out locally rather than with solutions imposed from outside. It places an important value on coping skills and on innovative measures born of necessity. The position contrasts with one in which knowledge is assumed to reside in the heads of outside 'experts' without, however, denying the potential role of outsiders in helping communities see and experiment with new ways to enhance early childhood development.

Respecting local cultures and reinforcing local ways can be termed a 'constructionist' rather than a 'compensatory' view. If community participation is real, programming will, by definition, be constructive and respectful of culture.

6 *Programmes should be financially feasible and cost-effective.*

Clearly, programmes must be possible to implement within recognized resource constraints, and they should be economically feasible beyond an initial period when costs may be borne by an outside source. The economic 'feasibility' of a programme, however, is only partly a matter of available funds – it is also a matter of priorities and of how funds are divided up. If a programme has been assigned a high priority, it can be afforded and made feasible by giving up something of lower priority.

Costs can vary considerably depending on the programme option chosen. It makes sense that every effort should be made to avoid using expensive imported technologies, materials, or personnel when these are not needed. Often locally available resources would produce equivalent results at lower cost.

The reader may notice that this guideline is not couched in terms of 'low-cost' programmes. The object is not to seek the lowest possible cost for a programme. Some cost-cutting measures will also lead to a cut in effectiveness. A low-cost project that has little or no effect is a waste, more so than a programme with higher costs that is an effective programme.

Within each of the five approaches are higher- and lower-cost options. A centre-based care programme in which 15 children are cared for in the home of a neighbourhood woman, trained as a paraprofessional, assisted on a rotating basis by mothers of the children in the centre and supported by a system of community health posts is likely to cost considerably less per child than a centre-based care programme gathering 60 children together in a special building, and employing a director, a professional preschool teacher, several aides, a cook, and a guardian, and stocked with store-bought furniture. Or, a mass media model of caregiver education may be able to reach many individuals with messages at a very low cost per person, as compared with a more labour-intensive, higher-cost (but potentially more effective) programme of discussion groups.

A higher-cost programme model may turn out to be much more effective than a lower-cost model. However, if the high cost is so prohibitive that it restricts a programme to only a few privileged individuals, it will not allow application on a large scale and may have to be discarded as unfeasible, even though it is cost-effective. Therefore, to make the best use of resources, it is critical to seek options that are relatively low in cost and high in effectiveness. These and related issues will be dealt with in Chapter

15. The observation that the lower the cost, the greater the extension of the programme can be with the same amount of available resources, brings us to the final guideline included in our programming approach.

7 *Programmes should try to reach the largest possible number of children living in conditions that put them at risk.*

Because the need is so great in most countries of the Third World, programmers should give priority to those programmes that offer the best prospect of reaching the most children who are at risk, with an effective solution. That means looking beyond demonstration and pilot projects to the possibility of implementation on a large scale.

The 'scale' of each approach may be pictured simplistically as running from very low coverage to a figure of 100 per cent. Determining what constitutes 'scale' is, however, not that simple. First, one must determine what population is to be reached. That may be very different from the total population of all children under age six, of all pregnant and lactating women. Not all individuals may need to be reached. And the number of children who need programme support may be different for different actions affecting early development. For instance, 100 per cent coverage may be both desirable and necessary for an immunization programme, but a programme of early stimulation may not be necessary for a significant proportion of that same population because they are already receiving adequate stimulation and nurturing.

We will argue in Chapter 14 that scale can be achieved in several ways, only one of which is by expanding a single model or programme to reach all the desired population. Another way is by adding together the results of several different actions, each based on a different model, and each reaching a different segment of the population. Scale emerges as the puzzle pieces are brought together. Taking this latter view of scale by 'association' or 'addition' allows high coverage to be increased by encouraging a series of smaller programmes as well as by launching uniform national initiatives. Adopting this approach to scale is crucial if we are to reconcile the desire for community participation with the desire for broad coverage.

These seven guidelines, taken together, provide a litmus test for programmes. The test can be applied to any or all of the complementary approaches at each of the developmental stages.

Having set out a broad framework to guide us, we turn now to some examples of what kinds of programmes can be organized within each of the five complementary approaches. Later chapters will deal with the programme characteristics set forth as guidelines in the framework.

NOTE

1   This chapter draws liberally on the contents of *UNICEF Programme Guidelines, Volume 5*, a manual prepared by Robert Myers and Cassie Landers for UNICEF, particularly chapters 1, and 4–9.

REFERENCE

Myers, R. and C. Landers. *Early Childhood Development: UNICEF Programme Guidelines, Volume 5,* New York: UNICEF, 1989.

Part III

A state of the practice

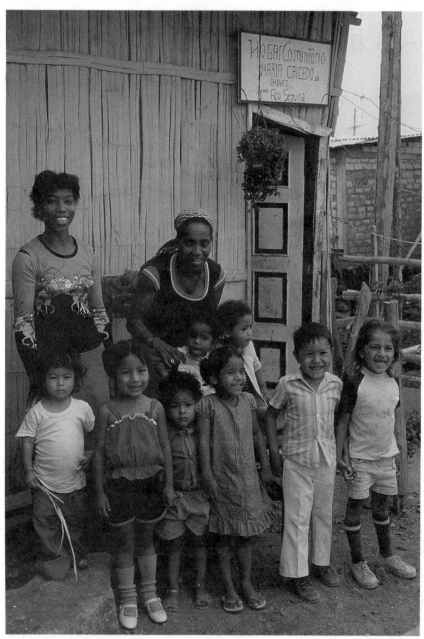

A home day-care programme, Guayaquil, Ecuador

Chapter 6

Some examples of what can be done

The reader may, at this point, say, 'This is all very academic. You have presented a set of interesting ideas and concepts, and advocated that attention be given to five complementary programme approaches. But what do these approaches look like when they are translated into action? What can I do that will be relevant to my particular setting? What examples are available from the Third World from which we can learn? What works and what needs adjusting? In short, what is the "state of the practice?"'

WHAT ARE THE PROGRAMME OPTIONS?

Fortunately, there is no lack of programme examples available to those who wish to look beyond survival to enhancing the well-being of 'the twelve who survive'. And most of these are not formal or expensive preschool options with fancy quarters and equipment and highly trained teachers. We shall describe some of those options in the following two chapters, discussing also potential advantages and disadvantages. We shall organize the discussion according to the five complementary approaches set out in Chapter 5 and in Table 6.1.

The intention in this chapter and the next is to provide the reader with a feel for the broad range of options that exist and to stimulate creative thinking about programme options that might be tried out that are not traditional and expensive 'preschools' and are not the more shallow forms of 'social marketing' and 'parental education' that tend to prevail. The examples will be presented briefly, with references given for readers who might wish to pursue one or more in detail. Not all examples will be 'model' cases; it is possible and advisable to learn from examples that have not worked well – in addition to learning from those that are 'exemplary'.

As examples are presented, we shall try to examine them in relation to the guidelines proposed in Chapter 5, i.e. with respect to their attention to the integration of programme components and actions, community participation, flexibility, local ways, scale and cost.

Table 6.1 Early childhood development: complementary approaches and programme options

Approaches	Options	
1 Delivering services in centres	1.1	Integrated child development centres
	1.2	Home day care
	1.3	Health or nutrition centres
	1.4	Child-care centres
	1.5	Formal/non-formal preschools
2 Caregiver support/ education	2.1	Home visiting
	2.2	Parental and adult education/support
	2.3	Open audience mass media
	2.4	Child-to-child
3 Community development	3.1	Changing the environment
	3.2	Strengthening organization
4 Strengthen institutions	4.1	Training and motivating people
	4.2	Improving facilities/equipment
	4.3	Adjusting and upgrading technology
	4.4	Improving organization and management
5 Strengthen awareness/ demand	5.1	Social marketing
	5.2	Selective advocacy
	5.3	Group discussion

ATTENDING TO CHILDREN IN CENTRE-BASED PROGRAMMES

Most discussions of early childhood development continue to be focused on the first of the five general programme approaches presented in Figure 6.1 – on attention to the child in centres created for that purpose. These programmes attend to children outside their homes, usually in a group, and for varying periods of time. They provide an 'alternative environment' for the child. The main beneficiary is the child and the success of the programme is measured in terms of what the programme does directly to improve a child's health, nutrition and/or psychosocial development. Often, the contribution of governments or other organizations to child development is measured in terms of the number of children who are participating in such centres. To do so is to leave aside the other four, less direct, forms of contributing to enhancing child development.

It is evident that centre-based approaches to child development can have an important, and sometimes impressive, impact on the development of children. It is also clear that there are many occasions on which child care outside the home is necessary (see Chapter 11 discussing child care and women's work). Our intention, therefore, is not to suggest that centre-based care is bad or unnecessary. Rather, we would like the reader to recognize centre-based attention as one among several approaches to enhancing early childhood development. And we would like to suggest that there is a range of possibilities for organizing centre-based programmes. That is particularly important as one thinks about mounting child development initiatives on a large scale. It is particularly important as one thinks about the responsibilities that families have played and will continue to play in the upbringing of their children.

There are several potential advantages to centre-based programmes:

- Grouping children creates the possibility of using child care as an entry point for primary health care promotion, prevention and monitoring. It can, for instance, facilitate immunization. If centres are big enough, it is possible to have specialized personnel of several kinds associated with the centre, facilitating integration of services.
- When attention is provided directly by programme staff, it is relatively easy for programme implementers to know whether or not a child is actually receiving various components of care (food, stimulation, health monitoring, etc.). That is not the case with the more indirect approaches in which programmes place reliance on parents and other caregivers.
- For children aged three to six, centres bring children together in a kind of organised social interaction that is not possible in most homes. During these ages, children need to interact with other children and may profit from consistent attention of an adult who is not their parent. They need exposure to skills and ways of thinking (and sometimes a language) that will help prepare them for primary schooling. Centres can help to meet these needs in ways that homes sometimes cannot, and which go beyond the informal groupings that children can form in most communities.
- Centres provide visibility that is useful politically, both to get programmes going and to sustain them. Formal, centre-based programmes are harder to remove than informal programmes focused on the home.

But centre-based programmes also have potential disadvantages:

- Grouping children increases the chances of their exposure to communicable diseases, requiring therefore special attention to potential health hazards.
- The availability of centres can erode family responsibility for care and development of their children.
- Attention to the child outside the home can raise conflicts between the home and the substitute environment.
- If the child returns to a home that is very different from the centre, improvements made in the centre may not continue.

– Centres can also undercut important cultural elements conveyed at home.

Whether it is useful to support a particular centre-based programme will depend on the following:

– Who is to be served;
– How the programme's content will respond to particular needs of the children and families served; and
– How the programme is to be organised and carried out – its quality, cost, extent of community participation, etc.

Variations of the centre-based approach

Direct attention to children by centre-based staff can be organized in many ways, only one of which is in the kind of formal preschool described at the outset of the chapter. We can distinguish at least five different kinds of programme options within this general programme approach:

– Integrated child development centres
– Non-formal, home day-care programmes
– Health or nutrition centres
– Child-care centres in the workplace
– Preschools

Integrated child development centres

Integrated child development centres seek to promote comprehensive development by combining early education with nutrition, health and, sometimes, other services at the centre. Some centres are designed from the outset as comprehensive centres offering several services. Others evolve from child-care programmes that add on additional services in such locations as a health post or a nutrition centre or in a preschool (see below). In some cases, an integrated centre forms part of a community development programme. We will emphasize here programmes that have attempted an integrated approach from the outset.

A Colombian example

In Colombia, a 1974 law mandated the creation of Centres for Integrated Attention for Preschool Children (CAIPs) to serve the children of public and private employees, the self-employed, and the unemployed. Funds for organizing these centres were obtained through a 2 per cent payroll tax on all public and private institutions. The Colombian Institute for Family Welfare (ICBF) received the funds from the tax and was charged with implementing all components of the programme (Pollitt *et al.* 1980).

The centres provided (and still provide) children up to six years of age with health, nutrition, and educational services for their physical and socio-psychological development. Each centre provides paediatric services and offers three meals a day, five days a week. With some exceptions, the centres care for children during an eight-hour period.

With the construction of new buildings to house the programme (or rental and renovation of existing buildings), and with the need for administrative, technical and supportive staff to run the centres, the CAIPs were found to be relatively expensive, even though the payroll tax proved to be an excellent source of funding. As might be expected, the extension of the programme was limited by the cost. Most of the participation was by children aged three or older and most of the CAIPs were found in urban areas. Many centres had little or no parental participation.

Against this background, the ICBF began to experiment with other, less expensive forms of caring for children in centres that would also involve greater community participation. The outgrowth of these experiments is reported in the next section dealing with non-formal home day-care programmes.

An Indian example

The massive Integrated Child Development Service (ICDS) provides a comprehensive and relatively inexpensive example of an integrated, centre-based programme. The ICDS, started by the Indian government in 1975, is intended to improve the quality of life for poor children, ages 0 to 6, and their mothers in urban slums, rural and tribal areas (UNICEF 1984). In 1989, it was estimated that ICDS reached 11.6 million children, 0 to 6 (Hong 1989).

The Service functions primarily through *anganwadi* centres (literally, courtyards) run by anganwadi workers (AWW) who gather together somewhere between 20 and 40 children for approximately three hours each weekday for supplementary feeding and for preschool educational activities. *Anganwadi* workers are paraprofessionals selected by the Central Government (not the community) according to uniform criteria based on education and experience, and are given pre-service training by existing academic institutions and non-governmental organizations. In addition to providing the early education and supervising the supplementary feeding, the AWW are charged with helping to monitor growth, distribute vitamin A, maintain immunization records, and, sometimes, to educate mothers. (Critics would say 'burdened' instead of 'charged' because of the many duties.) In these activities, the anganwadi workers are assisted by a helper and supported by a child development programme officer.

Although it is considered a community-based programme, it, as many other community-based programmes, is implemented centrally and with limited local participation. It also shares with many other programmes a series of challenges with respect to the employment of community workers who receive low pay because they remain outside the formal bureaucracy. The integrated approach has been maintained despite efforts by some national and international groups to focus programme activities on either health and nutrition, or on the preschool activities. In addition, ICDS has been more effective in reaching children aged 3 and up than it has been in reaching children below age three.

The ICDS can point to some successes. Attributed to the programme are reductions in infant mortality, severe malnutrition, morbidity, and school repetition (Tandon 1986; Chaturvedi 1987). The programme is the largest of its kind in the world and has continued to grow, suggesting that with sufficient political will and organization, a centre-based and centrally run programme of integrated development can be extended to a significant proportion of the population at an estimated cost of US$10.00 per child per year (Hong 1989), and with some effect.

A Brazilian example

A different kind of integrated, centre-based model comes from Brazil where children, aged 4 to 6, from poor areas of cities, come together during weekday mornings in groups of about 100 children. The name of this programmes indicates its origin as a nutrition programme: The Preschool Feeding Programme (PROAPE). From the start, however, an integrated view was adopted so that in addition to food and vitamin supplementation, the programme included supervised psychomotor activities and a health component (check-ups, dental treatment, vaccinations, and visual exams).

In one variant of the PROAPE model (Ministerio da Saude 1983), children are attended by a trained preschool teacher, assisted by volunteer mothers (or other family members) who participate on a rotating basis. In another, three trained paraprofessionals are paid 70 per cent of a minimum salary for the 3-hour work day and assisted also by volunteer mothers.

Evaluations of the PROAPE model have generally proven to be positive, as compared with other centre-based models also in use in Brazil (Franco 1983; Ministerio da Saude 1983). Indeed, we will draw on results from this model in Chapters 10 and 15, to demonstrate cost effectiveness (in terms of the cost savings, because participation substantially reduced the repetition rate in the first years of primary school). Here, our main purpose in referring to PROAPE is to present an innovative centre-based programme that differs from the stereotyped preschool programme described at the outset.

Home day care

One of the least 'institutional' forms of centre-based care and education is home day care (sometimes called family care, neighbourhood day care or child-minding). Home day care refers to an arrangement in which a woman (no examples with men have been found) cares for, in her home, several young children, including children who are not her own. The caregivers are often neighbours who also have young children of their own at home and who are not formally trained caregivers. The child-care arrangement may be informal and private and essentially custodial; or it may be formal, linked to other services, training, and on-site assistance for the caregivers. Payment for the service may be 'in kind' or in money. Too often the care provided may be purely custodial, with little or no stimulation or psycho-social development content.

This model of child care and development provides a useful alternative to formal child-care centres. Care provided in a home for a small number of children can ensure a safe and healthy atmosphere and also respond to the child's developmental needs for love, security, interaction, and exploration. Home day care is often both low-cost and community-based. It is likely to build on an existing practice – neighbours taking care of children – and it is likely to draw on local wisdom about how that should be done.

Several cautions should be noted in conjunction with the home day care approach:

–   Home day care is often favoured for the family-like atmosphere it provides for a child. However, the care given by someone who is not the child's mother and who must mind other children as well is not the same as the care given a child in his or her own home. If the numbers are large in a home day-care arrangement, the homey atmosphere is quickly lost. The larger the number, the more management skills a home day-care person will need.

–   Home day-care programmes are often of low quality because they do not include the training and supervision necessary to supplement traditional wisdom and to upgrade and maintain quality. Conditions may be unsafe and attention to children minimal. The possibility of poor quality is exacerbated if care in the home is not linked to supporting services outside the home.

–   The low cost of home day care may be a result of exploitation of women caregivers or a result of skimping on supervision and support services. This may mean unhappy caregivers, low-quality service, and a purely custodial programme with few benefits (and even some disadvantages) for the child.

A Venezuelan example

A home day-care programme was established in Caracas, Venezuela, in 1974 to provide mothers working away from home with access to child care. The programme built upon informal child-care arrangements developed by families in the poorer neighbourhoods in which the programme was put into effect. The government-financed programme sought to upgrade and to extend the existing arrangements. Day-care mothers, who had to be at least 18 years old, received a small stipend (paid partly by the Government and partly by the mothers using the service) to attend to no more than five children under the age of six for 12 hours a day in their homes. Care included an established routine of health, nutrition, and educational services. The programme equipped homes, which had to meet safety and hygiene requirements, with some furniture and materials.

To implement the Venezuelan programme, the Children's Foundation, a quasi-governmental organization presided over by the wife of the president, worked with government agencies, including those responsible for housing, public works, health and social services, social security and nutrition. A technical-support team, consisting of a social worker, health worker and a teacher serving groups of 20 homes, helped the day-care mothers to carry out their task. A neighbourhood coordinator was responsible for each group of 60 homes. According to an evaluation of the Venezuelan programme:

> The day care mothers provided the children with the necessary custodial care, are alert to their basic needs, abide by the stipulated schedule, know the norms governing the programme, have basic knowledge of the areas of health, nutrition, and child development, prepare and serve meals, protect the children against dangerous situations, take care of the children's personal hygiene and give the children a home-like environment until the arrival of their mothers.
>
> (de Ruesta 1978, p. 20)

Though less expensive for the government than formal day care in large nurseries, this particular day-care programme was still relatively costly. The programme grew to include 1,260 day-care homes in 42 neighbourhoods in Caracas. However, with a change of government, political backing for this particular home day-care system disappeared. Some day-care mothers continue to provide services on their own, but the programme as such no longer exists.

This example is notable, first, for its quality and a positive effect on the children, and, second, for its failure to cover a larger portion of the population in need, because of relatively high costs and the lack of continued political support.

Other Colombian examples

Parallel to the growth of the larger, more formal, integrated centres in Colombia that were described previously was a set of experiments in home day care. For instance, two home day-care programmes developed in the city of Cartagena, arising from the needs of working mothers in marginal areas (UNICEF/New York 1979). Several women from the community were willing to provide care in their homes for up to ten children, between the ages of two and four years. After the mothers were trained, a programme worker helped them monitor children's health, provide meals, establish a safe and sanitary environment and provide cognitive stimulation.

From this initiative grew another: to extend the day-care coverage, other members of the community volunteered to provide care during the morning in their homes for between 10 and 25 children under the age of four. The children, selected by the volunteers, received a morning snack obtained through the Family Welfare Institute. The volunteers were provided also with rudimentary training in child care, basic health, and skills for working with young children. No formal evaluation was made to determine what the programme benefits may have been to the children.

In these cases, the cost of care was kept low by relying on volunteers and by increasing the number of children cared for in a home. The fact that the programme was available only in the mornings meant that it did not meet the child-care needs of working women in the same way that the 12-hour programme in Venezuela did. Despite the lack of an evaluation there was a strong feeling that a home day-care mother could not handle the upper limit of 25 children.

From these and other home day-care experiments in Colombia has evolved a large-scale day-care programme called Homes for Well-Being (Hogares de Bienestar). Within 28 months of its beginnings in February 1987, the programme expanded to cover nearly 800,000 children throughout the country. It is expected to reach 1,500,000 children by 1992 (Sanz de Santamaria 1989). This programme also builds on the idea of 'volunteer' mothers who take children from the community into their homes. These 'community mothers' are chosen from within the community by other parents. They are provided with training in subjects related to child care and basic needs such as hygiene and preventive health, nutrition, and play or recreation. They are also given access to loan funds at very favourable rates in order to be able to upgrade their homes to meet minimum child-care standards, and they are provided with the necessary furniture and some play materials.

Although they are considered volunteers, the community mothers are compensated through a system of what are called 'scholarships'. In addition, the Family Welfare Institute, which oversees the programme, helps to meet 80 per cent of each participating child's daily nutritional requirements by distributing a nutritional supplement and by helping procure foodstuffs at below-market prices through a network of community stores.

Each of these home day-care centres is expected to accommodate a maximum of 15 children. Realizing that it is difficult for one person to care for 15 children during a full day, help is built in by expecting parents of the participating children to assist in the centre with cooking and child care one day of every 15. In addition, children under the age of one year are not accepted, except in very unusual circumstances.

This large-scale programme is still young and has not been evaluated formally. Informal indications are, however, that the model has considerable merit and is workable – if the basic model is allowed to vary somewhat from place to place in response to community needs. The per-child cost of the programme is estimated at one-fifth that of the more traditional programme of day care in large centres. Hours are more flexible. The programme coverage is greater. The programme generates some income for the community mothers, and it allows other women in the community to seek full-time employment. Moreover, the community economy is aided by assuring that procurement and local services related to the programme are provided through community enterprises and individuals.

An Ecuadorian example

In Guayaquil, Ecuador, a home day-care system is one component within a larger programme providing basic services for an urban area (UNICEF/ New York, March 1983; Mejia 1989). That programme brings together primary health care, nutrition, communication and activities to help women generate income. Day-care mothers care for up to ten children in their homes, from infancy up to six years of age. As in the Colombian and Venezuelan projects, mothers receive training and are helped to upgrade their homes. In this instance, the mothers of participating children form a committee to oversee the programme. Each week a different committee member is responsible for purchasing food for the children. The day-care system is linked to other supportive services (such as health) and supervision is provided. The project, although remaining small, seems to provide adequate care for children. Moreover, as caregiving mothers receive a minimum wage, the project has presented some women with an income-earning opportunity.

Nutrition or health centres

Another type of centre-based programme of early childhood care and development occurs within nutrition or health centres. Included in this category of centres should be those that attend to pregnant women. Often, such attention is minimal and, when it is given, it is (and should be) focused on diet and health considerations affecting the woman. Nevertheless, check-ups during pregnancy, particularly those during the third trimester, can provide the opportunity for discussing how to deal with the newborn so as to foster psychomotor development as well as growth. This is rarely done, even though this period in a child's development is known to constitute a 'touchpoint' when parents are anxious to know what to expect and do when a baby is born. It is a time when they are receptive to new knowledge.

More examples of developmentally oriented programmes come from the field of nutrition than from health, perhaps because the supplementary feeding process and nutrition recuperation lends itself more than does health attention to incorporating other components of direct attention to children. Health centres are visited only from time to time while nutrition centres usually involve daily attention over longer periods.

One of the sadder sights that a visitor to a nutrition centre may see is a row of inert toddlers propped against a wall or sitting lethargically and immobile on a straw mat, waiting to be fed. Or, infants in a nutrition recuperation centre may lie all day in a crib, with no stimulation other than at feeding time or when an attendant happens to pass by. These rather grim situations can be remedied, at very little cost, and with sometimes dramatic results. Stimulation can be added into these programmes both by training the regular attendants and by incorporating other individuals (who may serve on a volunteer basis) to play with the children.

A Jamaican example

A nutrition recuperation centre, located within the Tropical Metabolism Research Institute of the University of the West Indies, undertook a programme of educating attendants and providing them with incentives to improve the amount and quality of their interaction with the malnourished children (Grantham-McGregor 1983). As a result, children improved much more rapidly, both in terms of their weight gains and in their cognitive development. This small, highly targeted programme did not involve parents or communities at the outset. However, it evolved into an ongoing programme, reaching a larger number of at risk infants through a programme of home visiting (see Chapter 9).

A Kenyan example

As part of a Family Life Training Programme, nursery schools were set up in rehabilitation centres (UNICEF/EARO 1979). The schools catered first to the siblings of the malnourished children and then to other children of the community. Associating the nursery schools with the rehabilitation centres was seen as a means, in addition to caring for children, of providing education to families that would help to change the beliefs and practices that produced malnutrition.

A Peruvian example

Child-care centres have grown up in conjunction with community kitchens (Fujimoto and Villanueva 1984). Community kitchens are collaborative, community-based efforts located in marginal urban areas, designed to: (1) free up women's time by collectivizing the time-consuming process of cooking meals; (2) improve the diet of the community and reduce malnutrition; and (3) reduce food costs through wholesale buying and the receipt of subsidized food through food supplementation programmes. A group of women unite to do the buying and cooking, taking turns preparing meals for all in the group. These meals are either eaten in a group or, more frequently, taken home.

The idea of attaching a child-care centre to the community kitchen grew originally because mothers who were preparing the meals brought their small children with them and therefore needed some form of care and meals for their children. Adding a child-care centre was desired also to ensure that young children would not only receive a daily ration of food, but could also receive some early stimulation and education.

Child-care and development centres at the workplace

Another type of centre for young children is the child-care centre found at the workplace. The setting may be a factory, a marketplace, or a production cooperative run by women. Most such centres have been established first to provide custodial care for children of working women.

Care may be required by law, or it may be a response to workers' needs. Many countries have laws requiring companies employing more than a specified number of women to provide child-care facilities at the work site. We will deal with the relationship between these programmes and the needs of working women in more detail in Chapter 11. Meanwhile, here are several examples of centre-based programmes at the workplace.

A Senegalese example

In rural Senegal, women who were part of an *Animation Feminine* centre proposed, in 1962, to the *animatrices* operating the centres that a programme be started where children could be cared for while women worked in the fields (Bashizi 1979). The purpose of the children's centre, as proposed by the women, was 'to resolve the problem of caring for their young children while they and their older daughters undertook the difficult task of planting out the rice'. Entrusting the children to older sisters who were still too small to work in the fields was a solution that did not provide sufficient guarantees of safety; and leaving them on the edge of the rice fields meant they would be exposed to all the vagaries of the climate as well as to poisonous snakes.

The *animatrices* agreed to establish the day-care programme as long as the women's centre did not have to pay for the programme. To meet this demand, mothers rotated responsibility for planting and tending a community garden from which the children could be fed while they were in the centre. Also, parents pay a fee for the programme in the form of money, rice, oil, or dried fish. The centres function from 8 a.m. until 7 p.m. The first centre in 1962 operated for two and one-half months during the most difficult part of the agricultural season – when the rice crop is transplanted.

Over the years, the day-care centres spread so that they serve several thousand children. Administratively, they are the responsibility of the *Département d'Animation Rurale, Promotion Humaine.* Community developers within the *Département* quickly saw that these centres could be used as a base from which a variety of social services could be offered. They began to offer training to community volunteers, adult education courses in nutrition, hygiene, disease prevention, water purification, and treatment of such diseases as malaria and conjunctivitis. This programme provides an excellent example of ways in which a child-care and development centre has served as a catalyst and location for more general development activities that help the community at large.

An Indian example

The Mobile Creche Program, operating approximately 50 centres in New Delhi and Bombay, specializes in caring for children from one of the poorest sections of the Indian society – the children of migrant construction labourers. These centres take care of about 4,000 children on any given day. Mobility is built into the programme as a direct response to the special needs of families engaged in an occupation which takes them from site to site. The child-care centres are set up in whatever accommodation is available at a particular construction site, such as basements, tin sheds, or tents. When work at one construction site is completed and families of the labourers depart for a new site, the child-care workers also move, as soon as a new programme has been negotiated for the new location.

Begun in 1969, with the opening of one creche in New Delhi, the programme was initially the charitable effort of two concerned women who provided a supervised playing and resting place and some food for children while the parents were working. Since then, the programme has expanded to provide services for infants and toddlers (from 0–3 years of age), for children aged 3 to 6 who enter a nursery school (*balwadi*) programme, and for elementary school children from ages 7 to 12. In practice, however, the groupings are not rigid and there is considerable freedom of movement.

Included in the programme's content is the provision of lunch or nutritious snacks, regular visits by doctors and treatment of diseases and malnutrition. Emphasis is also given to children's cognitive and psychosocial development and one of the goals is to prepare them for the formal school system. The creches have also evolved into community centres which address the needs of parents and offer classes in nutrition and hygiene for the mothers, adult literacy training, and training in vocational skills.

In the programme, equipment is low-cost and locally provided. Culturally familiar materials are used. The paraprofessional day-care workers are trained on the job by a process of exposure, observation and participation, working under the guidance of experienced field workers who have some professional experience and participate in ongoing training. Creche workers receive salaries and are recruited from the local communities. Most are young women who may be part-time students or otherwise unemployed.

Although limited in scale, this integrated, low-cost and effective centre-based programme has consistently met the twin objectives of attending to the child in a holistic way while also serving the needs of the working mother at her workplace (Swaminathan 1985).

An Ethiopian example

In Ethiopia, a comprehensive child development programme was established to provide safe care for children whose mothers were part of a fruit-growing cooperative. Although women had the right to become income-earning members of the Melka Oba Producers Cooperative, it was difficult for them to do so because their domestic duties left little time and energy, and because they felt work in the cooperative was at the expense of their children. To remedy this situation, a programme was established that brought together introduction of appropriate technology to reduce work burdens, a creche and preschool to care for children, and services to provide health care and family life education (UNICEF/Ethiopia 1985).

The child-care centre is administered by a Children's Affairs Committee of the co-op. The co-op pays the salaries of the child minders who are trained to carry out health, nutrition, and other activities. Children attending the centre range from 45 days to 6 years of age. An innovative feature of the programme is provision of work credits to women for time off to breastfeed their infants and to parents to take younger children to the preschool. As a result of these initiatives, disease-related deaths among children aged 1 to 5 have been reduced and women's participation in the cooperative has increased (Hargot 1989).

This pilot project is being replicated in other districts of Ethiopia where cooperatives exist, but would not be an appropriate model for most of the country.

A Ghanaian example

The Accra Market Women's Association needed to set up a child-care programme for their children while they were involved in buying and selling (UNICEF/WHO 1982). Working with the City Council, the Department of Social Welfare, the Ministry of Health, and the Ministry of Water and Sewage, a building near the market was refurbished so that it could serve 200 children, from infancy through age 5½. Administered by the Regional Health Officer, the programme has a strong health and nutritional focus. Mothers are encouraged to come to the centre to breastfeed. Children are provided with a morning snack and a full lunch. For children to participate, they must have a physical examination and appropriate immunizations. Once a month a public nurse inspects the facilities, provides immunizations as needed, and completes children's medical charts. Good cooperation between the market women and supporting agencies has made this market centre a success. The model is replicable, although coverage is focused on relatively few children.

Preschools

As indicated at the outset, early childhood programmes have often been associated with formal preschool training in a classroom-like atmosphere in which relatively expensive materials are used to prepare children for primary school. Whether privately owned or overseen by a Ministry of Education, such preschools typically employ professional preschool teachers whose training has been scholastic, are not linked to broader participatory programmes of community development, do little to involve parents, and often give little attention to health and nutrition.

With few exceptions, programmes of formal preschool education are expensive (primarily because salaries of professional teachers are high, relatively). This model is not found on a large scale in the Third World. Where formal preschools are found, they tend to be concentrated in urban areas and to cater to middle-class children or government employees. In some countries, they serve as a selective device for entrance into favoured primary schools, thereby beginning a process that favours middle- and upper-class children (Gakuru 1983). In short, the formal preschool model is not well suited to most countries of the Third World.

Preschools need not be so narrowly conceived. They may, for instance, employ paraprofessionals rather than professionals, use local materials, incorporate health and nutrition components, involve parents and other community members in a variety of ways including assistance in the classroom, and be incorporated into an integrated child development scheme. Several examples of these programmes are described below. They are often labelled 'non-formal' because they are rarely part of the formal structure of government service delivery, relying instead heavily on community and volunteer help. In their organization and conduct, however, they are often structured and formal.

A Kenyan example

More than 650,000 children were attending (in 1989) non-formal pre-schools (called nursery schools) that originated in the self-help movement known as *harambee* (Otaala 1981; Njenga 1989). Evolving in part from a need to provide care for children while their mothers work in the fields, the preschools serve children mostly between three and six years of age. Parents see benefits not only in academic preparation but also in health care for their children. The Ministry of Education, with some assistance from international organizations, now supports the preschools through in-service training, supervision and a programme to develop curricula and material tailored to the local community. Although the preschools have many formal characteristics (hours, curriculum, materials), they are non-formal in character, remaining firmly rooted in and controlled by the communities which are responsible for building schools and employing the paraprofessionals who operate them.

A Peruvian example

In the early 1970s, a Peruvian programme of community preschools, called PRONOEI (*Programas No-formales de Educacion Inicial*), took shape that, by 1985, was serving more than 500,000 children, mostly in rural communities. In the PRONOEI model, a group of approximately 30 children between the ages of three and five are brought together four of five mornings a week for three-hour periods. A paraprofessional trained in a series of very short-term courses supervises activities designed to improve the children's physical, mental, and social development. A snack is provided.

Community participation takes several forms. The paraprofessional is chosen by the community and serves in a 'volunteer' capacity, receiving a small monthly sum called a 'gratuity'. On a rotating basis, mothers cook a snack or noon-time meal, sometimes adding community contributions of food to the subsidy provided through a national nutrition supplementation programme. The community also participates by providing the space in which the preschool is held, either building a separate building or donating an existing space. A parents' committee oversees the preschool and matters related to the programme are discussed in town meetings.

In some locations, the preschool serves as a catalyst for broader community development efforts, including some income-generating projects, school gardens, water and sanitation projects (Myers *et al.*, 1985). Where this has been done, the programme could just as well be classified under the community development approach to early childhood care and development. The PRONOEI model, on average, was found to cost approximately half of what formal preschools cost. The costing of this model will be discussed further in Chapter 15.

A Brazilian example

The two non-formal preschool examples described above are very similar in form and content. Departing radically from the two is a preschool experiment carried out in Santa Catarina, Brazil, that is non-formal in a more fundamental respect (Pro-Crianca 1986). The preschool has no fixed location; rather, it is carried out in the streets and public areas of the community. The teacher supervises and guides a group of children, aged four to six, who move from place to place, learning as they go. Each day, the teacher and children set goals and choose activities they will do together. Although focused on the social and intellectual development of the children, the project also educates the community by demonstrating activities that stimulate and educate children – things parents can do with their children outside the project hours. This model obviously requires a creative teacher and a hospitable climate. It would be difficult to replicate on a large scale. (The experiment was conceived, however, as part of a much broader early development programme that includes support for home day care, formal preschools, and informal programmes of preschooling in rural areas.)

What should be clear from the foregoing is that there are many ways of organizing centre-based services attending directly to young children. In the following chapter, this same variation will be sought for the four other complementary approaches: educating/supporting caregivers, promoting community development, strengthening institutions and creating awareness and demand.

REFERENCES

Bashizi, B. 'Day-care Centers in Senegal: A Woman's Initiative', *Assignment Children*, Nos. 47/48 (1979), pp. 165–71.

Chaturvedi, E., B.C. Srivastava, J.V. Singh and M. Prasad. 'Impact of Six Years Exposure to ICDS Scheme on Psycho-social Development', *Indian Pediatrics*, Vol. 24 (1987), pp. 153–60.

Franco, M.A.C. 'Da Assistencia Educativa a Educação Assistencializada – um estudo de caracterização custos de atendimento a crianças carentes de 0 a 6 anos de idade', Brasilia: Centro Nacional de Recursos Humanos, 1983.

Fujimoto, G. and Y. Villanueva. 'Going to Scale: the Peruvian Experience with Early Childhood Programmes', a paper presented to the Second Inter-Agency Meeting on Community-based Approaches to Child Development, New York, October 29–31, 1984. Lima, Peru: UNICEF and New York: The Consultative Group on Early Childhood Care and Development.

Gakuru, O.N. 'Education and the Formation of Social Classes: The Case of Pre-School Education in Kenya', in K. King and R. Myers (eds), *Avoiding School Failure*. Ottawa: the International Development Research Centre, 1983.

Grantham-McGregor, S.M., W. Schofield and L. Harris. 'Effects of Psychosocial Stimulation on Development of Severely Malnourished Children', *Paediatrics,* No. 72 (1983), pp. 239–243.

Hargot, E. 'Case Studies of the Melka Oba-Yetnora Cooperatives in Ethiopia', a paper prepared for the Consultative Group on Early Childhood Care and Development, New York, May, 1989. Mimeo.

Hong, Sawon. 'Integrated Child Development Services. Early Childhood Development: India Case Study', a paper prepared for the Global Seminar on Early Childhood Development, Florence, International Child Development Centre, June 12–30, 1989. New Delhi: UNICEF, June, 1989. Mimeo.

Mejia, J. 'Women's Work and Child Care. Case Study: Basic Urban Services in Guayaquil, Ecuador', a paper prepared for the Consultative Group on Early Childhood Care and Development, New York, June, 1989.

Ministerio da Saude (MS), e Instituto Nacional de Alimentação e Nutrição (INAN), 'Analição de PROAPE/Alagoas com Enfoque na Area Econômica', Brasilia, MS/INAN, 1983.

Myers, R., *et al.* 'Pre-school Education as a Catalyst for Community Development', an evaluation prepared for USAID/Lima, January, 1985. Mimeo.

Njenga, A.W. 'The Pre-school Education and Care Programme: A Kenyan Experience', a paper prepared for the UNICEF Global Seminar on Early Childhood Development, Florence, International Child Development Centre, June 12–30, 1989. Nairobi, Kenya: Institute of Education, June, 1989. Mimeo.

Otaala, B. 'Day Care in Eastern Africa: A Survey of Botswana, Kenya, Seychelles and the Republic of Tanzania', Addis Ababa: United Nations Economic Commission for Africa, 1981. Doc. ST/ECA/ATRCW/81/23.

Pollitt, E., with the collaboration of R. Halpern and T. Eskenasy, *Poverty and Malnutrition in Latin America.* New York: Praeger Publishers, 1980.

'Pro-Crianca: Attention to Children in Open Spaces', a paper presented to the Afro-Latin American Seminar on Innovative Alternatives for Attention to the Child, Florianopolis, Brazil, December 1–6, 1986. Mimeo.

Ruesta, M.C. de y A. Barrios de Vidal. 'Evaluación de Programa Hogares de Cuidado Diario: Estudio Ejecutivo', Caracas, Venezuela: Fundación del Niño, Noviembre de 1978.

Sanz de Santamaria, A. 'Programa Social: Hogares Comunitarios de Bienestar', a paper prepared for the Global Seminar on Early Childhood Development, International Child Development Centre, Florence, June 12–30, 1989. Bogota, Colombia: Instituto Colombiano de Bienstar Familiar, June, 1989.

Swaminathan, M. *Who Cares?* New Delhi: Centre for Women's Development Studies, 1985.

Tandon, B.N. 'Status Paper for India'. Prepared for the meeting on: Day Care as an Entry Point for Maternal and Child Health Components of Primary Health Care, Paris, the International Children's Centre, May 24–26, 1986. New Delhi: the All India Institute of Medical Sciences, 1986. Mimeo.

UNICEF/East African Regional Office (EARO). 'Basic Services for Children in Eastern Africa', final report of an IYC symposium held in Nairobi, Kenya, March 19–22, 1979. Nairobi: UNICEF/EARO, 1979.

UNICEF/Ethiopia. Annual Report, 1985.

UNICEF/India. 'Integrated Child Development Services', New Delhi: UNICEF, 1984.

UNICEF/New York. 'The Infant and the Young Child – A Focus for Assistance and a Stimulus for Family Improvement', *Urban Examples*, No. 1 (May, 1979).

UNICEF/New York. 'Primary Health Care in the Slums of Guayaquil', *Urban Examples* No. 4 (March, 1983).

WHO/UNICEF. 'Alternative Approaches to Day Care in Africa', WHO/UNICEF Workshop, Nairobi, Kenya, December 6–12, 1982. Nairobi: UNICEF, 1982.

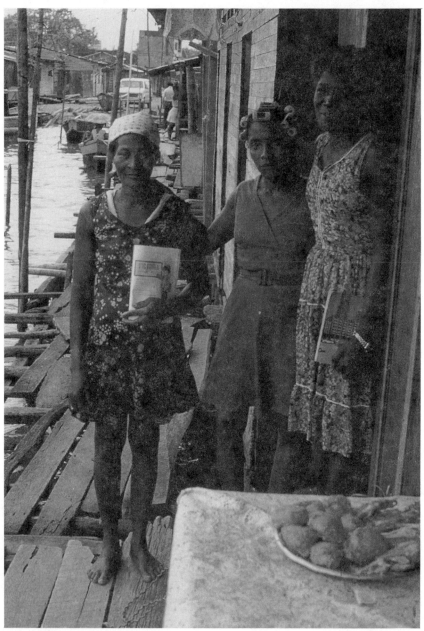

Home visiting, Buenaventura, Colombia

Chapter 7

Beyond centres and preschools: additional examples of what can be done

It is raining in the small Indonesian village, but the village volunteer is prepared to make her home visit just the same. In addition to the training she has received and the 'cartoon curriculum' that has been prepared for her to use with mothers, she has been provided with an umbrella with the word 'PANDAI' on it. PANDAI is at once an acronym for words meaning child development and mothers' care and a word which means clever or smart in the Bahasa language. The volunteer, or *kader*, had been working in the health post, but research results (Satoto 1989) suggested that a home-based intervention would work better, so she is now visiting children and their mothers in their homes once a week. She is focusing her attention on the mother rather than on caring for or teaching the child directly.

Whereas the examples in Chapter 6 provided a range of alternatives within the general approach of centre-based programmes for children, this chapter will elaborate and provide examples for four other, complementary programme approaches. As set out in the overall programme strategy (see p. 87) these are: providing caregiver support and education, promoting community development, strengthening institutions, and creating awareness and demand.

EDUCATING/SUPPORTING PARENTS AND OTHER CAREGIVERS

Programmes emphasizing education of parents and other caregivers reach the child indirectly – through the caregiver.[1] They complement and re-inforce service programmes that provide direct attention by programme staff to the health, nutrition, and developmental needs of the young child. Parenting education programmes provide encouragement and information that will allow more effective use of existing services. However, the main purpose of parent education programmes is to strengthen the self-confidence of parents and to empower them with knowledge and skills that will enhance their own ability to foster physical, mental, social, and emotional development in their young child.

Potential advantages and some cautions

Working with parents and other caregivers to enhance early childhood development, whether pursued separately or in conjunction with existing centre- or community-based approaches, is a potentially powerful strategy with a number of advantages:

- *Caregivers as well as children can benefit.*   Programmes to support and educate caregivers provide something of value to the caregivers as well as to the children. This value may be reflected in attitudes or actions that improve the physical well-being of the caregiver (for instance, greater awareness of the value of preventive health actions) as well as the child, and/or they may result in a caregiver's feeling more confident, and willing to take control of her, or his, own life as a result of feeling success and accomplishment in the caregiving task. This feeling of success is increasingly recognized as crucial to the general processes of both child development and of broader social development (Wood 1989; Engle 1986).

- *Family responsibility is reinforced.*   In most societies, the family maintains the primary responsibility for raising children. Programmes of child care and development should build upon, not undermine, family responsibility (except in the most extreme circumstances). If planners and programmers place their emphasis exclusively on attention to children in child-care and child development centres, responsibility can shift away from the family, to these institutions (much as has happened with later education), sometimes with negative results.

- *Existing service programmes are better utilized.*   Even when children spend part of their time outside the family at a child-care centre, the principal force for socialization continues to be the home. There, parents and other caregivers can provide, or fail to provide, the immediate intellectual, social, and emotional interaction and support needed for child development. What happens in the home can support or contradict what occurs outside in service programmes, adding to their effectiveness or rendering them ineffective.

- *Empowering parents helps to sustain improvements over the long term.*   Permanent improvement in the state of development of young children will require changes in the knowledge, attitudes, and child-rearing practices of the primary caregivers. These changes will not result from temporary programmes providing only direct services to children. On the contrary, providing children's services tends to re-inforce in primary caregivers a passive, rehabilitative approach rather than an active, preventive one. Parenting education offers a potentially effective way to sustain children's gains in early development, even if a particular programme or child-care centre disappears.

- *An integrated approach is fostered.*   Bringing together the diverse components of health, nutrition and psychosocial development can be done efficiently and effectively in parent education programmes – more easily than integrating a set of vertically organized services.

– *Broad coverage can be achieved at low cost.*   Some forms of parenting education lend themselves to broad coverage at relatively low cost, particularly in comparison with the building and maintaining of centres. Indeed, parenting education for early childhood development is the most feasible low-cost approach to programming on a large scale.

Several clarifications or cautions should be added:

– *To be most effective, parent education should be timely.*   There are 'touchpoints' (Brazleton 1982) when parents and other caregivers are particularly receptive to knowing about the child and acting on their knowledge. The period of pregnancy and the time of birth are two such points. Important events in the early life of a child, defined by developmental advances or established by cultural tradition, also provide particularly receptive moments for increasing caregiver awareness. Education at these moments is more likely to energize caregivers, provide a feeling of success and make a difference in a child's development than education at less receptive times.

– *Education should consider what people need and know.*   Too often parenting education is based on fixed and preconceived messages that do not incorporate the wisdom of traditional practices, even though doing so would increase effectiveness. It is important to recognize that many parents, even in so-called disadvantaged environments, are competent and effective caregivers. Their own competence, early socialization, and access to common wisdom provide a basis for child care and development that is well adapted to the needs of the particular situation. Moreover, the demands of childrearing are often shared by grandparents or other members of an extended family, whose help and valuable insights demonstrate strengths inherent in traditional culture.

Taking seriously the idea that a rich store of parental competence, knowledge, and experience exists in any community means that parenting education cannot be viewed simply as a process in which outside 'experts' transmit predetermined messages to caregivers who are assumed to lack knowledge. (Indeed, competent caregivers may be the best 'teachers'.) Rather, parenting education, to be effective, must identify and support common wisdom and local practices that foster a child's healthy growth and development, even while introducing new ideas.

– *More than information is needed.*   And more is needed than information that is timely, culturally appropriate, and presented so that it can be easily understood. Although many programmes have successfully transmitted knowledge about early childhood development, it is apparent that behavioural change requires something more. Programmes must provide (or build upon existing) interpersonal contacts and organizational structures that help to interpret information, and that reinforce and sustain changes in attitudes and behaviours (Rivera 1987; Manoff 1984). The section on 'educational communication' will pick up this theme.

–   *Support for caregivers is at least as important as education or information.*   The support that comes from interpersonal communication and groups, mentioned above, is one kind of support. But the idea of support for caregivers goes beyond social and psychological support to the sharing of household tasks, including caregiving. Programmes that help to involve fathers more in caregiving and household tasks are strengthening the support system.

–   *Parenting education should be viewed as one among several complementary strategies.*   Because it is possible to reach a relatively large number of people through existing communication channels at a relatively low cost, there is a tendency to look to parental education as a panacea. However, parents can seldom do everything needed for care and development on their own. They need personal support at critical times (from their social networks and from communities) and they need access to services as well. Long-term change requires changes in the larger environment as well as in the micro-environment of the family.

Variations on the theme

Just as there are many variants of the centre-based service model providing direct attention to children, there are many variants of an approach providing caregiver education and support. Education can occur in the home or outside. It can occur on an individual basis or in groups. It may be realized through face-to-face interaction or through long-distance techniques, using the media. It may be didactic or based principally on demonstration, observation, and imitation. Programmes will vary also in terms of their goals, the underlying theory guiding developmental activities, the contents and materials used, the participants, the training and background of the communicators, and the frequency of the contacts or messages.

We will provide examples of programmes representing four very different ways to support and educate parents and other caregivers. These are:

1 By visiting homes
2 Within programmes of adult education and literacy
3 Through the use of communications media, with open audiences
4 Through child-to-child or youth programmes

Home visiting

Home visiting provides a flexible approach to educating caregivers that reinforces learning through periodic visits, allows adjustments to specific circumstances, permits demonstration and observation followed by practice and immediate feedback, promotes private, free discussion that might not be possible in a group setting, and deals with the child in context rather than as an abstract entity. These features make it a potentially very effective form of parental support and education.

During visits to the home, some attention to the child may be given directly by the visitors, but, in contrast with centre-based programmes, the attention is brief and more by way of example so that caregivers will learn than as a substitute form of attention. The emphasis of a home visiting approach is on the parent or caregiver rather than the child.

When compared with centre-based alternatives, the cost of home visiting programmes may be relatively low. However, when compared with other forms of parenting education, home visiting can be expensive and/or time- and labour-intensive, making it difficult to extend coverage on a large scale, given scarce resources. If home visiting is more effective than other parental education programme approaches, because of the individualized attention, the extra investment may be justified. Moreover, costs will vary significantly depending, for instance, on whether or not an established system of home visiting already exists (agricultural extension or health, for instance), into which additional components can be incorporated. Expense depends also on the number of families for which a visitor is responsible, the frequency and duration of the visits, the degree of concentration or dispersion of participants, the qualifications (hence the pay level) of the visitor, and the kind of supervisory structure established. Selective attention to families that are particularly needy can also reduce costs.

Because communication during home visits is direct, the success of this approach depends heavily on the personality of the visitor. There is a need to avoid the image of a visitor temporarily substituting for a parent who, rather, must be viewed as the expert in her own home. Visitors should be prepared for situations in which husbands object to 'intrusion' into the home or where grandparents or mothers-in-law have a main say in upbringing, so as not to come into conflict with them.

Experiences with home visiting in many settings suggests that the approach works best if:

- it is combined with periodic group meetings;
- it involves all family members, not just mothers;
- visits focus on concrete problems and actions (not vague or abstract points);
- solutions are worked out jointly and in response to particular situations, not beforehand and by 'formula'.

Experience also demonstrates that paraprofessionals can be very effective in the role of a home visitor.

An Israeli example[2]

The Home Instruction Programme for Preschool Youngsters (HIPPY) was designed to help young children become more responsible, responsive, and successful school pupils and to promote awareness by mothers of their own strengths and potential as home educators (Lombard 1981). Initiated in 1969 as a research project, HIPPY was aimed at children from ages three to six years from educationally disadvantaged sectors of Israeli society. Behind the experiment was the idea that a programme could be built around the power of selection and training of paraprofessionals as home visitors. The programme has spread within Israel and has been adapted for use in India, Chile and Turkey (for the Turkish example, see Kağitçibaşi *et al.* 1987).

The HIPPY programme involves visits to homes every other week and a commitment from mothers to allot a certain period of time each day with their child for working through a packet of activities. The packet concentrates on language and discrimination skills and on problem solving. Simple story-books, and worksheets suggesting games and other activities, each lasting from five to ten minutes, are included in the packet. Home visits rely on role-playing to instruct the mother in the use of the material; the mother and the visitor take turns playing mother and child. If the mother is illiterate or for some other reason cannot cope with the material unaided, an older sibling may assume the teaching role in the mother's presence.

In addition, each mother attends a bi-weekly meeting with her aide and with 10 to 15 other mothers in the aide's group. Together they review the use of materials, discuss problems, share information and offer suggestions for solutions that have been found to work from each mothers' experience. Activities are also carried out related to the women's roles as women.

Each participating family pays a nominal fee amounting to about 10 per cent of the average cost of the programme per family. The rest of the cost is subsidized by The Hebrew University and the Ministry of Education and Culture. Materials are all relatively inexpensive and could be made if funds are limited. The method has more recently been applied to home instruction for young mothers with their first-born babies, ages one to three, adopting a broader approach to child development than the cognitive emphasis that characterized the original HIPPY programme.

A Mexican example

In 1982, a national programme of non-formal education of parents and community members was launched by the Secretary of Public Education

(SEP). As originally conceived, a system of successive training would occur in which (1) coordinators contracted by the SEP and each responsible for two states worked together with representatives in their states to (2) train individuals responsible for a particular sector within the state, each of whom, in turn, would be responsible for (3) training and supervising activities of 16 community-level promoters elected by community committees. Promoters were (4) to provide an intensive training course (30 hours over 15 days) to a group of approximately 30 parents. Following the intensive course, the promoter's task was to provide continuing advice and training through periodic home visits to the participating families, and through weekly meetings. In addition, there was a hope that (5) the initially trained parents would work with neighbours so that, by training one parent, the programme would reach approximately five children aged under six. Promoters are helped in meetings and in their home visits by a set of materials that includes a handsomely illustrated Parent's Guide, focusing on cognitive and psychomotor development.

Although this programme has had some successes and has been carried out at a very low per child per year cost, it has encountered difficulties as well, from which lessons can be learned. In the long chain of training it is difficult to retain quality. The need for greater supervision and motivation is present. In some locations, home visiting was not well received because husbands were concerned about visits made by male promoters. The original idea that parents should be trained in groups and have weekly meetings did not work in places where there was no tradition of community meetings. Where that was the case, the home visiting part of the programme took on greater importance. In addition, parental involvement with neighbours' children occurred infrequently. The estimate has been revised so that parents are expected to provide information affecting only two children, in all probability their own.

Adult education: group approaches

There are many examples of group approaches to parenting education. Most of these have evolved as a component added on to an existing health, nutrition, or other social service programme. Some, however, have begun as independent parenting education programmes covering a broad range of topics. Some have even focused on special groups of caregivers other than parents, such as adolescents (Trinidad: Pantin 1984) or elderly people (Jamaica: York 1985).

Many adult education programmes already exist, functioning at a national level with broad coverage and involvement. These programmes vary widely in terms of their focus on literacy, second-chance schooling (at both primary and secondary school levels), health or nutrition information, or provision of technical skills. Each of these programmes provides a potential opportunity for incorporating information about early childhood care and development, and at relatively little extra cost. The main costs lie in the development of educational and training materials.

In addition to the potential coverage and cost advantages associated with the possibility of incorporating child-care and development material into ongoing adult education programmes, this programme option can draw on the power of a group to aid understanding through discussion, to provide additional examples, and to apply a kind of pressure to act on what has been learned. Many adult education programmes do not take full advantage of the potential of a group; they tend to be lectures in which information is told to people rather than processes of discovering and constructing new knowledge in a group.

The Indonesian example, revisited

The Indonesian project described as the lead-in to this chapter has many antecedents. Over a period of approximately 15 years, a network of community-based programmes has grown, beginning with population and health goals, then extending to nutrition, and more recently including the mental and social development of children. In 1982, in conjunction with periodic weighing of young children and the distribution of food, the Bina Keuarga and Galita (BKG) project (Getting It Together ... 1984), initiated by the Associate Ministry for the Role of Women, began working to enhance the knowledge, awareness, and skills of mothers and other members of the family, thereby enabling them to provide an appropriate developmental environment for their children under age five.

Field workers – women from the community being served – were provided with training in child development and methods for working with adults. Usually, these women were chosen because they are 'positive deviants', that is, they have been successful in promoting the development of their own children in spite of adverse circumstances that put the children 'at risk'. These community workers organized workshops at the nutrition centres where mothers would participate in group discussions, share experiences, set easy activities that they can do with their children at home, and make toys. In addition, a toy library provided mothers with toys to take home and use in between workshops. This effort is now being comple-mented by the home visiting programme described at the outset (Satoto and Colletta 1989).

A Chinese example

A parental education initiative in the People's Republic places new emphasis on the family as an agency of socialization and on the skills of parenting (Chinese Parents ... 1987). 'Parent schools' (200,000, by one

1989 estimate) have grown up rapidly, at least in part because of concerns about how to deal with children in the one-child family. Most of the parent schools are attached to kindergartens, primary or middle schools or hospitals. In addition, neighbourhood committees provide programmes for newlyweds or potential parents.

Existing service institutions collaborate in organizing the parenting programmes, in part as a way of strengthening their own relationship with the parents. However, they are helped in their task by the All-China Women's Federation (ACWF), which takes a lead in mobilizing communities to establish the parent programmes. Specialists or staff from the local institutions provide the lectures in a curriculum which usually consists of between four and six classes spread over a term. Topics treated are determined by the findings of intersectorial groups brought together by the ACWF to examine existing research, identify local resources, and define needs of parents and children. Thus, each curriculum is different, based on a local determination of needs. General materials are provided by the ACWF in support of these localized initiatives. In some cases, parent libraries have been set up in a special room within the primary school where parents can come to read and study during the time between meetings. Participants are given a parenting education certificate if they have participated in all or most of the meetings.

A Colombian experiment

In a marginal area of Bogotá, a parenting education programme was set up as an alternative to home visiting, under the explicit assumption that visiting in the home would undermine a mother's position and confidence within her own home (FEPEC 1979). This experiment recognized the mother as an 'expert' with respect to her own child, and avoided bringing other 'experts' into the home. In the parenting project, mothers (or principal caregivers) met once a week in a community centre where they discussed common problems and received information about health, nutrition, and psychosocial development.

An innovative feature of this project was creation of a baby book containing messages *from* the baby *to* the mother about developmental accomplishments and about the needs, at particular times, for health checkups, immunizations, etc. These highly personalized books, covering the first two years of a child's life, provided an individual record for the child at the same time that it educated the caregivers and served as a basis for discussion at meetings. Although this particular model was not picked up and used widely within Colombia, the idea of a booklet providing a record for the young child and containing messages for caregivers has spread both within and outside the country.

A Jamaican example

In Browns Hall, a rural Jamaican community, an experiment in parenting education was undertaken by the Regional Pre-School Child Development Centre of the University of the West Indies. The experiment:

> grew out of ... a commitment to credit the strengths in parenting of the rural women with whom we worked. Observed parent education approaches – however well-intentioned – often appeared to overlook or disregard these strengths; to approach parents as passive receivers of new information and advice. In the Browns Hall group experience, the primary format was women sharing their own ideas, strengths, mistakes, opinions, advice about raising their children and grandchildren as well as their experiences with their own parents. They agreed at the outset to the publishing of a booklet on parenting as a goal – a goal they perceived as helping their children, grandchildren and others when they become parents. They do not always 'practise what they preach'.
>
> (Brown, 1984)

Using the mass media and alternative forms of communication with open audiences

Mass media approaches to educating parents and other caregivers include the use of print, radio, and television. Alternative forms of communication include use of such devices as community blackboards, travelling theatrical groups, and travelling salesmen or 'pitchmen' to deliver information.

Although the effectiveness of print is limited where illiteracy is high, pictures and cartoons can be used effectively to communicate messages. Photo novels have proven also to be effective means of reaching marginally literate populations. Access to television is increasing rapidly. In poor urban areas of many cities, coverage is now very high, and satellites have brought television to large numbers in the rural areas of some Third World countries, making it a potentially important medium for public education. At present, television is still biased towards reaching the economically and socially favoured sectors. Radio continues to be an effective means of adult education in many locations.

While there is no naturally preferred communication channel, research studies and programme evaluations have identified characteristics of 'messages' that seem to underlie successful communication efforts. For example, the communications literature suggests that a mass media approach will more effectively transmit knowledge if the messages are:

- directed towards a specific audience;
- sensitive to the abilities, belief structures, and value systems of the intended audience;

- perceived to be of high priority;
- presented in a format that avoids lecturing, incorporates messages into dramatic stories and into events with everyday significance, and uses popular language.

A Venezuelan example

One of the most noted examples in recent years of the use of mass media for family education comes from Venezuela. *Proyecto Familia,* begun in 1980, was intended to promote the intellectual development of children from birth to six years of age by providing informal education to mothers, both through direct contact and through the mass media. In urban Venezuela, television is said to reach 96 per cent of the population; in the most rural areas, radio reaches more than 80 per cent. To take advantage of this coverage and the existing communications infrastructure, *Proyecto Familia* produced an impressive number of television and radio pro- grammes and spots as well as slide presentations and films.

This creative effort was put into effect with strong political backing and produced some excellent materials, but an evaluation in 1984 concluded that, overall, the effort constituted 'a promise yet to be fulfilled' (UNICEF 1985). Fulfilment was limited in part by the fact that the mass media were not linked to a system of interpersonal contacts. In urban areas, television viewers were able to identify the name *Proyecto Familia* but there was no evidence that the approach had changed practices. After an initial run, it became difficult to convince commercial television stations that the messages should continue to be shown. In rural areas, there seemed to be somewhat better success. Radio messages were better accepted by local stations in search of programme material and were broadcast more often. The messages were also partially linked to a system of interpersonal communication involving both rural extension workers and health personnel in primary health care centres.

Other examples

- In Chile, a book dealing with *Early Stimulation* became a best-seller (Bralic *et al.* 1978).
- In India and Mexico, soap operas have been created with the plot built around social messages.
- In India, Indonesia, and Bolivia, puppet theatres have been used to educate parents (CHETNA 1987; UNICEF 1984, 1985).
- In Mexico cartoonists have volunteered their talents for comic strips or posters providing basic information about the early development of children (personal communication, Maria Eugenia Linares 1988).

The caution offered at the beginning of this section that 'more than information is needed' is particularly applicable to this programming option. The use of the mass media has the potential for reaching a large number of people at relatively low cost. But the simple transmission of messages through the media may not be the most effective way to support and educate parents. Receiving and even 'understanding' messages to the point of repeating them back to an evaluator does not mean the information is internalized or will be acted upon; changes in attitudes and practices require a form of education that reinforces open, impersonal messages with interpersonal forms of communication. We shall return to this observation as we discuss the complementary programme strategies of promoting community development and of advocacy.

Child-to-child

In most parts of the world, the care of younger children by older siblings is part of a time-honoured and traditional system for helping to meet childcare needs. Where such care occurs naturally, the practice can be reinforced and improved by teaching the young caregivers about the need for vaccinations, the use of oral rehydration techniques, and by encouraging talking, cuddling, playing, and proper feeding practices.

Teaching these sibling caregivers about health, nutrition, and other actions to improve development is a potentially effective approach for several reasons in addition to the possible impact it might have through immediate application. First, these caregivers will soon be parents themselves and the parental education will help to prepare them for that time. Second, older children can provide information about new practices to peers, parents, and other community members. Third, in conjunction with their education, they can carry out direct actions in the community, identifying health problems or organizing to clean up the environment, or setting up a playground.

For all these reasons, a programme approach, labelled the 'child-to-child' approach, has been developed focusing on health and developmental education for older children, usually in the upper years of primary school. Child-to-child programmes have spread rapidly since the idea was articulated in the late 1970s and now exist in at least 48 countries (Somerset 1988). For the most part, these are found in primary schools, although child-to-child programmes are also affiliated with health centres, nutrition programmes, social service programmes, the Scouts and other youth organizations, several programmes dealing with children in difficult circumstances (refugees, street children), and programmes for the disabled.

The content stressed in child-to-child programmes differs from place to place but generally encompasses some combination of health care, nutrition, accident prevention and mental and social development, with occasional attention also to sanitation and problems of disability. Emphasis is usually placed on an active and participatory form of learning and teaching. Activities and materials are often developed locally and include stories, songs, skits, puppetry, and posters. In many places this process has been inspired and guided by the London-based child-to-child programme affiliated with the Institute for Education of the University of London.[3]

A Jamaican example

This experimental project to teach primary school children basic health and developmental concepts was begun in Jamaica in 1979 by the Tropical Metabolism Research Unit of the West Indies (Knight and Grantham-McGregor 1985). The project aimed at improving the knowledge and practices of the participating children and those of their parents or guardians as well. A rural area was chosen for the project in which poverty was widespread, family patterns were unstable, housing standards were poor, health services were minimal and illiteracy was high.

School teachers were trained and a space was made in the regular curriculum of children in grades 3, 5, and 7 for activities related to immunization and disease, dental care, diet, toy-making and how to play with younger children. An action-oriented approach to teaching and learning led to role-play, group discussions, songs, and skits. About 30 hours over the course of the year were devoted to such activities, with important effects on the knowledge and actions of the primary school children. Effects were also found on the knowledge of parents or guardians and on the teachers.

This small-scale, relatively low-cost experiment was extended to an entire district and has subsequently been integrated into the primary school curriculum for the country.

An example from Botswana

In the child-to-child programme in Botswana older children ('little teachers') from the first three standards of primary school help prepare younger children ('preschoolers') for school entry while, in turn, enhancing their own cognitive and affective development. Beginning in 1979 with two schools, the programme has spread to 28 schools reaching approximately 5,000 children. To guide the little teachers, lesson booklets focusing on four major themes were developed dealing with feelings, health, the village and preparing for school (Somerset 1988).

Originally, the child-to-child activities took place outside the school, with little teachers visiting homes of their preschoolers. Now, the preschoolers also visit the schools periodically, making supervision by the school teacher easier. After in-school lessons, the pair continues to work at

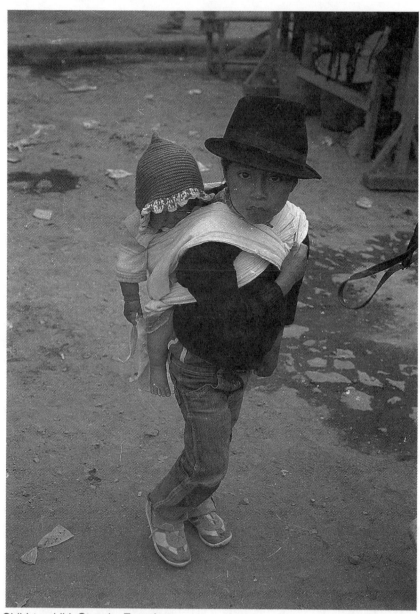

Child-to-child, Otavalo, Ecuador

home. At the insistence of parents, considerable time is devoted to learning letters and numbers and simple songs, much as might occur in a formal and cognitively oriented preschool.

An Indian example: the Malvani Project

In 1978, an ambitious project was started by doctors and paramedical workers responsible for primary health care in a low-income area on the outskirts of Bombay (Somerset 1988). Their objective was to change the awareness of the community regarding preventive health care and community hygiene. One way of accomplishing this objective was to train primary school children as 'communicators', equipping them with the skills and knowledge to affect changes in their own as well as the community's health. The 600 children trained in this initial phase of the project identified and brought to the centre 1,330 individuals with scabies, vitamin deficiency and tuberculosis. They also worked to introduce in the community the idea of oral rehydration.

In recent years, the project moved from the health centre to the school in order to reach more children. Staff members from the community health clinic visit the schools twice a week to instruct students with respect to such health topics as immunization, vitamin B complex, anaemia, tuberculosis, malaria, and leprosy. The activities include outings, plays, public performances and community surveys. These children have been instrumental in identifying anaemic individuals and in increasing immunization rates in the community.

From these diverse examples of support and education of caregivers, we turn now to a third complementary approach to early childhood care and development: promoting community development. In so doing, we take an additional step back from the child, focusing now on that level of the environment with which the child interacts that is represented by the community in which the child grows and develops.

PROMOTING COMMUNITY DEVELOPMENT

In the long run, general improvements in child survival, growth and development will depend on improvements not only in the home but also in the community environment that protects, nourishes, socializes and challenges the young child. A comprehensive programme of early childhood development must, therefore, include attention to community conditions.

Variations on the theme

'Community development' means different things to different people, varying both in terms of goals to be reached and of processes for reaching them. For many people, community development, much like national development, is a matter of improving the material conditions of life, including the level of income, health, food, shelter, and sanitation. In this view, it makes little difference whether the improvements occur as a result of a self-help initiative proposed and carried out by the community itself, or because an organization outside the community decided that community improvements were necessary and went about the task of building a road, installing a water system, immunizing, etc.

But community development can also refer to changes in the knowledge and organizational base that allow communities (and the individuals that comprise them) greater decision-making power and control over their own lives. In this view, the process by which community development occurs is as important as the specific goals of development. As part of development itself and as a means favouring development, the process must include participation by community members at all stages, including initial decisions about goals and actions to be taken.

In communities where there is a strong tradition of mutual help and solidarity, community development along this dimension is already well advanced. In such cases, there are two challenges as the community seeks material improvements and as it relates to the broader society in that process: one for the community itself, and one for those who would help the process along from outside. The challenge for the community is to open itself to technical advice and support from outside without giving up its control over decisions and its solidarity. For extension agents and doctors and other 'promoters' arriving from outside, the challenge is to recognize, respect, draw upon and strengthen (or maintain) the existing level of social and organizational community development rather than distorting it.

But most communities do not have a strong self-help tradition; nor are they helpless; they fall somewhere between a close-knit, well-organized communal group able to take decisions, mobilize resources, and negotiate successfully with the larger society, and a fragmented, disorganized community incapable of action on its own and ready to fall prey to outsiders. In these communities, the challenge is to mobilize for action in such a way that organization and solidarity and initiative will increase; in other words, so that the community will be 'empowered' to continue its own development.

If we were able to do a tabulation, we would probably find that most programmes falling under a community development label take as their principal goal improving the material conditions of life. We would probably find also that most efforts to mobilize for action follow a process in which the mobilizers or developers arrive with a ready-made solution to problems that may or may not be important to the community. Communities are sold the idea and donations of time and labour are sought from members to make the programmes go. But the real moving force may be a technician from a ministry of rural development or an extension agency or a health ministry or another organization anxious to involve the community in building a drainage ditch or a health post. In the process, little attention is given to drawing upon and strengthening the knowledge and organizational base of the community.

Potential advantages

A community development approach favours continuity and sustainability of programmes. The kind of participatory community development we have sketched above helps to provide the continuing organizational and environmental conditions that individual parents and families need in rearing their children. By strengthening both the material conditions of a community and the capacity for self-help, community development reduces dependence of a community on outside resources. At the same time, it increases the ability of the community to negotiate with the larger society, moderating the possible effects of periodic political and economic changes.

Child-care and development programmes within a community development context help communities in general, not just children. The same conditions that affect the survival, growth, and development of children affect the well-being of adult members of a community. Moreover, community-based discussions of early childhood can provide an excellent stimulus to broader community development for several reasons:

- Children are a kind of non-political rallying point. Doing something to benefit the children of a community may be easier, initially, than taking on such community development issues as land tenure or jobs, for instance.
- Child development, taking a holistic view, allows discussion and action in several areas, all directed to a similar cause. One need not separate out nutrition from health from stimulation and education.
- Most parents have a strong vested interest in the future of their children. They want them to succeed; that means more than surviving and being healthier; it also means being more intelligent. Most parents are motivated and willing to make some sacrifices to carry out activities that are directed to that end.
- Early childhood development sometimes provides a way for women to become involved in community affairs that would not otherwise be open to them. While recognizing that this may reinforce traditional, 'reproductive' roles of women, it also opens the door to new roles and to broadened community leadership.
- Through successes with the children, family and community members build confidence in their abilities to take on other problems.

But the real beauty of both the community and parental approaches is that adults also benefit in the process.

A cautionary note

Early childhood development should not be treated simply as a 'residual'. Within a community development approach that includes actions to enhance early childhood development, there is a tendency to think that changing conditions by, for instance, building a health post and establishing a women's income-generating programme will automatically take care of early childhood development. This is a partial truth. Obviously, modifying conditions that have put children at risk (even those modifications imposed from outside), will have an effect on the early development of a child. In addition, because child development is an integral process, it is likely that physical, mental, social, and emotional dimensions of development will all be affected to some degree. But a caution is in order.

Experience strongly suggests that *unless specific attention is given to the development of a child's abilities to think and reason and speak, to relate to others, and to feel, these developmental dimensions will be forgotten or slighted.* The broader, holistic view of child development requires that communities attend to changes that respond to a child's needs for affection, interaction and stimulation, security provided through consistency and predictability, and play allowing exploration and discovery. In brief, a community development approach to early childhood development should include these considerations as part of the developmental dialogue and as part of the emerging agenda for action. At the same time, attention to this dimension does not deserve to be imposed any more than others.

Examples

In the examples that follow, we shall not include examples of the multitude of experiences with programmes of general community development directed towards changing only the material conditions of communities. We shall focus, rather, on initiatives that have been taken by communities as part of an existing self-help approach or that have helped to build local participation and organization, not only as a means to other ends, but as an end in itself. And we will select examples in which child care and/or a stimulation or education component of child development has been included explicitly as part of a community development programme.

There are least three different ways of fostering community development and early childhood development at the same time:
1 Building on already existing local initiatives.
2 Promoting a process of participatory diagnosis.
3 Using the communications media to support both child and community development.

Building on existing organization and community initiative

An example from Zimbabwe

The National Early Childhood Education and Care programme of Zimbabwe, although begun by the Ministry of Education and Culture in 1980, became the responsibility of the Ministry of Community, Cooperative Development and Women's Affairs. The administrative location within a ministry charged with community development was logical because the original programme was built up around local initiatives; many rural communities had started some form of early childhood care and education activity on their own. These self-help community projects gathered children under trees, in huts, or wherever a space was available.

> A typical programme consists of upwards of 85 children, with only one or two mothers (generally untrained), caring for the children. Parents have little or no resources to pay for the programme; many use the bartering system to support their child's participation. What this means is that most teachers receive little or no pay for their work.
>
> The ECCE programmes are administered by Parent Committees who are responsible for hiring the teachers, establishing school feeding, and overall administration. The equipment that is available has been fashioned by parents, taking advantage of materials found in the area. In general, equipment, furniture, salaries of teachers and helpers are provided by parent and community donations.
>
> (Evans 1985)

With government involvement and some help from international funding, the programme has reached into more than 4,000 rural communities. A multisectorial community development effort has grown around the centres, involving health, sanitation, sports and recreation, and others. Community development projects include literacy, income generation activities, small-scale food production in community gardens (which provide food supplements), community education and sanitation programmes (for instance, the building of latrines at preschool sites by youth brigades). Preschools are used for early detection of disabilities, growth monitoring, and immunization.

Slowly the programme is being formalized as it is upgraded and spread. In a recent development, a very modest salary was introduced for the caregivers. A curriculum handbook is now available in four languages as is a handbook on how to make toys. Control was passed back to the Ministry of Education and Culture in 1988, perhaps signalling another step in formalizing the programme. (This, however, places control within one sector and it remains to be seen whether a broader 'integrated' approach can be maintained.) Yet the community continues to be involved and the

Zimbabwe programme, more than most others, can claim that it is community-based.

An example from Thailand

In selected communities in the north-east of Thailand, a programme has been operating for about ten years in which an early childhood development centre is linked to a system of local loans for small income-earning projects. In the participating communities, community centres for child care and education had been set up as community projects, but not all children within the age group attended because a modest fee was charged that some could not afford. An international funding organization, working through the Thai government and in communities selected as the most needy, approached communities with a proposition to pool funds so that all children could attend.

At the same time, a loan fund was established with two purposes in mind: to help communities economically (in projects in which they chose to invest rather than in imported ideas for income earning) and to seek a sound financial basis for keeping the early childhood programme open to all community children. A community committee made decisions about the loan fund and members were helped by the cooperating agency to administer the community fund that was set up to receive the money paid back by borrowers. Over a period of approximately seven years, the community fund grew to an appreciable size so that the proceeds from administration of the fund could be used in the future to maintain the early care and education programme. At that point, the international institution then moved on to another community. As of 1987, more than 100 communities had 'graduated' from the programme, strengthened in the process (personal field notes, visit to Christian's Children's Fund, Bangkok, April 1987).

Other examples

- Kenya, with its *harambee* movement, and Tanzania, in connection with *ujamaa* villages, have evolved early childhood programmes that are community-based efforts and part of broader development efforts. As in Zimbabwe, many of the child-care and education centres began as community self-help initiatives, run by parents, with equipment and locales provided by the community.
- The Peruvian example of a non-formal centre-based programme described earlier was, in its extension from the original site in Puno to several other states, titled 'preschool as a catalyst for community development'. In conjunction with the spread of the PRONOEIs, income-generating projects, nutrition supplementation, and water

projects were set up in some areas. The system of parental committees and the employment of a local teacher also give this initiative many of the appearances of a community-based effort (Myers *et al.* 1985).

– In Burkina Faso, preschools are being used to mobilize communities to action in programmes of water, sanitation and other basic services (Kabre and Beyeler-von Burg 1987).

Promoting a process of participatory diagnosis

A truly participatory approach to community development (and to programming for early childhood development within that framework) requires participation at all stages of a process, beginning with the definition of the problem. This is rarely done. And the stage most likely to get left out is the diagnostic, problem-definition stage.

When community members are involved in a diagnosis of the problem, there is a strong tendency for their participation to be restricted to collecting information that is then given to technicians who return to their bureaucratic cubicles to work out solutions. A more just and mobilizing process requires a different kind of relationship and participation. It requires a dialogue involving community members – with their knowledge based on experience and on an internal diagnosis – and 'outsiders' with their scientifically derived knowledge and with access to additional resources. Mounting such a participatory diagnostic process, in partnership, is at once a mutual exploration, a mobilizing force, and a form of negotiation with the larger community. From that dialogue will come the definition of needs and resources, and a set of actions that are feasible within the constraints of both the community and supporting organizations.

This collaborative process reverses the usual approach in which, for instance, a health post or a child-care centre is offered to a community, without determining whether or not this represents a priority, and then used as an 'entry point' for additional actions. In most instances this is relatively harmless because low-income, marginal communities have many needs, all of which are important. And many if not most communities have learned how to take what is offered and turn it to their own purposes, sometimes subverting the original purpose of the project along the way. Such subversion should not be necessary, however, and is almost always wasteful. Moreover, and this is the most important, the imposition does not foster control by communities over decisions or resources, nor does it allow 'ownership' of a project.

More specific attention will be given to this topic in Chapter 12, at which time examples will be presented.

Communication for group action

The concept of educational communication builds upon ideas associated with 'popular education'. It also stems from a re-examination within the field of education during the 1970s directed towards improving communication by making it more participatory. This approach to education and communication emphasizes active involvement by the participants in an educational exchange (as contrasted with the passive receipt of information). It begins with particular needs of the participants, drawing upon, reinforcing, and extending their experiences and popular wisdom, rather than beginning with a set of predetermined messages created outside. The effectiveness of educational communication is judged more by the strengthening of a group process and its translation into collective action to meet needs (which can include early childhood development needs), than it is by the successful acquisition of a certain body of knowledge (Rivera 1988).

A Chilean example

The Programa Padres e Hijos (PPH) experiment in southern Chile combines long-distance education with a system of local promoters. A private centre for educational research and development, working with a local radio station, began the programme in 1979. A set of 12 topics representing local expression of needs related to development of children aged four to six provides a starting point for the programme. These topics (which included such locally identified subjects as alcoholism) were converted into radio broadcasts presented once a week at a time when families in 50 communities reached by the radio station gathered together to listen. A discussion led by a local promoter follows each broadcast. Each theme provides the focus of discussion and activity for a month. To stimulate discussion, the promoter, chosen locally, also presents pictures that depict common incidents from the people's lives, helping relate the topic to a child's development and learning. The group discusses what they can do to apply during the week what has been learned during the group session. They are provided with some materials to take home.

Over the years, the PPH programme has spread slowly, now reaching approximately 200 communities. Additional themes have been added and the programme has incorporated other components related to productive activities. The success of the PPH programme lies both in the effect it has had on the relationships among people in the community and in its impact on the children (Richards 1985). The radio broadcasts are used as ways to promote reflection by community groups on problems affecting their children and, not incidentally, themselves. The engendered interpersonal communication led to both understanding and action. Simply transmitting messages by radio could not have had the same effect, although it would have been much less expensive.

Taking a community development approach to early childhood development will require more patience, flexibility and labour-intensive activity
than many bureaucracies are willing or prepared to accommodate. It will
require also working in a decentralized fashion and (as well be set out in
Chapter 14) looking at 'scale' as the sum of many smaller programmes rather
than as the uniform extension of one programme model over a wide area.

A first step in organizing a community development approach may be to
reorient and strengthen the institutions that will be responsible for carrying
out such an approach. This leads us to our fourth complementary strategy,
'strengthening institutions'.

STRENGTHENING INSTITUTIONS

Three complementary approaches have been discussed in the preceding
sections, one involving direct attention to children, and the other two
involving improvements in the immediate environments (family and
community) that affect a child's development. But the course of child
development is influenced also by social institutions, including those
related to health, education, religion, and work. For any or all of the first
three approaches to be effective and sustained, the institutions responsible
for carrying them out will need to be strong and supportive.

Institutional strength lies in:

- capable and motivated people
- adequate facilities and materials
- available and appropriate technology
- effective organization and management.

Capable and motivated people

The most direct and important interaction of the child with the broader
institutional environment occurs through interaction with the *people* who
are part of the social institutions that touch the child's life – with the
doctors and health promoters and herbalists, with home visitors or extensionists, with preschool teachers or child-care workers, with priests or
koranic school teachers, etc. Strengthening the ability of these individuals
to promote child development must be, then, an important part of a
comprehensive strategy of early childhood development. That means
support for training and for institutions that provide training. In some
circles, the phrase most used for this dimension of a strong institution is
'human resources'.

Consistent with our holistic view of the child, we do not restrict training
for child development to training that will help preschool teachers or child-
care workers do their job better. That is certainly part of the picture, and an

important one. But training is needed also for paediatricians and midwives and others. Moreover, training for all those who work with children should reach beyond the particular field of the individual involved to promote a broad view of development. Early educators need strengthening of their ability to detect health problems and to create a healthy environment. Health personnel need strengthening of their ability to support psycho-social development as they deal with both the child and the parent. Nutritionists need to be able to support the social and developmental outcomes of feeding as well as the nutritional ones.

Training may be directed to many different kinds of people (professionals and paraprofessionals, supervisors and directors, implementors and evaluators, etc.). It may emphasize training by peers or 'experts', involve different balances of training on the job and preservice training, and vary widely in its content and in the methodology used. Different forms of training will be more appropriate for different purposes. We shall not try to detail these differences, but will stress that, when considering ways to strengthen institutions influencing early childhood development:

- there are many alternatives to long, expensive, formalistic, and academic preservice training of preschool teachers.
- the closer to the job the training can be, the better. This means that training cannot easily be divorced from supervision.
- the more active and participatory the training, the better. Students often learn more from each other than they do from a 'teacher'.
- in the same way that education of parents should begin with an understanding of parental needs and knowledge, training of individuals in social institutions should start with what people know and need to know, reinforcing existing knowledge while adding to it.
- the choice of those to be trained may be restricted in unfortunate ways if too great emphasis is placed on formal qualifications (e.g. certain school certificates).
- 'Professionals' may be as much in need of retraining as non-professionals are of training, because of the narrow and relatively academic training that certified them as professionals.

There is another dimension to strengthening the human resources of social institutions: maintaining motivation. A well-trained and capable person may not be motivated to do a good job. Motivation may come from many sources including the pure pleasure of doing a good job, service to community, the chance for recognition, interaction with others in the workplace, the possibility of moving up to a better position, the money earned on the job, or, preferably, some combination of these.

Experience suggests that in the early stages of projects and programmes it is much easier to obtain and maintain enthusiasm than in the latter stages. It is harder also to motivate individuals in a very large and bureaucratic organizational setting. Thus, as programmes – whether directed to the child, the parents, or the community – grow and age, the issue of motivation becomes greater. As motivation slips, institutions weaken. Accordingly, one important approach to strengthening institutions is to improve incentives.

Examples

- In Thailand, a concerted effort is being made to incorporate into the curriculum of doctors and of health workers a child development component focusing on the psychosocial development of the child (*Child Development Newsletter* 1988).
- In Kenya, a national programme to upgrade paraprofessionals has evolved that is decentralized and that places emphasis on in-service training (Njenga, 1989).
- In India, supervisors of a child-care programme in Gujarat have requested training in interpersonal relations and in the organization of meetings so that they will be able to work better with groups of day-care workers, with the local management committees, and with parents in group meetings. The training is looked upon not only as something that will help them in their work, but in daily life as well (personal field notes 1990).

Adequate facilities and materials

For any programme to run well, at least a minimum of materials, equipment and facilities are needed, both at the level involving interaction of the child with materials and at the level that allows a programme to function. As with training, the variation in the kinds of facilities and materials is immense, from a school in the open air as described above to the extraordinary preschool facilities for 700 children one may encounter in the People's Republic of China, complete with its own bakery. A long discussion of materials and toys would not be appropriate here, but we will make several general points and provide an example.

- A lack of facilities or materials can be seen as an opportunity rather than an obstacle to programming for early childhood care and development. Communities can and do rally to find, or construct, locations and furniture, and to create learning aides. This participation may involve something as simple as the children bringing their own small chair or bench with them to a centre each day until a way can be found to equip the centre with benches, as was done in the so-called 'bench schools' in Cartagena, Colombia.
- The process of creating toys and other learning aides can be incorpor-

ated into the training process of caregivers of all kinds – whether in formal or informal centre-based programmes or by groups of mothers. The process is participatory, helping to build group involvement, and can be a low-cost way of producing materials as well.

- In the construction of facilities and the equipping of programmes, careful attention should be given to forms that are culturally accept-able. It is difficult to rationalize constructing cement buildings with glass windows that open and close, and with metal roofs painted a garish orange, in a humid and hot climate where mud and thatch and open spaces for windows are typical and functional. Imported battery-driven toys hardly seem appropriate when there are no replacement batteries available. To some readers these examples may represent the unthinkable but, unfortunately, they are real examples and similar cases are not difficult to find.
- It is possible to create local industries to produce the equipment and materials needed for early childhood development programmes. This approach may take the form of local cooperatives generating income for village carpenters or women's groups, or can be linked to a programme of work for disabled or others against whom there is often discrimination in employment, or can be organised as a national industry.
- Facilities and equipment and materials should conform to some minimum standard, even if produced by parents. They should be safe (for example, simple blocks can be made from wood discards, but should not have slivers; paint should be lead-free, etc.). Although this proviso sounds easy, it is difficult to follow when production is not centralized, and it sometimes leads to increases in cost that are not feasible (such as the need to import lead-free paint).
- A very large number of publications exist demonstrating ways to create inexpensive but appropriate play spaces (e.g. Kishigami and Hiroko 1988) or to make toys from locally available (often throw-away) materials (e.g. Carlile 1988; UNESCO 1988).

With these points in mind, the process of strengthening institutions in support of early childhood development may be more one of strengthening the capacity of local production than of donating or purchasing materials or constructing buildings.

An Indian example

An example that illustrates how materials can be created for early child-hood programmes at low cost and as part of a training programme comes from Karnataka State in India. There, a 'cognitive kit' of 25 items has been developed (Swaminathan 1986). Each item of the kit is related to a concept, or set of concepts, that an early childhood programme can help to evolve. Each item can be made from inexpensive materials by an early education teacher. The 25 items, which are directed towards health and nutrition as well as psychosocial concepts, are presented in Table 7.1.

Available and appropriate technology

Technology refers to both the materials and methods employed and to how they are organized. Just as there are significant choices to be made in health between emphasis on a hospital system employing certified doctors and nurses using sophisticated diagnostic methods and materials, and a primary

Table 7.1 A cognitive kit

In the Cognitively Oriented Programme for Preschool Children, run by Indira Swaminathan in Bangalore, India, training for grassroots workers includes construction and practice in the use of a kit of low-cost, easy-to-prepare materials. Included in the kit are the following:

- Rag dolls, male and female (to enhance self-concept and instil hygiene concepts)
- Jigsaw puzzle boards (3 varieties – environment, number, and colour)
- Books (picture books – 10 pages used as a single-page book; tracing maze shapes – 10 kinds of shapes)
- Manipulative and construction materials (rubber-band construction board)
- Puppets (glove, string, cone, and hand puppets)
- Health kit (stethoscope – made from rope and bead; thermometer and Red Cross symbol; badge)
- Musical instruments (xylophone and rhythm materials; drum made out of a mud pot)
- Toss bag (3 shapes and sizes)
- Mobiles (from waste material)
- Board games (9-piece matching board; nutrition gameboard; health gameboard)
- Card games (dominoes – 15 pieces; colour/number; position discrimination game; classification cards – 5 sets)
- Jute roller-board (with sponge piece to make designs; also usable as a puppet screen)
- Colour filters (3 colours, merging of colours)
- Spiral toy (spiral wire with bead – as science material)
- Rope (3 metres, used for dramatic and eurhythmic activities)

health care system in which paraprofessionals work in more rudimentary conditions, there are significant choices to be made in the technology of early childhood development. Large, well equipped day-care centres contrast with a neighbourhood home day-care approach. Community-based self-help programmes employing paraprofessionals and using local materials contrast with formal preschools run by 'certified' personnel. When pursuing an institution-strengthening approach, it may be necessary to make decisions about which type of technology will be emphasized in the process. Examples of different possibilities have already been given.

The Indian example presented above illustrates not only the production of materials at low cost, but also an interesting combination of technologies. The materials being used by paraprofessionals are simple; in that sense the technology is simple. But the method employed is derived from Piagetian principles that might be equally well applied by a highly trained teacher in a fancier classroom using fancier materials. The training process, then, involves introduction of a particular method, or technology, as part of the process of strengthening the institution that will apply it – in this case, the ICDS.

Institutions concerned with early childhood care and development may also need strengthening with respect to the technology of:

- measurement and evaluation (necessary for description and diagnosis, screening, monitoring children and for planning, monitoring, and evaluating programmes);
- communication and information (the use of the mass media as well as of the more traditional forms of communication);
- organization and management (see below).

Examples

In the People's Republic of China, a simple technology has been devised for use by caregivers in monitoring and teaching health habits to preschoolers. On arrival at the centre, each child is checked in four ways: by looking (does the child appear to be ill, with a runny nose or a lethargic look); by touching (is the forehead warm, for instance), by asking the parent or caregiver who brings the child; and by making a physical check (of pockets or fingernails, for instance). If a child seems to have a health problem, a colour-coded card is given that alerts the teacher and leads to a more thorough check later.

In Latin America, at least 12 countries have incorporated a set of child development indicators into the cards that are being used to monitor immunizations and child growth (Atkin 1989).

In Indonesia, a series of cartoon messages has been developed for use in the caregiver education programme (Satoto and Colletta 1989).

Organization and management

Child development programmes can be centrally controlled at a national level, supported by the district level, locally controlled at the community level, or controlled by multiple sources, including private organizations. All these levels and organizations may need strengthening in their ability to carry out effectively the particular programmes falling to them. Where responsibility is shared, ways will need to be devised to ensure, if not 'integration', at least convergence and collaboration (see Chapter 8). This may involve creating special agencies or committees to oversee implementation.

We have already stressed the need to strengthen community organization, suggesting that that goal should be an intrinsic part of programming. However, strong community organization brings with it an associated ability to initiate requests and to enter into negotiations with district and national levels in the process of planning and implementing programmes. This requires adjustments in the broader social organizations, including adjustments in the types of individuals recruited and their training. Organizations will need people who can facilitate, accompany, and respond to community initiatives rather than people who plan, inform, and impose ideas from the centre. There will need to be changes as well in information systems and flows, in accounting procedures, and other accepted forms if a bottom-up, decentralized, and participatory approach is to be followed. Helping an organization to make these shifts may be as important as helping to streamline procedures as programmes grow larger.

Other areas in which organizational strengthening may be needed include:

–   the legal bases for organizational action;
–   the ability to provide supervision. This is a particularly weak part of many large-scale efforts of programme implementation, starting from the unfortunate premise that supervision is more inspection than it is training on the job.

In brief, there are many areas in which institutional structures will need to be strengthened if they are to carry out programmes of direct attention, of caregiver education, and of child care and development embedded within broader community development schemes. A comprehensive strategy must include activities at this level.

CREATING AWARENESS AND DEMAND

Helping to shape a child's environment at all other levels (social institutions, community, family) is a set of overarching social beliefs and attitudes and values. These are embodied in different ways in politicians and policymakers, bureaucrats and community leaders, professionals and para-professionals, and caregivers of all kinds. These can be supportive of good care or, with changes of time and circumstances, can become obstacles to proper care. As new information and practices and ways of caring for children emerge, there is often a need to help people become aware of what is good about old ways (that should not be abandoned) and what is good about new ways (that should be incorporated).

Several terms that are being used to describe in different ways the process of strengthening awareness and demand are: advocacy, social marketing, social mobilization, and ethos creation. The most ambitious of these is the idea that one can actually create a new ethos − a new way of thinking about children and care and development at a broad level.

Whatever the term used, it is clear that political and social commitment are crucial elements in creating and sustaining child-care and development services and activities. Often support must be built among politicians and policymakers who set guidelines, make plans, and control budgets. Bureaucrats and professionals will often need to be convinced to try new ways and to look beyond time-worn and expensive models to alternative approaches. Without a commitment from these groups, most programmes can easily be undermined.

At least as important as the fairly well defined groups to whom advocacy efforts might be directed is the social awareness and involvement of the population at large. If there is little understanding of new ideas and no demand for services that build on these ideas, programmes will fail or continue to limp along. As we have suggested in the early section on the support and education of parents and other caregivers, there is a tendency to seek that understanding and commitment simply by providing information − by 'marketing' a new idea. There are many examples of the successes of a social marketing technique (Manoff 1984) in the social as well as the commercial realm. And the communication channels may range from spots on television to photo novels or comic books to the use of travelling puppet theatres or community 'blackboard newspapers'.

But, again, sustained changes in attitude and behaviour require something more than information. An incentive to apply information, and social support for the innovative process are also important. The insertion of information in an active and participatory process seems to be the most effective road to bringing about change, whether at the level of a head of state or at the community level. At the level of planners, participation in evaluations, workshops, informal meetings, or field visits is more active and potentially effective than formal presentations by experts.

In attempting to reach out beyond selected groups that help set the guidelines, make policy, and organize implementation, to the general population, a strategy of 'social mobilization' is increasingly called upon. Essentially, social mobilization means getting as many people involved in activities related to early childhood care and development as possible. That is often done by creating an event (a national vaccination day, a National Children's Day, a marathon dedicated to hunger, a sporting event or concert, etc.), then seeking the participation of organizations that have the power to mobilize. These include the schools, the churches, labour unions, entertainers, political parties, women's groups, scouts and other youth organizations, and the press.

Despite some dramatic successes, social mobilization efforts often stop short of truly mobilizing people because, when the event is over, there is a lapse into inactivity. If a deeper mobilization is to occur, the activities must become part of the consciousness and actions of the mobilized organizations. They must become part of the curriculum of the schools, of the advice given to young couples by religious advisors, of the list of merit badges for scouts, etc.

At a still deeper level, there needs to be organization for political action at local levels that will help to change the physical and social conditions contributing to the problems of child survival and development. Such social mobilization is sometimes threatening and always harder to achieve than either information dissemination or organization around a particular task or event.

Strengthening awareness and demand, then, can be approached at various levels and with many groups (political leaders; civil servants; university and professional groups; community organizations and movements; private voluntary organizations and non-governmental organizations; newspaper, television and radio reporters; promoters, teachers and extensionists; the staff of donor agencies, etc.). In addition, the range of options for organizing advocacy efforts and for communicating with the desired audiences is almost infinite, limited only by local conditions and imagination.

Examples

In Brazil, an extraordinary effort was organized in conjunction with the writing of a new constitution, not only to incorporate in the constitution specific articles dealing with the rights of children, but also to bring children's issues to the attention of the population at large. The creative strategy included such devices as arranging for children to make presentations to the national congress.

In Jamaica, a 'Children's Lobby' has been created, the purposes of which are:

– To help sensitize the Jamaican community to the needs of children.
– To support and amplify the voices that speak in the interest of the child.

- To monitor public plans, policies, and events relating to children for the purpose of keeping the wider community informed on issues that will impact on the family and the child.
- To encourage child, parental, and community input to government planning and policy implementation for children's services.
- To stimulate, discuss, collect, and disseminate research data as well as provide information to the public on new thinking and/or models to improve the quality of service to children in Jamaica.

At a regional level in Latin America, an advocacy effort has effectively mobilized the extensive network of the Roman Catholic Church to pay greater attention to the needs of young children. That activity included working with the regional officials of the church to create materials for use in orientation workshops for parish priests. (This example might have been placed under 'strengthening institutions' as well.)

The annual publication of *The State of the World's Children* represents an attempt at global advocacy, as do such activities as the Children's Summit (September 1990) and the Convention on the Rights of the Child.

The purpose of this chapter has been to set out a broad range of programming activities directed towards enhancing early childhood care and development. In order for the approach to be comprehensive, it will require complementary activities providing direct attention to children who need that attention in centres outside the home. It will require support and education of parents and other immediate caregivers. It will require work on longer-term solutions through community development activities intended to change conditions in a child's environment that help to cause problems. It will require strengthening the institutions that promote child care and development. And, finally, it will require convincing people at all levels that improved care and development is not only needed, but is possible to attain, with results that will be of benefit to the entire society.

NOTES

1   We are not including in this discussion education or training for professional or paraprofessional caregivers working in centres. Here the emphasis is on the home, the extended family, and the primary environment in which a child grows and develops (rather than the 'alternative' environment provided in child-care and development centres). Training for these alternative caregivers is considered to be part of strengthening institutions, the fourth of the complementary approaches.

2   Examples other than the two cited here can be found in Issue No. 4 of *The Coordinators' Notebook* (April 1987), from the Consultative Group on Early Childhood Care and Development, New York, UNICEF. Included are examples from Jamaica, Ireland, and the USA (both the Parent-to-Parent programme and the Portage Project which has been adapted to various Third World settings).

3   For a fuller discussion of child-to-child programmes and for additional examples, the reader is referred to Hawes 1989; Somerset 1988; and Otaala *et al.* 1988.

REFERENCES

Atkin, L. 'Early Growth and Development: A Review of Latin American Measures and Methods', Mexico: Instituto Nacional de Perinatologia, a paper prepared for the Consultative Group on Early Childhood Care and Development, April, 1989.

Brálic, S., I.M. Haeussler, M.I. Lira, H. Montenegro and S. Rodríguez. *Estimulación Temprana.* Santiago, Chile: UNICEF, 1978.

Brazleton, T. Berry. 'Early Intervention: What Does It Mean?' *Theory and Research in Behavioural Pediatrics,* Vol 1 (1982), pp. 1–34.

Brown, J. 'The Experience of Parenting: Brown's Hall'. Kingston: the Regional Pre-School Centre for Child Development, September, 1984.

Carlile, J. (ed.) *Toys for Fun: A Book of Toys for Pre-School Children.* London: Macmillan Publishers Ltd, July, 1988.

CHETNA. 'Workshop in Creative Drama and Puppetry', *CHETNA News* (April–June 1987), pp. 6–7.

'Chinese Parents Go Back to School', *People,* Vol 14, No. 4 (1987), p. 25.

d'Agostino, M. 'The Early Childhood Development Centres in Benin', *Notes, Comments . . .,* No. 181, UNESCO/UNICEF/WFP Cooperative Programmes, Paris, May, 1988.

Engle, P. 'The Intersecting Needs of Working Women and their Young Children: 1980 to 1985', a paper prepared for the Consultative Group on Early Childhood Care and Development, 1986. Mimeo.

Evans, J. 'The Utilization of Early Childhood Care and Education Programmes for Delivery of MCH/PHC Components', a paper prepared for presentation at a meeting of the World Health Organization, Paris, May 25–29, 1985.

Fundación para la Educación Permanente en Colombia (FEPEC). *Educación No-Formal y Desarrollo Infantil.* FEPEC/CEDEN, 1979.

'Getting It Together for Children', *UNICEF News,* No. 119 (1984), pp. 26–7.

Hawes, H. *Child-to-Child: Another Path to Learning.* Hamburg: UNESCO Institute of Education, 1989.

Kabre, M.B. and H. Beyeler-von Burg. *Children Lead the Way in Burkina Faso.* Ouagadougou: UNICEF and the International Movement ATD Fourth World, 1987.

Kağitçibaşi, C., D. Sunar and S. Bekman. 'Comprehensive Pre-school Education Project: Final Report', Istanbul, Turkey: Boğaziçi University. A report prepared for the International Development Research Centre, November, 1987.

Kishigami, C. and S. Hiroko. 'Design Ideas for Pre-school Centres and Play Spaces', *Notes, Comments . . .,* No. 184. Paris: UNESCO/UNICEF/WFP, September, 1988.

Knight, J. and S. Grantham-McGregor. 'Using Primary School Children to Improve Child-rearing Practices in Rural Jamaica', *Child: Care, Health and Development,* No. 11 (1985), pp. 81–90.

Lombard, A. *Success Begins at Home.* Lexington, Mass: D.C. Heath and Co., 1981.

Manoff, R. 'Social Marketing and Nutrition. A Pilot Project', *Assignment Children,* 65/68 (1984), pp. 95–113.

Manoff, R. *Social Marketing. New Imperative for Public Health.* New York: Praeger, 1985. ·

Myers, R. *et al.* 'Pre-school Education as a Catalyst for Community Development', an evaluation prepared for USAID/Lima, January 1985. Mimeo.

Njenga, A.W. 'The Pre-school Education and Care Programme: A Kenyan Experience', a paper prepared for the UNICEF Global Seminar on Early Childhood Development, Florence, International Child Development Centre, June 12–30, 1989. Nairobi, Kenya Institute of Education, June 1989. Mimeo.

Otaala, B., R. Myers, C. Landers and L. Otaala, 'Children Caring for Children: New Applications of an Old Idea', a review of programmes and approaches prepared for the Consultative Group on Early Childhood Care and Development, New York, 1988.

Pantin, G. *The Servol Village.* Ypsilanti, Mich: The High/Scope Press, 1984.

Richards, H. *The Evaluation of Cultural Action: An Evaluative Study of the Parents and Children Program (PPH).* London: Macmillan, 1985.

Rivera, J. 'Comunicación Educativa para el Desarrollo Infantil: Conceptos y Estrategias', a document prepared for UNICEF, Regional Office for Latin America, Bogotá, August 1987. Mimeo.

Satoto and N.D. Colletta. 'A Low Cost Home-Base Intervention Using a Cartoon Curriculum. The Indonesian "PANDAI Project"'. A paper presented at the International Conference on Childhood in the 21st Century, Hong Kong, July 31–August 4, 1989. Indonesia, the Medical School, UNDIP, Semarang, 1989. Mimeo.

Somerset, H.C.A. 'Child-to-Child: A Questionnaire Review and Studies of Projects in Three Countries', a paper prepared for the London University Institutes of Child Health and Education, 1988. Mimeo.

Swaminathan, I. In *The Coordinators Notebook*, No. 2 (April 1986), p. 16. New York: The Consultative Group on Early Childhood Care and Development.

'The Implementation of Child Development in Thailand', *Child Development Newsletter*, Vol 1, No. 1 (August 1988), Bangkok, Thailand.

Wood, A.W. 'Community Mobilization', a paper presented to the International Conference on Childhood in the 21st Century, Hong Kong, July 31–August 4, 1989. The Hague: the Bernard van Leer Foundation, August, 1989. Mimeo.

UNESCO. *Games and Toys in Early Childhood Education.* Digest No. 25. Paris: UNESCO/UNICEF/WFP, 1988.

UNICEF/Bolivia. Annual Report, 1984.

UNICEF/Indonesia. Annual Report, 1985.

UNICEF/New York. 'An Evaluation of Venezuela's Proyecto Familia', New York: UNICEF, the Programme Division, November, 1984. Mimeo.

UNICEF/New York. 'A Promise Yet to be Fulfilled', New York: UNICEF, 1985. Mimeo.

York, R. 'Learning about Children: A Manual for Training Elderly Citizens', Kingston, Jamaica: University of the West Indies, Regional Child Development Centre, 1985.

Part IV

Combining programme concerns

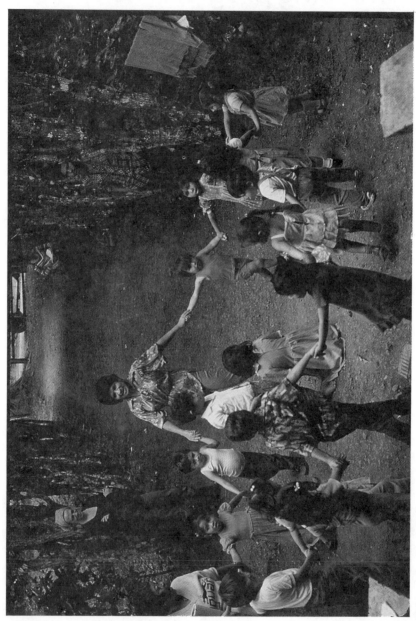

'All together', rural Nicaragua

Chapter 8

Integrated programming: an elusive goal

... a child is born without barriers. Its needs are integrated and it is we who choose to compartmentalize them into health, nutrition or education. Yet the child itself cannot isolate its hunger for food, from its hunger for affection or its hunger for knowledge. The same unity extends to the child's perception of the world. The child's mind is free of class, religion, colour or nationality barriers, unless we wish it otherwise. It is this intrinsic strength in the unity of the child, that we need to exploit, for building a better world, and a more integrated development process.

(Alva 1986)

THE RHETORIC OF INTEGRATED ATTENTION

Beginning with the 'unity of the child', or the 'whole' child whose needs are integrated, there seems to be widespread agreement that programmes to increase survival and foster normal development should be integrated. Indeed, calls for integrated attention to the young child are often made in documents of governments and international organizations. For instance:

The needs of the young child are interdependent and therefore any measures for his or her advancement must be based on a holistic approach to child development and be implemented within the framework of an integrated structure.

(Government of Sri Lanka 1986, p. iv)

UNICEF should use its multisectoral strengths to encourage multisectoral collaboration in child development in order to incorporate the education–stimulation dimension into health, nutrition and custodial care activities and vice versa; it is a question not only of child survival but of the fullest possible development, according to existing knowledge, of the genetic potential of the human being.

(UNICEF 1984, p. 31)

However, as one moves from rhetoric to the implementation of specific projects and programmes, integration can prove to be elusive. It is not always clear what an integrated approach to programming for early childhood development means, operationally, or even conceptually. At a minimum, integrated attention to the child seems to include health, nutrition, education, and psychosocial development actions together in the same programme. Sometimes the needs of both mother and child are included, sometimes not. But how these should fit together, under what circumstances, and with what kind of 'integrated' organizational strategies is not so evident.

Often, a kind of territoriality develops as programmes are implemented. Primary health care centres are located in one area, nutrition projects in another, water and sanitation programmes in yet another and none of them in the same location as child-care centres. Even when there is geographic convergence, there may be more competition than coordination among the organizations involved. Health projects often lack a psychosocial development dimension and vice versa. Women's income-generating projects fail to incorporate child care and child-care projects fail to adjust to the needs of working women.

Why is an integrated approach so difficult? What gets in the way of combined programming and action? How can one make good on the rhetoric of 'integrated childhood development'? More specifically, how can child care bring together health and nutrition and attention to psychosocial needs, in order to take advantage of the synergistic effects that can occur? How can the demands of schooling and the preparation for schooling be approached together, and holistically, overcoming the bureaucratic barriers that separate 'preschool' from 'school' and both from health and nutrition? How can programmes be organized that respond simultaneously to the overlapping, and sometimes competing, needs of children and women in an integrated way? These specific topics will be be taken up in the chapters that follow.

Forms of integration

Part of the problem associated with integration, as it is applied to programming, is semantic. The word 'integration' is accompanied by false expectations. In line with its dictionary definition, integration conjures up visions of 'combining parts into a whole'. It suggests a relationship that is interdependent and much more permanent than can be achieved by simply setting parts, or programmes, side by side. Integration implies much more than just 'working together' in a cooperative relationship. It depends on mutual acceptance and is expressed fully in unity of purpose and organization. These requirements are difficult to meet in the everyday atmosphere of specialization and competition for scarce resources that characterizes bureaucracies and, indeed, much of life.

To get behind the word, and behind the rhetoric of integrated programming, it is useful to distinguish several levels at which integration may be sought in the process of programming. These are often lumped together, creating confusion. The form and feasibility of integration at each level is different. Integration may occur:

- at the level of ideas
- in planning
- in organization and implementation
- in the content of programmes
- in the actions of caregivers, families and communities

Let us examine briefly each of these levels, or points, in the programme process.

Integration at the level of ideas

The concept or idea of the child with a set of inseparable needs provides a fairly simple starting point for an integrated approach to programming. However, the idea that a child's needs are inseparable does not translate easily or automatically into the idea that programmes should respond simultaneously to the full complement of needs, i.e. to its hunger for affection and knowledge as well as its hunger for food, as stated in the initial quotation. As needs get translated into programming, they are separated out and put into a hierarchy. The idea of the 'total' child gets lost. Moreover, the scientific underpinnings for a truly integrated view are not always known or appreciated. Chapter 9 will try to strengthen that base.

Chapters 3 and 4 illustrated how growth and development are treated differently at the level of ideas by different fields: medicine, nutrition, psychology, anthropology, education, etc. Each field brings to the topic its own definitions, terminology, and biases regarding the variables, and the relationships among them that are seen as most important. In those chapters, an attempt was made to sort out areas of overlapping interest and to identify variables and relationships that seemed to permeate discussions, even those originating from different viewpoints. However, no attempt was made to provide an 'integrated model' that combined all the parts into a unified whole. Rather, different models were seen to serve different purposes.

One way that is often used in programme formulation to try to overcome narrow, specialized, and unintegrated thinking about early childhood is to bring together individuals from different fields in a multidisciplinary team. Often, however, the result is a set of parallel and unconnected ideas and analyses. There is little or no real integration of ideas. A multidisciplinary team only achieves conceptual integration to the extent that it helps members of the team understand and internalize the concepts that each brings to the task. Real conceptual integration takes place in the heads of individuals, not in the presentation of a set of ideas placed side by side. When real integration occurs, it is reflected in changes in the language of discourse and in the terminology found in programme documents. To effect these changes is no mean feat.

The above reservations notwithstanding, it is possible to see a process of integration at work at the level of ideas. At the simplest level, that integration is present in a view of the whole child with inseparable needs. Concepts and terms from medicine are being used and accepted in education and vice versa. As seen from the material in Chapters 3 and 4, serious and effective efforts are being made to cut across fields. The language of discourse is changing slowly. The main stumbling block to integrated programming is not at the level of ideas.

Policy and planning

Policies are set in very different ways according to the kind of governmental and organizational structure that is in operation. In most cases, however, general policies are set at the central levels of governments and organizations, with more or less participation of others. A national policy for children, at a general level, that incorporates elements from many sectors, exists in some countries. The crucial ingredient for such a policy seems to be a strong feeling by someone in power that it is a good idea. And, at this level, it does not seem difficult to incorporate a holistic view of the child. The more difficult task comes further down the line with planning and implementation in an integrated form.

The planning process often begins with ideas and actions proposed by individual 'sectors' or fields. The result is a health plan, a nutrition plan, an education plan, etc. The same is true for plans which are often made by special departments, such as women's affairs, with little integration of the components that affect the young child in a synergistic way. Rarely is there a plan for children.

In normal circumstances, each sector and department is not only convinced of the central importance of what it does, but is also competing for funds. It is only logical, therefore, that the plans presented will focus rather narrowly on what each sector or department knows, is charged with doing, feels strongly about, and can do best. But if planning for early childhood care and development is to be integrated, a meaningful and just way must be found to bring these pieces together. The method most often used is to assemble an inter-sectoral group, perhaps in a planning office, which is charged with adding together these specialized plans. But this will not necessarily result in an 'integrated' plan, any more than setting ideas side by side results in the integration of those ideas. The process should, however, help to be sure that no sector is left out.

There are at least two other approaches to planning that have greater potential for resulting in an integrated plan. One is to begin with a problem area that cuts across the usual bureaucratic lines – such as 'rural development' or 'child survival and development'. Each sector or department is then asked what it can contribute to working on the problem.

Another approach to planning is to begin by defining a specific population – for instance, children, 0 to 5 years of age, living in conditions that put them 'at risk'. Once a specific group has been chosen, the needs of the population and the contribution of each sector to meeting those needs can be defined. Again, each sector or department can be asked to focus its planning on that group, increasing the possibility that some form of meaningful integration can be achieved.

Focusing on a particular population also opens up the possibility of involving that group directly in the planning process. Planning from the 'bottom up', or, better yet, in a collaborative way involved technicians as well as community groups in a constructive dialogue, each bringing its own form of knowledge to the planning process (Bosjnak, in press). It facilitates also the process of linking planning to actions that are integrated.

Although achieving an integrated plan is difficult, it is certainly possible. India, for example, has a national policy for children and, we have seen in the examples, a plan for an Integrated Child Development Service. Another example, at the state level, comes from Santa Catarina in Southern Brazil, where the governor took the lead in setting an overall plan for children called *Pro-Crianza*. In this case, each sector of the government was asked to indicate, then improve upon, its contribution to child development. These contributions, taken together, constituted a plan.

Organizational and institutional integration

Although it is difficult to achieve integration at the level of ideas and in policies and plans, the real test of an integrated approach comes in the implementation of programmes. In that process, the unitary child is usually cut up into bureaucratic pieces. The health piece corresponds to ministries of health, with medical and public health departments of universities and professional organizations looking over their shoulders. A nutrition piece is itself chopped up into bits because, as noted by Berg (1987, p. 1), 'Nutrition is not a sector ... rather, it is a condition'. Nutrition activities are found in ministries of agriculture, health, and others. Ministries of education concentrate on mental and social development, rarely, however, in direct collaboration with health, nutrition, or social welfare institutions. Moral and ethical development is set aside for the church. Child care is usually the responsibility of several institutions, each working on its own.

The problem is complicated further by distinctions in the kinds of organizations involved in the delivery of early childhood programmes. Public sector organizations differ from non-governmental organizations. Among NGOs, the range is also broad, from churches to entrepreneurial organizations. Trade unions, funding organizations and professional associations are also involved and each functions in different ways from governments and from most NGOs.

Each of the areas and kinds of organizations mentioned above has its own formal and informal networks, publications, budget allocations, reward systems, and training programmes. Moreover, most bureaucratic structures charged with carrying out programmes of health or nutrition or education are vertically organized, each with its own personnel at several levels, each with its own geographic organization, each with its internal rules and regulations. It is extremely difficult, therefore, to 'integrate' institutional structures and to find a common language and a joint *problématique* providing a solid basis for cooperation and communication.

It would be possible to dwell upon the many organizational and institutional features that make truly integrated programming and implementation so difficult. However, these are well known and frequently analysed (see, for instance, Bradley 1982). Because these barriers to institutional integration are so widespread and persistent, we prefer to start from the premise that true organizational integration will seldom occur and that most attempts to force such integration will be counterproductive. At the organizational level, then, we take the emphasis off structural integration of organizations and institutions charged with implementing programmes in different fields such as nutrition and child care or development.

In what is more than a semantic distinction, our emphasis is on 'convergence'. Convergence means seeing that various services arrive at the same place. Convergence should occur in those areas where children and their families are most at risk. This requires cooperation and agreement in the planning stage about the groups of individuals most at risk. If combined with a strategy of planning from 'bottom-up', or collaborative planning, and with the strengthening of a knowledge base and organization at the community level, converging services will be brought together by the users in an integrated way. In addition, we place much more emphasis on integration of the content to be treated in programmes and on the training of individuals within communities and in the specific institutions who will use that content. These two points – integrating content and supporting integrated actions in the community – are treated below.

At the same time that we question the feasibility of structural integration in programme implementation, it is possible to identify strategies that have helped to overcome, or that get around, organizational barriers, facilitating convergence on particular groups and fostering cooperation among institutions that will never become structurally integrated.

Content

Integrating the content of programmes seems to be more feasible than institutional and organizational integration. Major structural changes in organizations are not needed. It is possible for an organization to incorporate into its own staff individuals who will have specialized knowledge from another field. A Ministry of Education can contract a medical doctor or a nutritionist, for instance, who can easily include information about health and nutrition in a suggested curriculum for non-formal preschools. But even when this is done, the organic relationship among these components is seldom recognized and emphasized. (An example that does recognize the organic relationship comes from Benin where educational activities are built around health and nutrition themes [d'Agostino and Masse-Raimbault, 1987]).

The process of working on the integration of various themes into one set of materials can itself be integrative. If a multidisciplinary team works on creating content for a programme, the act of creation can help to integrate the team.

In the minds and actions of caregivers, families, and communities

In the last analysis, integration occurs in the minds and in the actions of the people who surround the child as he or she grows and develops. Fortunately, in most of the world, integration at this level is not a problem; most people do not separate out mental and social well-being from physical condition.

The challenge is to find ways in programmes to strengthen and build upon the integrated concept of the child that is so prevalent, and to fill in gaps in knowledge without disrupting the holistic cosmovision that most caregivers have. Thus, strengthening integrated action by caregivers requires attention to local attitudes and beliefs, as well as to the interpersonal and organizational forms that provide support for growth and development-promoting actions.

Making the link

There are a number of strategies that can help to overcome, or bypass, organizational barriers to integration. Nine are listed and discussed briefly in the following paragraphs.

1 Build political will

If political will is present and strong, it can be used to bring together disparate and uncoordinated elements into a forceful programme of integrated child care and development. Building such will requires responding to both political and technical concerns. It requires sensitivity to the particular ideological stance of those in charge. It requires convincing key advisors and, in the long run, the people who sustain the politician in office, of the value of investing in early childhood.

To help build the necessary political will where that is not present, it may be necessary to place heavy emphasis on advocacy in the early stages of building a programme. Convincing key people of the importance of integrated (or convergent) attention to young children usually is not easy. It involves finding a rationale that is politically as well as technically convincing. More than just telling, it involves showing that programmes are technically feasible, either by travelling to see experiences elsewhere or by setting up a demonstration programme at home. Supporting the technical arguments, analyses in which differential figures for mortality, malnutrition, and other indices of children at risk are provided can also be part of an advocacy effort, helping to identify populations most in need. Such analyses can be carried out jointly and serve as one basis for combined effort that could lead to joint planning. Thus, analyses of current conditions should be looked at as more than a source of information; they can be part of a mobilizing process.

2 Stress 'convergence'

As indicated above, institutional integration may, in practice, be too much to expect in the implementation of programmes. The goal of integrated programming is to respond to the needs of the child in an integrated way, not to achieve integration of delivery systems. Convergence can be accomplished if various programmes attend to the same children and families. Even if the administration of the programmes is not integrated, the results may be.

Convergence is helped if there is a physical and/or social focal point. A building that is at once a nutrition centre and a child-care or preschool centre and a place that the doctor can visit and a location for parental education provides natural convergence of programmes. A social or economic grouping – such as a cooperative or local women's organization or labour union – can provide another focal point for convergence of services and self-help programmes.

Convergence is also facilitated if those upon whom the convergence is supposed to occur are participants in the planning, implementation, and evaluation processes.

3 Seek agreement on those most in need

To achieve convergence requires agreement at a high level about the population groups most in need of attention, and a mechanism for defining the areas in which they will be found. That may be as simple as designating one area of a country – north-east Thailand, for instance. Or it may involve a relatively sophisticated situation analysis in which pockets of rural and urban poverty are identified to which all programmes should be directed. Once such a definition has been made, special budget incentives might be made to ensure that the various organizations involved put their effort into those regions. Multisectorial and/or sub-regional groups can be set up to supervise programme implementation.

Although seeking such agreement might seem to be an easy thing to do, it too can encounter barriers. Almost inevitably, political interests and pressures come into play, not only in the form of favourite areas, but, in some cases where governments are accountable, in the desire not to show favouritism that might weaken a political position. There is need, then, for a relatively high level of political will.

4 Make planning a collaborative process

A collaborative planning process must be something more than simply joining together people with expertise from different sectors in an isolated planning department. It must be an active process involving people with current responsibilities in the different sectors sitting together to work out a joint plan. A technical planning office can both stimulate such a process and provide important inputs into it, but should not serve as a substitute.

Collaborative planning implies not only intersectoral planning, but also incorporation of those who are to participate in programmes into the process from the beginning. In so doing, it is crucial to recognize traditional wisdom as a valid form of knowledge, to be drawn upon in the planning process.

5 Focus efforts initially, then add on according to a stepwise plan

Although the clear intention of a plan or programme may be to provide combined attention, it may be advisable and necessary to begin with one component and to phase in others along the way. The desired convergence would be achieved over time. This compromise to an initially integrated effort may be necessary for financial as well as structural reasons. The component (nutrition, child care, etc.) which provides the starting point need not be the same in all places. If starting points are different they will result in temporary dispersion rather than convergence of efforts. It is, therefore, crucial that they be part of a plan that seeks convergence and is associated with a community-based strategy of educational communication (see below).

6 *Place coordination outside specialized agencies*

If a specialized organization such as the Ministry of Health or Education controls the coordination of an 'integrated' programme, it will often be difficult to achieve the converging, multifaceted attention that is desired. Efforts will be biased towards the component for which the particular agency in charge is specifically responsible. For all the reasons noted above, achieving the cooperation of other specialized organizations may be difficult.

There are, however, mobilizing and coordinating structures that are not as specialized and that can help to bring together the specialized organizations. Among the strategies that have been used in different places are:

- Placing coordination under a national women's organization with mobilizing power at several levels (China).
- Creating a Ministry for Rural or Community Development that takes responsibility (Zimbabwe).
- Establishing a Ministry of Programme Implementation with an independent life (Sri Lanka).
- Attaching efforts directly to the office of a national or state-level leader (Santa Catarina, Brazil, where a social development committee involving representatives from all pertinent ministries as well as labour unions and other groups was directly responsible to the governor and was charged with the coordination).
- Assigning responsibility to non-governmental organizations with recognized mobilizing ability (India, Gujarat).
- Decentralizing to a district level where ministerial lines tend to blur.

There are potential disadvantages as well as advantages in placing coordination outside specialized agencies. Unless the organizations to whom responsibilities are assigned have the power, staff, resources, and decision-making responsibility to carry out their charge, they are sure to run into resistance from specialized agencies, making their task impossible.

7 *Create interorganizational activities*

Although delivery structures and decision making may continue to be vertical and parallel, several mechanisms may facilitate communication and combined efforts. Without threat to the normal way of functioning, for instance, it is possible to:

- involve several organizations together in the diagnosis, planning and implementation of an experimental project.
- create interagency groups to work on a particular problem, with each asked to indicate what they can contribute to the solution of the problem.

- form an interagency group to create materials that would then be used by the several agencies.
- organize joint training programmes involving personnel from several specialized agencies.
- create a joint commission charged with overseeing a combined programme.
- publish a periodic bulletin to which each sector and/or organization contributes, telling of their progress with respect to overall goals and describing new initiatives.

8 Strengthen community organization/responsibility

Another integrating force that is not linked to a particular specialized organization or bureaucratic structure is the local community. If organization of the local community is strong, there will be greater chance not only that various programme components will reach the community (because demand and execution will be strong), but that real coordination will develop at the local level. Although many programmes speak of community participation and make some overtures in that direction, vertical structures and centralized decision making continue to predominate in most cases (Rifkin 1985).

9 Parent, family and community education: an educational communication strategy

Because the responsibility for integrating different components in responding to the multiple and interacting needs of the young child falls to parents and family members charged with the immediate care of the child, the most basic integrating strategy is one that is directed towards supporting and educating parents and communities in ways that will improve their ability to respond to the complete gamut of needs of their children. That requires more than social marketing which transmits messages to an audience (of 'receptors') through the mass media. It requires a concept of education that goes beyond the delivery of knowledge by certified teachers. It requires opportunity for interpersonal communication, to adjust ideas to local circumstances, to understand better new approaches, to appreciate the value of traditional strategies that are still useful, and to reinforce and instigate specific actions. An educational communication strategy, therefore, must have a strong organizational as well as informational component (Rivera 1987; Haffey 1986).

If several of the above strategies can be successfully carried out at the same time, it may be possible to overcome some of the barriers to combined programming and implementation. It may even be possible to avoid some duplication of effort in attempting to achieve a convergence of programme efforts directed to children most in need.

We turn, now, to a more detailed consideration of three areas in which combined programming is desirable, but often hard to achieve. In each case, we will review evidence indicating why the combined approach is desirable and evidence showing that a combined approach can have an effect.

REFERENCES

Alva, Margaret. 'Keynote Address to the South Asian Association for Regional Cooperation's Conference on South Asian Children', in *Children First*. New Delhi, India, 1986.

Berg, A. *Malnutrition, What Can Be Done?* Baltimore: Johns Hopkins University Press, 1987.

Bosnjak, V. *From the Margins to the Mainstream*. Manuscript prepared for publication, 1989. Author's copy.

Bradley, M. *The Coordination of Services for Children Under Five*. London: National Foundation for Educational Research, 1982.

d'Agostino, M. and A.M. Masse-Raimbault. 'Proceed with Caution ... Children Under Six', in *Children in the Tropics*, Nos. 170–171 (1987).

Government of Sri Lanka. 'Report on Early Childhood Care and Education in Sri Lanka', Sessional Paper No. III, Colombo: Department of Government Printing, May, 1986.

Haffey, J. 'Communication Technologies', in G.R. Wilson, S. Ofosu-Amaah, and M. Belsey (eds), *Primary Health Care Technologies at the Family and Community Levels*. Geneva: the Aga Khan Foundation and UNICEF, 1986.

Pugh, G. *Service for Under-Fives: Developing a Coordinated Approach*. London: National Children's Bureau, 1988.

Rifkin, S. B. *Health Planning and Community Participation: Case Studies in South-East Asia*. London: Croom Helm, Inc., 1985.

Rivera, J. 'Comunicación Educativa para el Desarrollo Infantil: Conceptos y Estrategias', a document prepared for the Regional Office for Latin America and the Caribbean, UNICEF. Bogotá, Agosto 1987.

Chapter 9

Relating health and nutrition to social and psychological development

Most of the world thinks about health in a holistic way. Physical, psychological, social and spiritual well-being are not separated. For instance, herbalists in Oaxaca, Mexico, gave the following description when asked, 'What does it mean to be healthy?'

> It is when a person is content, calm, with a desire to work and to eat. The eyes shine. It is when a person has no problems with family, neighbours, or authorities and it is to be well with God and fellow men. In general it is to feel happy.

The response to 'What does it mean to be sick?' was:

> One can see that a sick person has problems. They look tired, can't move along, are sad and desperate. They do not have peace in the family. When they look emaciated, the blood is giving out and now there is no peacefulness. It is when one smokes and drinks all the time or is desperate with fright.
>
> (Instituto Nacional Indigenista, p. 14)

Prominent in these descriptions are social and psychological dimensions of health that are often missing in modern medicine's focus on health as absence of disease. To be healthy, for Mexican herbalists, includes being happy and relating well to others. It means not being frightened and being right with God. Health and sickness are also linked to eating and to malnutrition, described in terms of being emaciated and with poor blood.

We do not know how modern, clinically trained medical doctors would respond to the same questions. One might speculate, however, that many, if not most, would begin their definition of health with a physical, biological description, and that this would be much more likely among the growing number of specialists than among general practitioners or community health professionals. They might or might not go on to include mental health and a social dimension. And, if included, mental health might be defined more as the lack of psychiatric problems than in a positive way. Sickness might or might not be linked to nutrition in the definition.

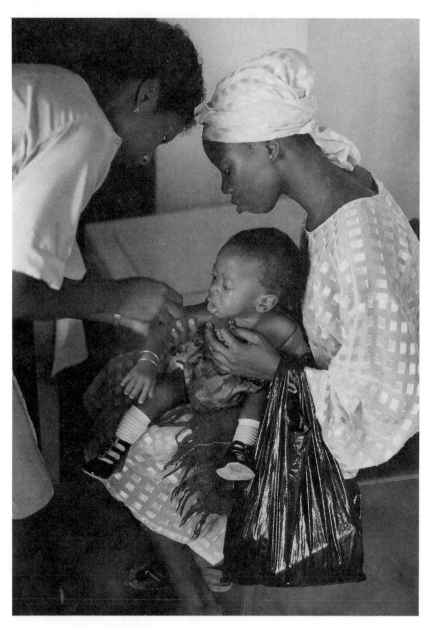

'Ouch', near Abeokuta, Nigeria

Reflecting the curative bias of modern medicine, health would probably be described first as the absence of sickness rather than as the positive, rounded state of well-being described by the traditional herbalists quoted above.

The tendency to break health into components and to emphasize physical health is in part a product of our age of specialization. It represents also the central place a biological model of disease has occupied as the medical profession has developed. These tendencies are evident in the training of medical doctors, worldwide. They are mirrored in the programming of national governments and international organizations seeking to reduce infant mortality and to combat disease. They have made combined programming and integrated attention to child survival and development needs a sometimes difficult task.

Health, nutrition, and psychosocial well-being

As a first step towards responding in a holistic and integrated way to the unity of a child's needs, a shift is needed in the way in which the relationships among health, nutrition, and psychosocial well-being are perceived. Figure 9.1 depicts the relationships as they are presently interpreted by most professionals and planners.

An interaction, or 'synergistic relationship', between health status and nutritional status is now broadly recognized, as indicated by the double arrow between H and N in the figure. Sickness increases the possibility of malnutrition and malnutrition increases the possibility of sickness.

However, the relationship between either nutrition or health and psychosocial well-being is ordinarily seen as a one-way relationship, running from N to PS or from H to PS. The debilitating effects of poor physical health on social and emotional development are recognized, but

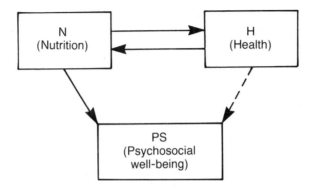

Figure 9.1 A common view of nutrition, health and psychosocial well-being

the reverse effect, of psychosocial development (or debility) on physical health, is given much less attention. Similarly, the effect of nutritional status on psychosocial development is accepted, and thought to occur primarily because malnutrition affects growth and development of the brain, or the energy level, of a child. Nutrition interventions are (appropriately) thought to affect a child's social and psychological, as well as physical, development. But psychosocial development interventions are not recognized as having an effect on nutritional status or on growth.

Although this formulation may seem a caricature to some readers, particularly those who see all these components as of one piece, the relationships depicted are reflected in major lines of action and in the implementation of programmes. Nutrition and health are found together in the basic documentation providing the foundation for major programme initiatives, but explicit reference to psychosocial development is not.

At the international level, for instance, combined attention to health and nutrition was recognized in the Alma Alta Declaration in 1978 (WHO–UNICEF 1978). In the UNICEF programme of child survival and development, health measures are combined with nutritional measures. At a national level, health ministries are often assigned responsibility for nutrition programmes that were once found within ministries of agriculture or in another part of the bureaucracy.

However, looking again at the Alma Alta Declaration, now with mental health and psychosocial well-being in mind, it is striking to see that the eight fundamental elements of primary health care do not include specific actions directed towards mental health (although 'mental development' has been added by some countries – for example, Kenya – in national formulations of what primary health care should include). Similarly, in UNICEF's programme of Child Survival and Development, the psychosocial development and well-being of children is assumed to be derivative from seven core programme actions (captured in the acronym, GOBI–FFF), none of which involves direct attention to social and psychological needs of infants and young children. Rarely do national plans or programmes include psychosocial components in a health or nutrition programme, whereas feeding or health attention are often included in pre-school programmes. These actions are consistent with, and supported by, the common view presented in Figure 9.1.

In brief, this limited view, in which social and psychological well-being is seen only as a by-product of good health and nutrition, undercuts the integration of psychosocial components into nutritional and health actions. It does not allow realization of the potential for improved psychosocial well-being to contribute to improvements in physical health and in survival.

Slowly, however, a new view of the relationships among health, nutrition, and psychosocial well-being is emerging. Figure 9.2 depicts the change. Synergistic relationships are pictured between psychosocial well-

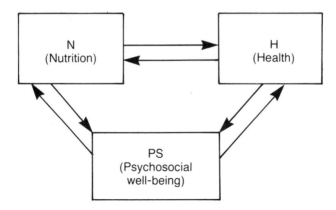

Figure 9.2 An emerging view of nutrition, health and psychosocial well-being

being and both health and nutrition as well as between health and nutrition.

If this newer formulation of relationships is accepted, then actions to strengthen social and psychological well-being must be included in health or nutrition programmes focusing on 'survival'. This viewpoint affirms that improvements in the social and psychological condition of caregiver and child can affect survival and physical development.

The following two sections of this chapter will provide evidence that the synergistic relationships pictured in Figure 9.2 do indeed exist. Suggestions will then be offered for specific ways in which psychosocial components can be incorporated into health and nutrition programming.

Health and psychosocial well-being: establishing the synergistic relationship

> Health is a state of complete physical, mental and social well-being and is not merely the absence of disease or infirmity.

> (World Health Organization Constitution 1946)

This broad definition of health, found in the Constitution of the World Health Organization, provides a basis for integrated programming. It corresponds more closely to the emerging view of relationships presented in Figure 9.2 than to the partial view of Figure 9.1. It also provides an interesting link to the holistic definitions of health by Mexican herbalists quoted at the beginning of this chapter.

But neither the WHO definition nor the herbalists' definitions specify causality or discuss interactions among the different dimensions of health. Both these sources of wisdom simply provide a rounded picture of health that includes social and psychological elements. One must go behind the descriptions to see how the relationships are perceived and acted upon. When that is done, it seems that modern medicine has some catching up to do, with its own broad view expressed in the WHO charter and with the herbalists.

The wisdom embodied in traditional medicine (see, for example, Negussie 1988; Coppo 1988) and the practices and traditions of various currents of non-Western medicine (e.g. Wu 1982) provide strong evidence supporting the idea that one's state of mind and one's social relationships strongly influence one's physical health. Even in Western cultures, popular concepts such as 'mind over body' or 'the will to live' are often heard and seem to be widely believed. A category of illnesses is labelled 'psychosomatic'. Moreover, medical anthropology, behavioural medicine, and psychiatry all suggest a close connection among social, mental, and physical well-being. But these sources of knowledge have not made much impact on mainstream medical science. In spite of these popular and academic supports for an integrated and interactive view, the separation of physical from mental and social health in concept and action continues to occur.

Fortunately, however, popular wisdom and medical science are beginning to come together. Research examining psychosocial 'stress' as it affects the functioning of immunological systems is providing evidence that '... directs attention to interactions among social and psychological as well as biological factors in the etiology, course, and treatment of disease' (Jemmott and Locke 1984, p. 78).

Summarizing an extensive review of research, Jemmott and Locke contend that:

> ... the bulk of empirical evidence indicates that people who have been exposed to a high degree of recent life stress have greater degeneration of overall health, more diseases of the upper respiratory tract, more allergies, a greater risk of hypertension, and greater risk of sudden cardiac death and coronary disease than do people who have been exposed to a low degree of life stress. Other research indicates that life-style factors and poor mental health, quite apart from life stress, are related to physical health status.
>
> (Ibid. p. 79)

People are exposed to stress when they are placed in situations requiring some sort of change or adaptation in response to novelty, uncertainty, or unpleasantness. These situations can be acute and short-lived or moderate and prolonged. Social and psychological sources of stress include such conditions as overcrowding, parental rejection, family discord, separation, etc.

Stress is related to disease. However, stressful situations do not produce infection; rather, they create reactions that impair the ability of our immune systems to function properly. If we are under stress and exposed to a disease, we are more likely to get sick. The specific physiological mechanisms that underlie the relationship between stress and disease are being sorted out. Researchers are examining the effects of hormonal reactions to stress as they affect the immune system through such changes as the level of circulating antibodies, the ability of certain cells to destroy foreign organisms, and the ability of such cells to multiply. But while the specific mechanisms are being discovered, the general relationship is now well established.

For our purposes, perhaps the most interesting and pertinent part of the discussion linking stress to disease is the accompanying observation of individual differences and the search for reasons explaining these differences in how stress influences disease. The variation is not only related to the timing, duration and proximity of the source of stress, but also to *the adaptive capacity of each person.* That adaptive capacity, or resilience, is affected in turn, by such personal characteristics as self-esteem, self-efficacy, and the sense of control over external events, as well as by the degree of social support available (Krantz and Glass 1984; Rutter 1985; Gentry and Kobasa 1984). These are psychological and social characteristics that can be fostered and that begin to appear in the very earliest months and years of a child's development. They can be fostered by responding adequately to psychological and social needs (as defined, for instance, in Chapter 3, p. 41), assuring children the experience of success and a sense of love and social support. Moreover, these responses require something more than attending to a child's health and feeding a child.

Most of the recent psycho-neuro-immunological research work on the link between stress and disease has been done with adults (or with animals). There is little reason to believe that these same conclusions would not hold with young children, and some reason to believe that they may be even stronger (Jemmott and Locke, p. 82).

The knowledge that healthy social and psychological experience helps an individual to cope with exposure to stress certainly provides a valid reason for attending to social and psychological development in the early years, when self-esteem (or a sense of failure) begins to form. However, there are also more immediate implications of social and psychological attention to (or neglect of) young children. The survival and health of children aged 0 to 6 living in stressful conditions can be affected dramatically. Failure to provide children with the psychosocial support needed for their development is a source of stress and at the same time deprives children of the chance to learn to cope with stress. Neglecting psychological and social development means that these children will be more susceptible to disease and to death than children whose needs are being met. Indeed, some of the earliest work on 'separation' carried out by Bowlby demonstrates that, under particular conditions, separation of the child from a caregiver (usually the mother) to whom it had become 'attached' could, indeed, lead to death (Bowlby 1969).

In the preceding paragraphs, we have focused on the direct interaction between psychosocial development or well-being and physical health (or disease). In addition, however, recognizing the synergism between nutrition and health means that the effects of a child's psychosocial well-being on nutrition, to be discussed in the following section, will also have an indirect effect on susceptibility to disease and on survival. Thus, although health and nutrition are separated in our discussion, they must be viewed together in practice.

Nutrition and psychosocial well-being: establishing the synergistic relationship

Evidence has accumulated from diverse sources that physical growth is affected by the interplay between various psychosocial interventions (that respond to social and psychological needs by strengthening and enriching a child's environment and caregiver/child interaction) and nutritional interventions.

A vast and varied literature links nutritional status to mental development. (For more detailed reviews of that literature, the reader can consult: Pollitt 1987; Dobbing, 1987; McGuire and Austin 1987; Werner 1979; Zeitlin *et al.* 1990.) Less evidence is available relating nutrition to social and emotional development, but that too is growing (Barrett and Radke-Yarrow 1982, and Pollitt 1987, the latter for relationships between micronutrient deficiencies and behaviour). As suggested by Figure 9.1, the effect of nutrition on mental development has been established and accepted, although with some shifts in thinking about how that occurs.

Here, we will be less concerned with the effect of nutrition on mental development and more interested in 1) the interactive relationship between psychosocial well-being and physical growth of the young child, and 2) the synergistic relation between non-nutrition interventions that promote psychosocial development and nutrition interventions intended to promote growth. Evidence will be presented from:

- animal research on brain development;
- research on effects of touch on low birthweight and premature babies;
- studies of children who thrive in conditions that put them at risk;
- studies of children in nutritional recuperation centres; and,
- studies of planned interventions with children at risk or with moderate or mildly malnourished children.

The sum total of results from these extremely varied approaches suggests strongly that a synergistic relationship is at work. Taken together, the evidence makes an impressive case for combining nutrition and non-nutrition interventions in promoting both growth and psychosocial development.

1 Animal research on brain development

Working with animals allows control over environmental complexities in a way not possible with humans and permits study of the brain at death. A considerable body of animal research suggests that early stimulation and an enriched environment can have beneficial effects on survival, maturation, growth, responsiveness to stress, and behaviour (Newton and Levine 1988; Crnic 1983).

In controlled experiments the environment of well-nourished and of previously undernourished rats was 'enriched' by including in the environment playthings and other rats with which to interact. Comparisons were made with rats whose environment was not enriched. The results showed that an enriched environment can affect brain development and can partially compensate for effects of undernutrition on development and behaviour (Smart 1987). Specifically, when previously undernourished rats have been subsequently provided with adequate food and placed in different environments (enriched and impoverished), results show:

– compensatory effects of enriched environments on brain weight, forebrain length and width, and on the depth, area, synapses, synaptic disc diameter, and dendritic branching within the occipital cortex.
– that previous undernourishment did not impair the ability of the rats to respond to environmental enrichment.
– that brain maturation of the environmentally enriched but previously undernourished rats always remained below that of the environmentally enriched but previously well-nourished rats.

Clearly, both nourishment and enrichment have effects on the growth and development of the brain. An enriched environment produced compensatory effects, and an undernourished state did not allow the experimental animals to live up to their potential. Although the mechanisms producing these effects are still being discussed, it is clear that there is more to both achievement and growth promotion than increasing food intake, and that a varied and enriched environment helps.

The effects of touch on low birthweight and premature babies

One non-nutritional aspect of the interaction between caretaker and infant that seems to have an effect on physical growth operates through the sense of touch. To a large extent, research examining the effect of touch on growth and behaviour of infants stems from research with animals showing that handling, or touch, affects the level of growth hormone (Schanberg, Evoniuk, and Kuhn 1984). It is hypothesized that the touch system is part of a primitive survival mechanism found in all mammals which depend on maternal care for survival in their earliest weeks or months. Absence produces stress and seems to trigger slowing of metabolism (until the mother can return); hence its need for nourishment is reduced. This is functional in the short run but leads to stunted growth if prolonged.

Stimulating touch seems to promote growth and brain maturation and has an effect on activity and behaviour. In a recent intervention experiment, a group of premature babies in a United States hospital were lightly massaged and their limbs moved passively during three 15 minute periods per day for 10 days. As a result, the babies averaged a 47 per cent greater weight gain per day than other infants who were kept in incubators and were not massaged, even though the massaged infants did not eat more than the others. The massaged infants were also more active and alert during sleep/wake behaviour sessions, and showed more mature signs on a variety of behavioural tests. Eight months later, they did better than the others on tests of mental and motor ability and continued their advantage in weight (Field, Bauer and Nystrom 1986).

A study in south India (Landers 1989) showed that low birthweight babies who were massaged showed a remarkable catch-up in their weight and on a battery of developmental tests over a period of six months. This research showed a clear effect of mother–child interaction on both physical and developmental outcomes.

Massage is a common, but declining child-care practice found in many cultures throughout the world. Why the practice is so widespread is not known, but a reasonable guess is that it emerged from experience and became a socially institutionalized practice providing an effective and natural way to assist underweight babies to survive, grow, and develop in adverse conditions.

These research findings leave us with questions, but, independently of the work on attachment (Harlow and Harlow 1966), give support to such common Third World practices as carrying babies on the back and sleeping with babies, both of which are ways of maintaining physical contact and communicating through touch. What comes through clearly is that *caregiver–child interaction is very important for growth as well as mental development.*

Children who thrive in 'at risk' conditions

Most nutrition research has been directed towards discovering causes of malnutrition and identifying the effects of attention to malnourished children. More recently, another line has focused on children who grow up in conditions of poverty that often lead to undernourishment but who manage to be well-nourished. Why do some children thrive while others do not? What are the mechanisms of biological, social, and behavioural adaptability to nutritional stress that allow these 'positive deviant' children to grow and develop well?

Zeitlin, Ghassemi and Mansour (1990) review 16 studies which compare children who thrive with those who do not. They also examine a large body of related research. The authors consider three kinds of correlates, noting the importance of 1) sociodemographic and 2) physiological correlates of malnutrition, and then focusing on another cluster of variables – the 3) 'psychosocial and behavioural aspects of the mother–child interaction, their individual temperaments, and the social network supporting the dyad'. Their purpose was to learn from adaptive child-care and feeding behaviours and the social networks that support them.

The review examines energy metabolisms, growth-related hormonal adjustments, immune responses of the body, and psychological stress as related to positive deviance. A link is made between psychosocial well-being, nutritional thriving, and a healthy condition. The importance of examining psychological as well as genetic or physiological factors is explained as follows:

> The fact that some children are genetically more resistant than others adds to the unexplained variance in the results of psychosocial research, just as uncontrolled psychological factors add to the 'noise' in physiological research findings.
>
> (Zeitlin *et al.*, p. 33)

Zeitlin *et al.*, go on to say:

> Stressful caretaker–child interaction can be expected to increase protein requirements while tending to decrease the amount of food that the child consumes. Pleasantly stimulating interactions, on the other hand, enhance the child's tendency to exercise its developing organ systems and hence to utilize nutrients for growth and development.
>
> (p. 33)

In short, psychological stress has a negative effect on the use of nutrients whereas psychological well-being stimulates the secretion of growth-promoting hormones. 'These mechanisms help to explain how psychosocial factors, such as the affect between mother and child, are associated with adequate growth and development' (Zeitlin *et al.* p. 34).

Three major conclusions emerge from the overall review by Zeitlin, Ghassemi and Mansour:

1 Psychological and social well-being

> ... psychosocial factors associated with adequate growth amidst poverty are not specific to nutrition alone. The same characteristics that predict a good nutritional outcome also predict good cognitive development, health, and long-term development of the individual into a stable, productive member of society.
>
> (p. 34)

2 Attitudes and aspirations

Parents of positive deviants are more likely than others in their communities to be upwardly mobile, to discard fatalistic attitudes and to take initiative, adopting modern practices for themselves and their children, and to be more enterprising. They make a more effective use of health services, family planning, and educational facilities, and tend to ... bear fewer children, have higher aspirations for these children, and invest more resources in each child.

(p. 35)

3 Behaviours, technologies, and social structures

There are positive deviant behaviour patterns and technologies networks that are specifically adaptive in protecting the nutritional status and health of infants and young children.

(p. 36)

Positive caregiver–child interactions

From their review, Zeitlin *et al.* identified characteristics of caregiver–child interactions associated with adequate growth and development:

- Frequent physical interaction (holding, hugging);
- Rapid, consistent, and appropriate response to perception of child's needs;
- Speaking and responding to a child's vocalizations, both when holding the child and when the child is at a distance;
- Looking directly into the child's eyes;
- Showing affection by smiling and friendly behaviour rather than inflicting hostile or dominant behaviour;
- Permitting the child to initiate and guide interaction;
- Avoiding interaction that is too slow or too rapid and overstimulating;
- Giving clear instructions;
- Rewarding achievements;
- Reprimanding without being brusque, harsh, or severe;
- Avoiding forms of control in which the only objective is to demonstrate authority over the child;
- Creating a stimulating physical environment for the child.

A nutrition-related interaction related to positive deviance was found to be actively feeding toddlers instead of expecting them to feed themselves.

Although these observations need to be associated with age and elaborated to give a more specific idea of *how* and *what* to do, that is not our purpose here; rather, we are concerned with establishing the general principle that actions to improve psychosocial well-being will affect growth.

Social support

Figuring prominently in the identification of children that thrive in conditions of risk was the efficiency and quality of the network of social support available to caregivers. A supportive system (family or community) helped to moderate effects of overwork as well as of stress and depression. The importance of social support noted in the Zeitlin review is also a central finding in one of the most detailed positive deviance studies that has been carried out, following a group of multiracial children from different social backgrounds in the same Hawaiian community from the prenatal period to the threshold of adulthood. In their book, *Vulnerable but Invincible*, Werner and Smith (1982) identify protective factors within the child and the caregiving environment that differentiate high-risk children who are resilient from those who develop serious learning and behaviour problems. The major sources of support within the caregiving environment were (p. 134):

- Four or fewer children spaced more than two years apart
- Much attention to the infant during the first year
- Positive parent–child relationship in early childhood
- Additional caretakers besides the mother and care by siblings and grandparents
- Steady employment for mother outside the household
- Availability of kin/neighbours for emotional support
- Structure and rules in the household and shared values – a sense of coherence
- Close peer friends and availability of counsel
- Access to special services

These studies of 'positive deviant' children help to identify conditions and behaviours that permit some families to bring up well-nourished children in spite of the conditions of poverty in which they live. They draw upon and reinforce other lines of research demonstrating the interaction between nutritional and non-nutritional behaviours and between a child's characteristics and the environment in which the child grows and develops. Crucial features of that environment are the relationship of the child with its caregiver and the psychological and social support available to the caregiver.

Studies of children in nutritional recuperation centres

Whereas the studies of positive deviance compare children of different nutritional levels experiencing different environmental conditions, studies of children in recuperation centres examine what happens to children who are all seriously undernourished when they are exposed to a different type of environment. Two telling examples come from Chile and Jamaica where experimental studies were set up in nutritional recuperation centres. The studies compared a) the progress of children who received a treatment of stimulation and play as well as food with b) the progress of those who received only food (Chile) or who were well-nourished (Jamaica).

Chile

In the Chilean experiment (Monckeberg 1986), infants were fed, provided with psychosensory stimulation (for 30 minutes twice a day), with physical exercise (also 30 minutes twice a day), and with opportunities to play with attendants throughout the day. These children were compared with children with similar characteristics who received the same diet but no psychomotor or affective stimulation.

For the stimulated children:

> Not only was the weight gain different, but the physical growth was better and there was a significant difference after 50 days of treatment. The psychomotor quotient also exhibited the same pattern. While for the control group the average quotient was 65 (plus or minus 12) at the 150th day of treatment, for the experimental group it was 85 (plus or minus 7).
>
> (Monckeberg, p. 28)

These differences, for weight, psychomotor and mental development, were more pronounced for children who were less than 6 months of age at admission to the recuperation centre than for those between 6 and 12 months of age.

To explain the differences in recovery, Monckeberg hypothesizes that stimulation and affect trigger and help reinitiation of growth. He then makes reference to the links mentioned above relating resumed growth to biochemical processes and to the functioning of growth-promoting hormones.

Jamaica

The Jamaican study (Grantham-McGregor 1984) compared three groups of children. Two of the groups had been admitted to the hospital for nutrition recuperation and one group was well-nourished but was admitted for other reasons. In the recuperation programme, one group of malnourished children was also provided with psychosocial stimulation, the other was not. The stimulation consisted of instructing attending nurses to play with the children for one hour each day.

When children entered the hospital, both malnourished groups had similar developmental quotients and were significantly behind the control group. By the time they left, all three groups had improved, but the intervened group had improved the most and was no longer significantly behind the control group.

One of the more interesting features of these two studies is that they both followed up the children after leaving the recuperation centre. In the Jamaican case, that follow-up included an active programme of home visiting, using community health workers (CHW). The CHWs visited homes once per week over 24 months. Visits included reinforcement of the need for psychosocial interaction as well as monitoring of the physical status of the children. During this time the weight recuperation was maintained. The gains registered in psychological development were maintained as well, so that the children who had been played with in the hospital continued on a par with the comparison group of well-nourished children when followed over a period of 36 months.

In the Chilean case, no additional action was taken following departure from the recuperation centre. As contrasted with the Jamaican study, the Chilean follow-up led to the conclusion that the programme of stimulation succeeded in raising mental performance only for the period of the programme. A decline was observed when the children went back to their former environments. By way of comparison, in a small group of 35 recuperated children, who had been adopted after discharge by families of higher socioeconomic status, mental ability scores were normal, well above the scores quoted above.

Long-term effects of nutritional and psychosocial interventions with mild to moderately malnourished children

Yet another form of evidence supporting the importance of attending to both nutritional and non-nutritional conditions affecting growth and development comes from studies of intervention programmes carried out in conditions of everyday life where many children suffer from mild to moderate malnutrition. In several instances, interventions have been designed to try to sort out effects from nutritional supplementation and effects from non-nutritional interventions intended to improve psychosocial development.

In an extraordinary study (Super et al. 1987) carried out with families in poor neighbourhoods of Bogotá, Colombia, 280 Colombian infants at risk of malnutrition were randomly assigned to one of four experimental groups formed by the presence or absence of one, or both, of two interventions: 1) nutritional supplementation for all members of the family, from the last trimester of pregnancy until the target child was three years old; and 2) a twice-weekly home-visiting programme designed to promote early cognitive development, from birth of the target child until age three. All families received free medical care and were studied prospectively.

The following extract summarizes some results:

At three years of age, children who had received nutritional supplementation averaged 3 centimeters and 800 grams more than controls; the incidence of children with severe growth retardation was reduced by half. Home visiting had no overall effect on size but did reduce the number of severely underweight children.

At age six (three years after intervention) the Supplementation effects remained at about the same magnitude. Children in the Home Visit condition had become larger than controls, by 1.4 centimeters and 483 grams. Both interventions reduced the incidence of stunting and wasting. Dietary recall data suggest that changes in family functioning as well as biological mechanisms account for the observed pattern of results.

(p. 2)

The effects noted for the Bogotá experiment were greater for lower levels of father's education.

A host of other studies could be cited (see review by Pollitt 1987) to support the contention that nutrition interventions can have short- and long-term effects on some aspect of behaviour such as improved attention, heightened social responsiveness, reduced irritability and inability to tolerate frustration, higher activity levels, and increased independence. These behaviours are related to both cognitive and social behaviour in the long run.

What causes the effects listed above? How should these findings be interpreted? Pollitt (1987) suggests that, in much of the literature, interpretation has been built around a model based on the biomedical tradition of disease causation that did not take into account the social context in which development occurred or the previous and subsequent history of an individual. This static, linear model and interpretation contrasts with another model beginning with the premise that 'through its interactions with illness and adverse family and socioeconomic conditions, undernutrition increases the probability of diverting the trajectory of mental development ...' (Pollitt 1987, p. 19). It also differs from a view that 'effects may occur within a synergistic system where the malnourished infant is less successful at engaging caretakers in interaction and, in turn, is responded to less often and with less sensitivity, resulting in a failure to develop normal patterns of social interaction' (Lester 1979, as quoted in Barrett et al., p. 542).

Slowly, however, an interactive view is being recognized and used as a basis for designing as well as reinterpreting research results. For instance, in a recent study of 'food intake and human function' carried out in Mexico (as part of a three-country study including also Egypt and Kenya), the interactive model serving as the basis for analysis of cognitive performance and social conditions was as follows:

... one pathway by which low intake may affect development is through subtle effects on the young child's manner of interacting with his or her environment, including reduced activity, attentiveness and social responsiveness. These behaviors, which lead to reduced stimulation and hence reduced opportunity for more complex responses, may also affect the child's intake, perpetuating continued low intake because he or she does not 'demand' food. Similarly, development may be compromised by an interaction between child passivity and maternal time allocation in households where child care time is limited because the caretakers are pushed by economic necessity to long hours of work. In such a situation, low intake in the child interacts with the behavioral consequences of poor economic resources, with each component contributing to and reinforcing a less than optimal outcome.

(Chávez *et al.* 1987, p. 298)

Following this model, a measure of cognitive development for children at 30 months was related to measures of 1) growth (length), 2) caretaking (using the observed appearance of the child as a proxy for maternal caretaking), 3) current diet, and 4) socioeconomic status. In a series of regression analyses allowing a look at different combinations of the variables, cumulative growth was the dominant significant variable, but caretaking and SES were also significant. When all four variables were entered, length and child care continued to be significant.

The analysis lends strong support to an interpretation of development that looks at the interaction between the characteristics of the child and its environment, including interaction with the caregiver and with the conditions surrounding both the caregiver and the child. The researchers concluded that:

Social–environmental conditions of the household (as measured by socioeconomic status indicators and maternal caregiving) clearly affect development. The biological and behavioral experiences of the child, as reflected in growth, also affect development. The mechanism of these effects is probably synergistic. That is, child nutrition, health and activity ... have a synergistic relationship with respect to social and social–relational conditions, with respect to risk of poor or delayed cognitive development. The model is analogous to the dynamic interaction of infection and malnutrition, which have a synergistic relationship with respect to mortality.

(Chávez *et al.* 1987, p. 303)

Focusing on weight instead of cognitive development, and on infants, aged 0 to 6 months, a similar kind of interaction seems to be present.

Infants increased faster in weight from birth onwards if the exterior and interior sanitary conditions of their homes were better, and if the preschoolers and mothers of the household appeared cleaner...

(p. 327)

The implication is that nutrition interacted with an environmental condition related to better health and to better maternal care, as represented in the attention given to cleanliness of the house.

Summary

The review presented above provides evidence that satisfying psychosocial needs can have an effect on nutritional status through its effect on metabolism linked to stress reduction, and by helping to produce changes in the care demanded and provided. At the same time, nutrition is seen to have an effect on psychosocial development, operating primarily through its impact on attention, responsiveness, independence, irritability, and affect. Nutrition is one of a complex of factors operating to influence that development and associated behaviour.

The discussion suggests a kind of spiral effect in which food intake, providing energy and needed nutrients, increases the physical activity of the child and hence the child's ability to interact. In interaction, the child attracts attention of the caregiver and demonstrates its needs. The caregiver responds, providing food and affection, further energizing the child.

The spiral applies to the caregiver as well. A better nourished and healthier caregiver who is also free from social and psychological stress will be better able to energize and respond to the child, helping the child to demand more food, increasing the food intake....

But the spiral can move downwards as well as upwards, with an impaired ability of the child to elicit a response from the caregiver leading to reduced food intake, producing even further inability to interact leading to lower food intake, etc.

SOME STRATEGIC CONSIDERATIONS

1 Combine programme actions

The review of the literature has tried to show that satisfying social and psychological needs can have an effect on both nutrition and health. It should not be surprising, then, that the first implication for programming to be drawn from the evidence is that nutritional and health actions should be combined with other actions designed to improve the social and psychological well-being of the child. Doing so takes advantage of the synergistic relationships that have been identified.

Several other implications also emerge from the analysis regarding how one might go about taking advantage of the interactive relationship and set the spiral in an upward direction.

2 Support caregiver and child, not just the child or the mother

Researchers have emphasized that satisfying a child's psychosocial needs requires mutually satisfying caregiver–child interactions within a supportive and stimulating environment. Thus, programming should be directed towards the caregiver–child dyad (using the word 'dyad' captures the reciprocal nature of the interaction between caregiver and child) as well as to the caregiver (usually the mother) and to the child, viewed individually. Improving the nutritional and health condition of both is obviously important but, again, is not enough.

What can be done to improve the interaction? Caregivers can be helped to interact better with their infants, toddlers and preschoolers by at least two kinds of actions – strengthening the supporting environment and providing information to caregivers within a supportive structure.

3 Improve the supporting environment

The first, and probably the most important, type of action is one that will help to remove limiting conditions that prevent natural interaction from occurring. Most caregivers will be loving and attentive and responsive and stimulating if they are given the chance. But there are many pressures on resources, time, and psyche that produce stress in caregivers, affecting their interaction – other than stress induced by undernutrition. As suggested by Zeitlin *et al.*, there is an important need to look at the social support systems caregivers can count on – at whether there are additional hands and hearts available. Are there ways in which time taken for other tasks can be reduced? These concerns are in addition to efforts to improve the larger environment through changes in water systems, sanitation, and other features of the physical environment. They are in addition to providing opportunities for education, a move which has many indirect benefits for caregiving.

4 Work with caregivers to improve childrearing practices

A second set of actions would focus more directly on the caregiver. Without underestimating the natural parenting abilities of most caregivers or disregarding the many traditional practices that help foster a positive interaction between caregivers and their children, it is possible to see important ways in which working with caregivers could improve interaction and foster child development. Many mothers, for instance, are not aware of the ability of their newborns to see and hear and respond at birth, do not value play, see no harm in 'bottle propping' (leaving the child alone with the bottle instead of interacting during the feeding with a bottle), or are unaware of the importance of stimulating the child through touch, talking, and eye contact. In urban conditions, a teenage girl may not have had the socialization to child care she would have had in a rural area. She is in need of help with her parenting skills. In short, programmes of parental support and education that include discussions of nutritional and other childrearing information may be appropriate.

5 Treat feeding as a social and developmental process

Feeding is a childrearing practice that varies considerably from place to place and family to family. From the review of evidence emerges a natural link between nutrition and psychosocial development related to the fact that feeding is a social and developmental as well as a nutritional process.

In nutrition programmes, *how* a child is fed should be attended to – along with attention to screening for malnutrition and to *what* a child is fed. Feeding is at once a social activity with psychosocial development purposes as well as a nutritional activity with nutritional and growth purposes. The quality of the social and psychological interaction during feeding affects nutritional status both through a physiological effect on the child and through its influence on the amount of food the child demands and ingests. Still, as the analysis in the appendix to this chapter shows, these considerations are seldom included in nutrition manuals.

Interactions during breastfeeding or bottle-feeding, during the weaning process, and at meal times can encourage or discourage proper feeding while helping to satisfy important developmental needs.

These general suggestions for improvements in programming can find their expression within many kinds of existing health and nutrition programmes.

INCORPORATING PSYCHOSOCIAL DEVELOPMENT INTO HEALTH AND NUTRITION PROGRAMMES

Is it difficult to incorporate actions that will improve psychosocial development into health and nutrition programmes? Obviously, some programme approaches will lend themselves more easily than others to the task.

Training

Perhaps the most important way to begin the integration process is by reorienting the training of health and nutrition personnel. Approaching integration through training of professionals and paraprofessionals would not be costly in monetary terms. It would involve, first, a reorientation of training curricula and materials. That reorientation would require more than just adding a unit on psychosocial development to the curriculum; a re-examination of the full curriculum should be undertaken to see where

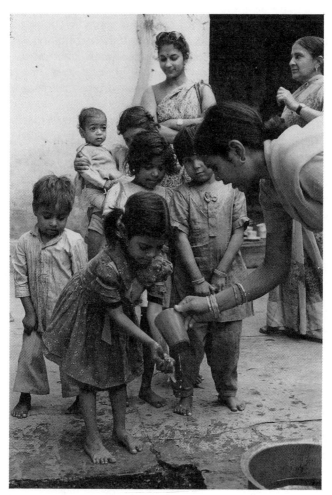

Forming health habits, Old Delhi, India

the integrative perspective should be included. A unit that deals with the physiology of disease and with immune systems, for instance, should include material about the effects of proper psychosocial well-being and the relationship of the ability to handle stress and the immune system. New materials would have to be created. All of this might be done with an inter-disciplinary committee. The second step in the reorientation would be to re-educate or retrain those responsible for training. That retraining could not be done on a crash basis; it would have to occur over time as the new and integrated perspective found its way into the mainstream of medical and health education.

Although this process of reorienting a field could be relatively inexpensive financially, it would require immense dedication, persistance, and tact. Even relatively small changes are often hard to introduce. There are certain obvious speciality areas in which the changes might first be explored: paediatrics, community medicine, home economics, or training traditional birth attendants (where there is already a sense of integrated thinking that can be reinforced, even as new ideas are being introduced).

But in the long run, integration requires broader attention. That means convincing prestigious individuals in the field that an integrated vision is important. It means working with professional associations to see that, within the association, for instance, there is a commission dedicated to reorienting training and, more broadly, to working on child development, including the psychosocial dimensions of development. The real cost is the cost of the time and energy necessary to make such a reorientation occur in a way that is not just a mechanical adding of yet another piece to a curriculum.

Let us turn now to considering where a psychosocial component might be introduced into more specific health and nutrition programmes.

Health programmes

As a starting point for suggestions about how programme components might be combined, let us take the eight essential elements of primary health care from the Alma Ata Declaration. The word 'medicine' provides a handy mnemonic device[1] for remembering those elements:

Maternal and child health
Education for health
Drugs and appropriate therapeutics
Immunization
Common disease treatment
Indigenous diseases; local prevention and control
Nutrition
Environmental sanitation and water

Provide maternal and child health (MCH) care

MCH programmes often do, but always should, include attention to the psychosocial well-being of mothers and children. The periods of pregnancy and lactation are two periods when women need not only medical supervision and advice, but also strong social and psychological support. These are also times when women, and families, are very open to learning about child care and development, when particular interventions can have greater impact on behaviour than at other times (Brazleton 1982).

If the formation of the health personnel (in formal education programmes or in traditional, non-formal ways) who attend the mother during this period has included attention to the psychosocial needs and development of mother and child during these periods, a major step towards integration will already have been taken.

In addition, however, there are specific actions or procedures that might help introduce a psychosocial component into maternal and child health programmes. For instance, measures can be recommended that facilitate 'attachment' of the child to the mother, at birth and in the neonatal period. Such simple procedures as giving the child to the mother immediately and beginning the process of breastfeeding as soon as possible not only have nutritional value, but help interaction and the expression of affect. One need not enter deeply into the literature on maternal–infant bonding (Klaus and Kennell 1982), or the continuing controversy over the scientific basis upon which bonding theory has been constructed (Chess and Thomas 1982; Lamb 1982) to appreciate that favouring early interaction is one potentially useful strategy for facilitating attachment. Nor should such simple suggestions lead to a naive belief that such procedures will have lasting effects if they are not reinforced and continued later on. Moreover, such suggestions must be placed in cultural context, with the understanding that different cultures and different economic circumstances dictate different forms of maternal thinking (Scheper-Hughes 1985).

It is possible also to consider introducing, within maternal–child health programmes, a form of health monitoring that will include the psychosocial health of mother and child as well as their disease and nutritional status. Instruments are available (e.g. Sri Lanka: Nikapota 1990; Latin America: Atkin 1989) and/or being tried out in many Third World locations (WHO 1990) that can facilitate this process. Over the next few years, one can expect additional advances that should further facilitate integrating this component into MCH and PHC.

Because our emphasis is on introducing psychosocial components into health programmes, we will not deal here with the reverse side of the same coin. It is obvious, however, that programmes of child care and development whose primary purpose has been to enrich the social and psychological condition of children, or, more narrowly, their preparation for school, will provide logical 'entry points' for MCH components of primary health care (see Evans 1986).

Education for health

Health education takes many programmatic forms, and is carried out in hospitals and primary health care centres, in schools and programmes of adult education, and with the population at large through campaigns using the mass media. In some cases, health education is conceptualized to include the psychosocial component, but in practice that component may be left out. For instance, the Child-to-Child programme, which is directed towards children aged 10-12, specifically includes activity sheets and other materials designed to help older siblings be supportive of younger siblings. In practice, however, most child-to-child programmes have neglected this component.

A worldwide campaign to provide basic knowledge that will help children survive and grow has been organized by UNICEF around a publication called *Facts for Life*. This initiative has evolved from the limited idea of producing an informative book meant to be an end in itself to a view of *Facts for Life* as a set of raw materials to be adapted and used in the best way possible to reach hard-to-reach people with critical information. One of the adaptations needed and being made in some places is to provide more information about the importance of parent–child interaction. (In the Spanish version, one message dealing with parent–child interaction was included among the 50 prime messages. This was so in spite of the fact that one section, including eight messages, was called 'child development'. The other seven messages in that section dealt with nutrition.)

Education for health provides one of the most logical openings for integrating the physical and psychosocial dimensions of health and of child development into one programme. As suggested in the previous chapter, it is often possible to combine programme components at the level of content even when it is not possible to achieve integration of organizational efforts across sectoral lines.

Drugs and immunization

For the most part, these two aspects of the primary health care strategy have been approached programmatically through campaigns and by seeing that the organizational apparatus is in place to ensure that drugs and immunizations are available at appropriate times and places to as broad a population as possible. These programme approaches do not lend themselves easily to incorporating psychosocial actions affecting child survival and development. On the other hand, child-care and early education programmes that focus on psychosocial development can facilitate immunization and provision of drugs, by motivating parents to attend to their child in a holistic way, by requiring that children be immunized before entering the programme, and by gathering children together, facilitating the distribution process.

Prevention, control and treatment of common and indigenous diseases

It is difficult to approach social and psychological development within programmes that are defined in terms of 'disease'. Even severe mental retardation will not be included in this component of primary health care because it is not a common disease. Nevertheless, it is possible and appropriate, as indicated by the scientific literature, to include psychosocial considerations as a complementary part of a preventive approach to disease. Traditional practitioners and family doctors have known and practised that approach for centuries. Recovering the broader approach marks a challenge for health services in general, and for primary health care in particular. And, as suggested earlier, it provides a challenge to reorient the training of health personnel.

Environmental sanitation and water

This important component of primary health care is usually handled by a separate organizational structure. Sanitation and water programmes do not lend themselves easily to incorporation of information about parent–child interactions, or about providing the child with a stimulating environment. However, were these programmes to be conceived as part of a broader effort to provide children with an environment that favours survival, growth, and development, then concerns about water and sanitation could be brought together with environmental measures to improve psychosocial well-being.

As with immunization and drugs, it may be easier to integrate this component into child-care and development programmes rather than the reverse. The drilling of wells has been coordinated in some places (e.g. in specific projects in Nepal and Burkina Faso) with the construction of community child-care or preschool centres. In many other instances, however, this has not been done.

Nutrition programmes

One of the most logical places of all to incorporate attention to psychological and social well-being, within the PHC lines set out in Alma Ata, is within nutrition programmes. Moreover, nutrition programmes are often handled separately from health programmes. Consequently, the discussion of this option will be somewhat more extensive than for others.

Perhaps the most visible form of nutrition intervention is food supplementation. Huge programmes of food supplementation have been mounted throughout the world. Often these are given a great deal of publicity for political reasons. Large 'give-away' programmes have been criticized on a number of grounds, with the criticisms also providing visibility. Indeed, there has been an unfortunate tendency on occasion to talk about nutrition interventions as if food supplementation is the only kind of nutrition action to be taken.

There are, however, many kinds of nutrition interventions in addition to food supplementation, some of which lend themselves better than others to combined programming and to incorporation of a psychosocial development component. The following sets out and discusses briefly a broad range of programme possibilities:

Increase food production

On a large scale, this strategy does not lend itself to combined action, focusing usually on the introduction of new and better seed varieties, on irrigation systems, or on other technological solutions that can be applied broadly. The strategy can be conceived as part of a broader and integrative programme, but in implementation is unlikely to include other components.

On a small scale, promoting community gardens in conjunction with operation of child-care centres could help to combine developmental and nutritional actions, but such actions are unlikely to make a major impact on food production.

Improve marketing mechanisms/adjust food prices/ subsidize purchases, including food coupons

These actions, intended to improve the nutritional situation of a population, are also broad and sweeping actions. At first glance, it is difficult to see how other dimensions of attention to the child might be integrated into them. If, however, marketing occurs through a system of centres in which prices are subsidized, these centres could also be considered as locations in which, for instance, oral rehydration packets could be distributed. They could also be locations where health consultations could be given; where child-care centres might be located; where information could be provided about other services; or where discussion groups might be formed.

Provide mineral and vitamin supplements

This action will benefit psychosocial development and behaviour to the extent that the supplements help to prevent disabilities such as cretinism (related to iodine deficiency) or xerophthalmia (vitamin A deficiency) and/or are linked in other ways to learning and behaviour (Berg and Brems 1986). Evidence is mounting, for instance, concerning the effect of iron deficiency anaemia on children's ability to concentrate and perform normally in school because they are weak and fatigued (Soemantri, Pollitt, and Kim 1985; Pollitt 1987).

Because of their nature, these extremely important interventions are likely to be attached to other programmes or to be handled centrally through such devices as fortifying bread or salt. They do not, therefore, normally provide the structure or opportunity for integration of other components into the action.

Provide food supplementation

Programmes of food supplementation are widespread. They may be directed to particular areas or communities or families or to pregnant or lactating women, or to infants or preschoolers, or to some combination of these. Some programmes involve provision of food in centres. In other cases, food is distributed for consumption at home. The amount and kind of food provided varies considerably. Sources of food may be imported or local. In short, food supplementation takes many forms.

Food supplementation programmes, particularly those involving imported food that is given away, are controversial. Critics contend that the programmes undercut incentive to cultivate and consume perfectly good local alternatives; that the amounts given are often too small; that the supplements are usually not supplements but are substitutes so that total food intake remains the same; that the programmes are hard to manage logistically so lend themselves to misdirection and corruption; that programmes lack continuity, undercutting the potential effect when discontinuity involves substantial periods during a given year when food is not provided, and creating a problem at the time of early programme termination for those who have come to depend on the source of food and have adjusted their bodies accordingly.

Supporters of food supplementation, while recognizing problems, point to real benefits that well-conceived and administered programmes can bring, both direct benefits in terms of better nutritional status, and indirect benefits in terms of the convening power of food which brings people together in groups so that other actions can be taken as well. And, novel programmes are being developed that do not create dependency on outside sources, that promote local cultivation, and that help overcome both logistic and social problems by supporting community efforts (the promotion of school and community gardens in Zimbabwe and Tanzania are good examples).

Examples can easily be found of both successful and unsuccessful food supplementation programmes. It is our purpose to enter into the controversy, but it is clear that there are better and worse ways of setting about providing food supplements.

Most important for our argument is the fact that many supplementation programmes do not incorporate complementary programme elements that would help to improve the health and psychosocial development of children at the same time that they improve nutritional status. Too frequently, children who are gathered for feeding sit listlessly, propped against walls of the nutrition centre, waiting for their food when they could be participating in activities that would stimulate them and help to make good on the nutritional assistance. Too frequently, caregivers bring young children and either leave them for a period or stand idly by while the children are fed when they could be participating and learning about proper care and feeding. Or, food is distributed without, for instance, taking the opportunity to talk with parents about nutrition and health problems or about what might be done to overcome the frequent diarrhoea contributing to malnutrition.

In brief, food supplementation can provide the opportunity for related and complementary actions helping to improve early childhood development.

Nutrition recuperation

Nutrition recuperation centres are a special case of the food supplementation action described above. These centres treat children with severe malnutrition. The children are usually below the age of three and usually live in the centres while they are being treated. Evidence quoted earlier from Chile and Jamaica shows clearly that the addition of a stimulation component to the recuperation programme speeds the process of gaining weight while providing psychosocial benefits as well. Still, many recuperation programmes fail to incorporate activities responding to children's psychosocial needs. Making the combination may involve some additional training for personnel responsible for recuperation or the addition of caregivers to hold and cuddle and play with the children. These might be volunteers as in the Chilean example.

This nutritional action lends itself to a combination of nutritional and psychosocial activities. Given the demonstrated benefits, the relatively low cost involved, and the fact that intervention does not even require cooperation across bureaucratic lines, failing to make the combinations seems unforgivable. If, however, follow-up actions cannot be organized, the extra efforts in the centre may have no lasting impact.

Growth monitoring

The practice of periodic weighing in order to identify children in need of special attention and to detect growth faltering spread over a wide front during the 1980s. Growth charts are now relatively commonplace. The person responsible for weighing, recording, and interpreting the weight data is sometimes a professionally trained individual, sometimes a para-professional, and, less often, a parent or caregiver. The occasion for weighing also varies, occurring during home visits, health check-ups, as part of a centre-based child-care routine, in conjunction with food supplementation programmes, in nutrition centres, etc.

Depending on the circumstances of the weighing, growth monitoring can provide an excellent opportunity to combine nutritional and psychosocial programming. This is done, for instance, in some projects in India and Indonesia.

Nutrition education

Experience with various forms of nutrition education is accumulating and along with it a considerable evaluation and implementation literature (van der Vynckt 1987). Some education is directed to parents, some to school-children, and some to the public at large. Nutrition education may be made part of a regular school curriculum, incorporated into home visits, made the subject of a special adult education course, or carried out through the mass media. If nutrition education is provided using a strategy of educational communication directed towards families and communities, involving interpersonal exchanges and strengthening organization, its potential for integration is enhanced.

For the most part, nutrition education focuses on diet, i.e. on what children should be fed. As indicated, however, feeding should be treated as a social process as well and attention should be given to how children are fed (see appendix to this chapter).

Nutrition education, to be integrative, does not require the integration of bureaucratic structures; rather, integration occurs in combining content from the other areas with that of nutrition. Moreover, the same audiences that nutrition education programmes are intended to reach are often the very audiences that health and education and others will take as their focus. This convergence of interests could become the basis for cooperative production of materials incorporating information about health and psychosocial practices into nutrition education and vice versa in an attempt to respond in an integrated way to the combined needs of the child.

Promotion of breastfeeding and proper weaning

In breastfeeding, a natural combination of a nutritional and psychosocial action occurs. Both of these features can be promoted but the failure to consider feeding as a social and developmental as well as a nutritional process has led to neglect of the psychosocial side. The same is true of the treatment of weaning where, however, the combination is not as direct as in breastfeeding.

From the above, it is evident that some nutritional actions lend themselves better than others to incorporating a developmental component. Nutritional recuperation, food supplementation, promotion of breastfeeding and proper weaning, nutritional education, and growth monitoring are the most logical candidates for incorporating psychosocial development activities.

A programme example

The following example (taken from Kotchabhakdi 1988) brings together several of the programme suggestions that have been mentioned earlier. It is a particularly instructive example for several reasons:

– It focuses on young mothers and other caregivers attending to children from birth to age two.
– It incorporates both nutrition and psychosocial education components into primary health care and a national programme of growth monitoring and targeted supplementary feeding.
– The educational programme is based on previous study of nutritional status, and of caregiver knowledge, attitudes, and practices.
– The addition of the developmental component was based explicitly on the idea that nutrition and development are synergistically related. It focuses on the mother–child dyad and interactions, with the assumption that '... improved mother–child interaction would have a positive effect on child nutritional status, acting through improvements in maternal understanding of the child's need and better feeding of supplementary food (ibid., p. 2)
– An evaluation accompanied the combined education programme and showed significant results.

The context   Analyses by the Ministry of Health in Thailand pointed to three major constraints to significant reduction in the level of protein energy malnutrition (PEM) in infants and preschool children: 1) the inadequate coverage of the health system, 2) the lack of community awareness of the problem, and 3) the inadequate multisectorial input to the nutrition programme. Studies had shown also that, by themselves, income-generating projects did not necessarily have an impact on the problem.

Accordingly, the government, in 1979, introduced a programme of community-based primary health care together with a programme of growth monitoring, accompanied by a supplementary food programme and nutrition education, all within a national plan for poverty alleviation.

Within this programme mix, nutrition education was directed towards the families with the most vulnerable infants and preschool children. An important part of that nutrition education was a psychosocial component focusing on caregiver–child interactions and on the physical and social environment in which children were being raised.

In north-east Thailand there are usually more than two generations living together in the same house or in the vicinity. The women, including the mother, aunt, grandmother, and sisters, are responsible for child care. However, these women must also do the housework and participate in agricultural and other income-earning activities. The physical and mental condition of the mothers may, therefore, account in part for the lack of interaction between mothers and infants.

Values, beliefs and practices   A study of childrearing attitudes and practices revealed several attitudes and beliefs affecting the caregiver–child interactions:

- Few mothers recognized the visual, perceptual or auditory abilities of infants.
- Mothers displayed little awareness of their own capacity to make a difference in their child's development by making use of existing resources to create a more nurturing environment.
- When introducing semi-solid foods as supplementary to breastfeeding, many mothers would discontinue feeding when the child turned away or thrust out its tongue.
- A misbelief about colostrum and early suckling was associated with failure to begin breastfeeding immediately following birth.
- Although mothers breastfed, they did so with little understanding of its nutritional or psychosocial benefits and were ready to change to bottle feeding.
- Children are often seen lying in a closed cloth cradle.

Identifying these beliefs and practices helped to provide a basis for the combined nutrition and development education programme.

The education programme   A series of five interactive videos was created. One of the five was specifically oriented towards child development, aimed at creating maternal awareness of her child as an individual with early perceptual ability, and at recognizing the importance of play and of mother–child interaction in that play and in supplementary feeding. A second video compared two 15-month-old boys, one malnourished, the other normal, identifying behavioural as well as nutritional differences. The remaining videos dealt with cooking of supplementary food, the value of breastfeeding, and the nutritional value of five food groups.

Health communicators in each village, who also served as distributors of supplementary food, were trained in the use of the videos which were presented several times in each village.

Evaluation and results   On the basis of interviews with mothers of children under two years, and of observations in the home, the evaluators concluded that:

- Maternal knowledge about, and attitudes towards, infants' ability to see were significantly more positive after seeing the videos.
- More open cradles were found during home visits.
- Compared with mothers in villages where the video was not presented, a significant increase was found in the percentage of mothers reported giving colostrum to their newborns and in the percentage committed to early suckling right after delivery.
- Significantly more mothers responded to 'tongue thrusting' or disinterest in taking food by repeated tries and by playing with the child until the child took more food, rather than just discontinuing feeding.

These results suggest that visual messages, provided in a way that permits discussion, can bring about significant changes in beliefs and practices surrounding feeding, seen as a social as well as nutritional practice. In addition, educational communication can produce changes in the ways in which a caregiver establishes the environment for child development and interacts with infants. The method and the associated behavioural changes do not depend on literacy.

A concluding note

From the reading of this chapter should come several messages. Among the most important of these are:

1 There is a two-way, interactive relationship between psychosocial well-being and health and nutritional status. That synergistic relationship is evident in the results of research cutting across a broad spectrum of scientific disciplines. Accordingly, health, nutrition, and psychosocial well-being should be approached together, whether the principal goal of a programme is survival or growth or social or intellectual or emotional development.

2 Although there are many barriers to combining health, nutrition and psychosocial development, there is also a variety of ways to get around these barriers – conceptually, in policy and planning, in forms of organization and in setting programme content.

3 Several kinds of health and nutritional programmes lend themselves to incorporating a psychosocial development dimension. These include programmes of maternal and child health care, health and nutrition education, promotion of breastfeeding and proper weaning, food supplementation, and growth monitoring.

4 Because the ultimate and most desirable integration of health, nutrition and psychosocial well-being occurs in the beliefs and actions of family members and other caregivers, programmes of educational communication which facilitate integration in action should receive high priority.

5 Good examples of combined programmes exist to show that combination is possible and to provide useful models of how to do it – in a variety of ways, under varying conditions, and at relatively low cost, with potentially positive outcomes.

Against this background, there is no good substantive reason why programme elements cannot be combined, given the will to do so. Excuses for not making good on the rhetoric of integrated attention to health, nutrition, and psychosocial well-being of the young child are weak. The rationale is strong.

To move beyond rhetoric to action requires a strengthened belief that combined actions are really appropriate and needed, the political will to pursue that belief, and some retraining of health and nutrition personnel who will carry out the integration.

APPENDIX

Feeding as a social and developmental process

There is an unfortunate tendency to consider feeding exclusively as a nutritional activity. It is, however, a social and developmental activity as well. Psychosocial considerations associated with breastfeeding, bottle-feeding and weaning are discussed briefly below and three nutrition manuals are examined for their treatment of the feeding process.

Breastfeeding

Breastfeeding provides natural and frequent opportunities not only for touching and holding, but also for cuddling, exchanging glances, and talking and responding to the baby. All of these can contribute to its psychological and social health and development and have an influence on nutritional status.

In spite of the obvious and direct relationship, the promotion of breastfeeding gives little, and sometimes no, place to this dimension. Pictures are published and distributed in which the breastfeeding mother is not in eye contact with the child. In the advantages mentioned, social and psychological advantages tend to be omitted. This occurs in part because the promotion falls to nutritionists. An interdisciplinary effort would produce a better result.

Bottle-feeding

In discussions of the problems that can be associated with bottle-feeding, emphasis is correctly placed on over-diluting, on the frequent use of unclean water to dilute the milk, and on the insanitary conditions surrounding the process of drinking the milk (insanitary nipples, dropped bottles, etc.). Seldom mentioned are the convenient (for the caregiver) but negative (for the child) social consequences of 'bottle propping'. A child that is left alone with the bottle does not receive the warmth or interaction that holding the child can give. To the extent that a bottle is substituted for the breast at an earlier and earlier time, this withdrawal of a support for psychosocial development becomes more important.

Weaning

Most of the literature dealing with the weaning process (defined as the period from the first introduction of supplementary foods to the period of halting breastfeeding and/or bottle-feeding of milk) is directed exclusively to when the process should begin, to what kinds of locally available foods provide the best supplement to milk, and to the amount of supplementary food needed. These are the most important nutritional concerns. Little or no attention is given to social dimensions of weaning such as separation and self-feeding.

Separation   Occasionally, in anthropological literature, references will be made to a process in which a child is abruptly sent away from the mother in order to terminate the weaning process. The psychological effects of this practice are not well understood and some controversy exists over whether or not (or under what conditions) the practice results in unnecessary trauma (Timyan 1988). Sometimes, maternal separation is automatically equated with deprivation, i.e. with removal of stimulation through touch, sound, and movement, with a break in consistency, and with discontinuity in meaningful relationships. That view is a gross oversimplification.

In a detailed review of separation during early childhood, based for the most part on research in the United States and Europe, Yarrow (1964) concludes that psychosocial effects will depend on:

– Age at time of separation;
– The quality of the relationship with the mother prior to separation;

-   The character of maternal care subsequent to the separation;
-   The character of the relationship with family during the separation;
-   The duration of the separation;
-   Subsequent reinforcing experiences;
-   The role of constitutional factors in the child (differences in basic sensitivities to changes in kind and intensity of stimulation);
-   The constancy (or similarity) of old and new environments.

The most sensitive time of separation may be the period from about six months to two years, when the infant is establishing stable affectional relationships, both with the mother and others in the immediate surroundings (Yarrow 1964, p. 122). This is the period when most weaning takes place.

Self-feeding   In the weaning process and when weaning is completed, emphasis is sometimes placed on the child's learning to feed itself. This may be an adequate and good practice in the sense that it helps a child to develop coordination. It may help develop independence as well. Sometimes, however, self-feeding is begun too soon and a child does not get the amount of food that it needs. And, again, the question of interaction should be taken into consideration. The equivalent of bottle propping in which a child is left alone to feed should be avoided. Indeed, the positive deviance findings reported by Zeitlin *et al.* suggest that active feeding was a positive behaviour. It is borne out by recent research (Zeitlin *et al.*, n.d.).

An analysis of three nutrition manuals: feeding as a social process

If psychosocial elements are to be integrated into nutrition programmes, an integrated perspective should be incorporated into manuals. Unfortunately, the propensity to divorce the treatment of social, psychological, and nutritional themes related to child development carries over into the production of manuals and other materials used in training and programme implementation.

Instances of both isolated and combined treatments will be described briefly below in discussion of three manuals. The first two examples illustrate a cursory treatment of the social dimension of feeding and of early childhood development as it is related to nutrition. The third example demonstrates a more integrated view.

A missing psychosocial dimension: two examples

1 One widely distributed nutrition field manual, now in its third edition, is the *Manual on Feeding Infants and Young Children* by Margaret Cameron and Yngve Hofvander (1983). This manual was prepared under the auspices of the FAO/WHO/UNICEF Protein Advisory Group.

The manual is intended primarily for professional groups who have some basic knowledge of nutrition, child health, home economics, etc. Early childhood development, as first mentioned in a paragraph on page five, is treated exclusively in terms of the development of skills related to the functioning of the brain. An initial chapter dealing with risks and screening includes brief mention of development 'milestones', treated as a screening device, much as a growth chart.

The only mention of the social dimension of feeding is in relation to breastfeeding where two pictures make the points that 1) quiet confidence assures successful lactation and 2) breastfeeding establishes a close and happy contact between the mother and child. The effect of this quiet confidence and contact on the nutritional status of the child is implied but not explicit. In one of the pictures, the mother is looking at her child; in the other she is not. A paragraph labelled 'social aspects of breastfeeding' does not include anything about interaction between mother and child. A summary of advantages of breastfeeding has nothing about interaction or about psychosocial development. A chapter dealing with the management of breastfeeding has nothing about holding, gazing, interacting or talking. The same holds for a chapter on 'replacement feeding'. Guidelines for weaning do not include anything about mother–child interaction (or its absence).

2 Another prominent manual is titled *Improving the Nutritional Status of Children During the Weaning Period, A Manual for Policymakers, Program Planners, and Fieldworkers.* This manual was produced for the Office of Nutrition of the United States Agency for International Development by Karen Mitzner, Nevin Scrimshaw, and Robert Morgan in 1985.

The cover of the manual shows a woman feeding a child, but with the child turned towards the camera and away from the mother. In a chapter dealing with collecting information about feeding practices, attention is given to what is fed and to whether food is properly prepared, but none is given to the actual feeding practice or to mother–child interaction. A section on 'Feeding Techniques' does not deal with interaction, except to say that by the time the child is two years old it should be given its own portion of the family food and be allowed to eat by itself. There is no treatment in the book of the interaction between mother and child in feeding.

Towards incorporation of a psychosocial dimension

In a more positive vein is *Nutrition and Families* (Ritchie 1983), originally distributed as a *Manual on Child Development, Family Life and Nutrition.* The integrated tone is set in the introduction as follows:

> Successful progress from childhood to adulthood depends to a large extent on whether families and communities can provide children with

good nutrition and a healthy environment, and with the necessary care, encouragement and education to allow full and normal growth of body, mind, and emotions. The close relationship which mothers form with their babies and young children is of great value in early life, when important steps in children's growth occur. In Africa during the early years when children are on the breast, they rarely leave their mothers and close ties exist. After babies are weaned, however, they are usually quickly replaced by younger brothers or sisters and it is difficult for mothers to devote the time, energy and resources needed for the best development of the weaned children.

(p. 1)

The first substantive chapter of the manual is devoted to 'Child Development and Growth', treating mental and social–emotional development and physical growth in an integrated way. The discussion of breastfeeding includes the following:

African mothers are accustomed to having infants in the same bed with them and no African mother harms her child by overlying him. Separate beds for normal children with normal mothers should not be encouraged. In addition to the nutritional advantage to the child of suckling at night, the sharing of a bed by mother and child provides the child with warmth and security ...

(pp. 85–6)

A discussion of weaning states:

A mother should not send her newly weaned child away from her or put him in the care of people who do not know how to feed him properly.

(p. 92)

Practical learning experiences include examination of childrearing practices and conditions contributing to good physical, mental, emotional and social growth of children, the preparation of play materials, as well as practice with measuring growth, food preparation and other explicitly nutritional exercises.

In brief, although a stronger position might have been taken with respect to the synergistic nature of developmental components and actions, this manual does a relatively good job of bringing together in one place the various dimensions of development. It illustrates that a thoughtful combination of psychosocial and nutritional components is possible within a nutrition manual.

NOTE

1   This was provided by Dr John Hillman.

REFERENCES

Atkin, L. 'Analysis of Instruments Used in Latin America to Measure Psychosocial Development in Children from 0 to 6 Years of Age', Mexico City: Instituto Nacional de Perinatologia, 1989. A paper prepared for the Consultative Group on Early Childhood Care and Development. Mimeo.

Barrett, D.E., M. Radke-Yarrow and R.E. Klein. 'Chronic Malnutrition and Child Behavior: Effects of Early Caloric Supplementation on Social and Emotional Functioning at School Age', *Developmental Psychology*, Vol 18, No. 4 (1982), pp. 541–56.

Berg, A. and S. Brehm. 'Micronutrient Deficiencies: Present Knowledge of Effects and Control', Technical Note 86–32, World Bank, Population, Health, and Nutrition Department, Washington, DC, 1986.

Bowlby, J. *Attachment.* New York: Basic Books, 1969.

Brazleton, T.B. 'Early Intervention. What Does It Mean?' *Theory and Research in Behavioural Pediatrics*, Vol. 1 (1982), pp. 1–34.

Cameron, M. and Y. Hofvander. *Manual on Feeding Infants and Young Children.* Third Edition. Oxford: Oxford University Press, 1983. Prepared under the auspices of the FAO/WHO/UNICEF Protein Advisory Group.

Chávez, A., H. Martínez, L. Allen and G.H. Pelto. 'The Collaborative Research and Support Program on Food Intake and Human Function: Mexico Project, Final Report', a report submitted to USAID, 15 November, 1987.

Chávez, A. and C. Martínez. *Growing Up in a Developing Community.* Guatemala City: Institute of Nutrition of Central America and Panama (INCAP), 1982. (Original in Spanish, published by Nueva Editorial Interamericana, S.A., Mexico, 1979.)

Chess, S. and A. Thomas. 'Infant Bonding: Mystique and Reality', *American Journal of Orthopsychiatry*, Vol. 52, No. 2 (1982), pp. 213–22.

Coppo, P. (ed.) *Medecine Traditionnelle, Psychiatrie et Psychologie en Afrique.* Rome: Il Pensiero Scientifico Editore, 1988.

Crnic, L.S. 'Effects of Nutrition and Environment on Brain Biochemistry and Behavior', *Development Psychology*, No. 16 (1983), pp. 129–45.

Dobbing, J. (ed.) *Early Nutrition and Later Achievement.* London: Academic Press, Inc., 1987.

Erny, P. *L'enfant dans la pensée traditionnelle de l'Afrique noire.* Paris: Le Livre Africain, 1968.

Evans, J. 'The Utilization of Early Childhood Care and Education Programmes for Delivery of Maternal and Child Health Components of Primary Health Care: A Framework for Decision-Making', a paper prepared for a meeting organized by the World Health Organisation on 'Day Care as an Entry Point for Maternal and Child Health Components of Primary Health Care', Paris, 26–29 May, 1986. Mimeo.

Field, T. 'Interventions for Premature Infants', *The Journal of Pediatrics*, Vol 129, No. 1 (July 1986), pp. 183–91.

Field, T., S. Schanberg, F. Scapidi, C. Bauer, N. Vega-Lahr, R. Garcia, J. Nystrom and C. Kuhn. 'Tactile/kinesthetic Stimulation Effects on Pre-term Neonates', *Pediatrics*, Vol. 77, No. 5 (May 1986), pp. 654–8.

Ganellen, R.J. and P.H. Blaney. 'Hardiness and Social Support as Moderators of the Effects of Life Stress', *Journal of Personality and Social Psychology*, Vol. 4, No. 1 (1984), pp. 156–63.

Garmezy, N. and M. Rutter (eds) *Stress, Coping and Development in Children.* New York: McGraw-Hill Book Company, 1983.

Gentry, W.D. and S.C. Kobasa. 'Social and Psychological Resources Mediating

Stress–Illness Relationships in Humans', Chapter 4 in W.D. Gentry (ed.) *Handbook of Behavioral Medicine*. New York: Guilford, 1984, pp. 87–116.

Grantham-McGregor, S. 'Rehabilitation Following Malnutrition', in J. Brozek and B. Schurch (eds), *Malnutrition and Behavior: Critical Assessment of Key Issues*. Lausanne, Switzerland: the Nestle Foundation, 1984.

Harlow, H. and M.H. Harlow. 'Learning to Love', *American Scientist*, Vol. 54, No. 3 (1966), pp. 244–72.

Instituto Nacional Indigenista, 'Memoria del Primer Encuentro de Medicina Indigena de la Mixteca "Oaxaquena y Poblana"', Santiago Apoala, Nochixtlan, Oaxaca, Diciembre de 1986.

Jemmott, J.B. and S.E. Locke. 'Psychosocial Factors, Immunologic Mediation, and Human Susceptibility to Infectious Diseases: How Much Do We Know?', *Psychological Bulletin*, Vol 95, No. 1 (1984), pp. 78–104.

Klaus, M. and J.K. Kennell (eds). *Maternal Infant Bonding*. St Louis: C.V. Mosby, 1982.

Kotchabhakdi, N. 'A Case Study: The Integration of Psychosocial Components of Early Childhood Development into a Nutrition Education Programme of Northeast Thailand', a paper prepared for the Third Inter-Agency Meeting of the Consultative Group on Early Childhood Care and Development, Washington DC, January 12–14, 1988.

Krantz, D. and D. Glass. 'Personality, Behavior Patterns, and Physical Illness: Conceptual and Methodological Issues', Chapter 3 in W.D. Gentry (ed.) *Handbook of Behavioral Medicine*. New York: Guilford, 1984, pp. 38–86.

Lamb, M. 'Maternal Attachment and Mother Neonate Bonding: A Critical Review', *Advances in Developmental Psychology, Vol. 2*. Hillsdale, NJ: Lawrence Erlbaum Associates, 1982, pp. 1–39.

Landers, C. 'Biological, Cultural, and Social Determinants of Infant Development in a South Indian Community', in K. Nugent, B.M. Lester, and T.B. Brazleton (eds) *The Cultural Context of Infancy*. New York: Ablex Press, 1989.

Locke, S.E. 'Stress, Adaptation, and Immunity: Studies in Humans', *General Hospital Psychiatry*, No. 4 (1982), pp. 49–58.

McGuire, J. and J. Austin. 'Beyond Survival: Children's Growth for National Development', *Assignment Children*, No. 2 (1987), pp. 1–52.

Mitzner, K., N. Scrimshaw and R. Morgan (eds) *Improving the Nutritional Status of Children During the Weaning Period, A Manual for Policymakers, Program Planners and Field Workers*, Washington DC: United States Agency for International Development, 1985.

Monckeberg, F. 'Nutritional Rehabilitation in Severe Early Marasmus', in *Proceedings of the xviiith World Congress of OMEP*, Jerusalem, Israel, July 13–17, 1986.

Myers, R. 'Programming for Early Childhood Development and Growth', a document prepared for the UNESCO–UNICEF Cooperative Programme. New York: the Consultative Group on Early Childhood Care and Development, June, 1988.

Negussie, B. *Traditional Wisdom and Modern Development, A Case Study of Traditional Peri-natal Knowledge among Elderly Women in Southern Shewa, Ethiopia*. Stockholm: University of Stockholm, Institute of International Education, 1988. Studies in Comparative and International Education, No. 13.

Newton, G. and S. Levine (eds) *Early Experience and Behavior*. Springfield, Illinois: Thomas, 1988.

Nikapota, A.D. 'Case Study for Sri-Lanka – Child Development in Primary Health Care', a paper prepared for UNICEF/Sri Lanka and the Ministry of Health of Sri Lanka, and presented to the Innocenti Technical Workshop on Psychosocial Development, Florence, Italy, 1990.

Pollitt, E. 'A Critical View of Three Decades of Research on the Effects of Chronic

Energy Malnutrition on Behavioral Development', a paper presented at the meeting of the International Dietary Energy Consultative Group, Institute of Nutrition of Central America and Panama, Guatemala City, Guatemala, August 3–7, 1987. Mimeo.

Pollitt, E. and E. Metallinos-Katsaras. 'Iron Deficiency and Behavior: Constructs, Methods and Validity of the Findings', in Wurtman and Wurtman (eds) *Nutrition and the Brain: Vol. 8. Behavioral Effects of Metals, and their Biochemical Mechanisms*. New York: Raven Press, 1990, pp. 101–46.

Ritchie, J. *Nutrition and Families*. Revised edition. London: Macmillan Education, Ltd, 1983.

Rutter, M. 'Resilience in the Face of Adversity, Protective Factors and Resistance to Psychiatric Disorder', *British Journal of Psychiatry*, No. 147 (1985), 598–611.

Schanberg, S.M., G. Evoniuk and C.M. Kuhn. 'Tactile and Nutritional Aspects of Maternal Care: Specific Regulators of Neuroendocrine Function and Cellular Development', *Proceedings of the Society of Experimental Biological Medicine*, No. 175 (1984), pp. 135–46.

Scheper-Hughes, N. 'Culture, Scarcity, and Maternal Thinking: Maternal Detachment and Infant Survival in a Brazilian Shantytown', *Ethos*, Vol. 13, No. 2 (1985), pp. 291–317.

Smart, J. 'The Need for and the Relevance of Animal Studies of Early Undernutrition', in J. Dobbing (ed.) *Early Nutrition and Later Achievement*. London: Academic Press, Inc., 1987.

Soemantri, A.G., E. Pollitt and I. Kim. 'Iron Deficiency Anemia and Educational Achievement', *The American Journal of Clinical Nutrition*, Vol. 42 (December 1985), pp. 1221–8.

Super, C., M.G. Herrera and J.O. Mora. 'Long term effects of nutritional supplementation and psychosocial intervention on the physical growth of Columbian infants at risk of malnutrition', Boston, Harvard School of Public Health, April 1987. Mimeo.

Timyan, J. 'Cultural Aspects of Psycho-social Development: An Examination of West African Childrearing Practices', a report prepared for UNICEF, Office for the West African Region, Abidjan, January, 1988.

UNICEF. 'UNICEF/WHO Joint Study on Proposals for Collaborative Action in Child Mental Health and Psychosocial Development', a paper prepared for the Executive Board of UNICEF. Doc: E/ICEF/L.1389, New York: UNICEF, January 19, 1979.

van der Vynckt, S. *Show and Tell*. Paris: UNESCO, 1985. Document ED/85/WS/12.

Victora, C.G., F.C. Barros and J.P. Vaughn. *Epidemiologia de Desigualdade, um estudo longitudinal de 6000 criancas brasileiras*. San Paulo: Editora Hucitec, 1988.

Werner, E.E. *Cross-Cultural Child Development, A View from the Planet Earth*. Monterey, California: Brooks/Cole Publishing Company, 1979.

Werner, E.E. and R. Smith. *Vulnerable but Invincible, A Longitudinal Study of Resilient Children and Youth*. New York: McGraw-Hill Book Company, 1982.

WHO–UNICEF. 'Primary Health Care', Alma Ata Declaration, 1978.

WHO, The Constitution, adopted by the United Nations Conference on July 22, 1946 and entered into force on September 1, 1948.

WHO, 'Progress Report on the Activities of Physical Growth and Psycho-Social Development (September 1988–April 1990),' WHO, programme of Maternal and Child Health, Geneva, Switzerland, 1990.

Wu, in A.J. Marsella and G.M. White (eds) *Cultural Conceptions of Mental Health and Therapy. Vol. 4. Culture, Illness and Healing*. Dordrecht, Holland: Reidel, 1982.

Yarrow, L. 'Separation from Parents during Early Childhood', *Review of Child Development Research*, Vol. 1 (1964), pp. 89–136.

Zeitlin, M., H. Ghassemi and M. Mansour. *Positive Deviance in Child Nutrition, with Emphasis on Psychosocial and Behavioural Aspects and Implications for Development.* Tokyo: The United Nations University, 1990.

Zeitlin, M., F.C. Johnson and R. House. 'Active Maternal Feeding and Nutritional Status of 8–20 Month Old Low-income Mexican Children', draft, n.d.

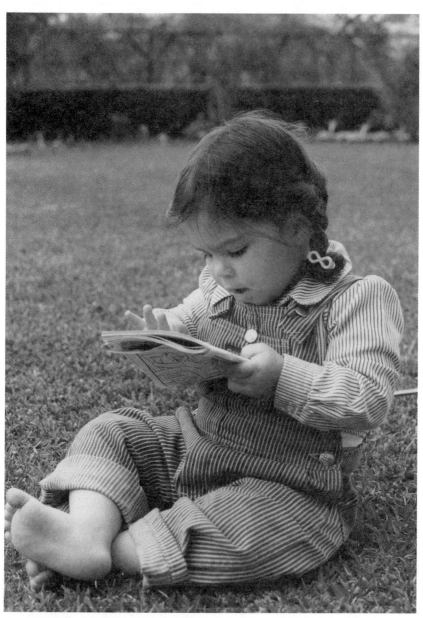

'Carolina plays at reading', Jalapa, Mexico

Chapter 10

Relating child development to schooling and beyond[1]

Child development is a continuous process set within the larger process of human development. Our focus has been on the early years – on the child as she grows and develops to age six. But physical, social, and mental development obviously do not stop at age six. Indeed, this is the age when most children are about to make an important adjustment in their life: they will go to school. The manner in which this change is handled and the resulting success or failure in primary school will affect all of later life, and carries effects into the next generation.

Schools are different from homes, often dramatically so. They differ not only in the physical setting and the people with whom the child will interact, but also in activities, expectations and rules of conduct and in ways of learning. Many of the millions of children entering primary school for the first time this year will be expected to speak in an unfamiliar language, to pay attention for long periods of time, to relate to a large group of children their own age, to use abstract symbols, and to do other things that are not part of their normal routine. Inability to cope with these differences will make the new experience difficult – even traumatic (see Table 10.1).

There are differences also between organizations and agencies responsible for schools and those that work with the child and the family in the home and community during the preschool years. This artificial division emphasizes rather than moderates differences and leads to uncoordinated programming that is not in the best interests of the children or of the respective institutions involved. The division disregards the fact that the child who leaves home is the same child that arrives at school and that previous experiences influence in important ways what happens upon entering school.

The articulation between home and school increasingly includes passage through one or more programmes explicitly or implicitly designed, among other goals, to affect the child's readiness for school. The impressive growth of preschool, child-care and other early childhood programmes in the Third World was documented in Chapter 2. These diverse initiatives –

Table 10.1 Comparing home and school learning environments

Home	School
– Parent-child relationship informal, loving	– Teacher-child relationship more formal, less personal
– Learning through imitation, trial and error, doing	– Learning through didactic teaching, memorization
– Flexibility in actions	– Regimentation
– Integration into immediate environment	– Separation of child from environment
– Adjustment to interests and needs of the child	– Child expected to adjust to needs of the school
– Emphasis on the concrete	– Use of symbols
– Active participation in events of household	– Passive role in events of school
– Learning in mother tongue	– Learning in national language
– Emphasis on language comprehension	– Emphasis on language production
– Emphasis on process	– Emphasis on results

Note: The above are obviously caricatures. Some teachers can develop personal relationships with the child, respond to individual needs and interests, emphasize process, etc. Some parents are not capable of providing the informal, loving relationship usually assumed for the home. In some cultures, socialization prior to entering school is very controlled, with emphasis on results and considerable attention to memorizing instructions, rhymes, etc. (so that a school attempting a more active learning method would conflict with the home, reversing what we have indicated above).

providing different combinations of education, health, nutrition, early stimulation, and sometimes other components, in programmes of direct attention, parental education, and community development – are the focus of this chapter. We shall pay particular attention to programmes as they affect psychosocial development.

One basic argument of this book is that programmes of early childhood development can be a good investment. One test of that lies in whether children who participate in such programmes are better prepared for schooling, and are more likely to enter school and to do well than those who have not participated. The potential effects of early childhood programmes on school-going capture the attention of policymakers and planners seeking ways to increase educational performance and to reduce costs through reduced repetition and dropout. And, parents often expect these programmes to give their child a 'head start', easing the transition from the social world of the home to that of the school and the larger society. Whether or not intervention programmes really have the schooling effects hoped for is, therefore, a critical question.

Clarifications

1 *Goals other than schooling are also important.* We will examine studies that look at effects on school-going and performance. But effects on schooling are obviously not the only, and may not be the most important, effects of early childhood programmes. By focusing here on schooling effects, we do not mean to exclude or give less importance to other goals of early childhood development such as improving children's physical health, providing child care for working parents, rehabilitating children who are disabled, inculcating particular values, and generally improving children's quality of life. Our position in the rest of the book should make that clear.

Moreover, we shall argue that the appropriate way to approach this topic is *not* in terms of the usual concept of transition to school. Rather, we should see the school as one of several learning environments in which a child functions (including the home). In most cases a child does not leave the home to enter school but remains very much a part of a family. Conceptualizing the entry into school as a 'transition' *from* home *to* school puts undue emphasis on school and tends to devalue the home as a place for learning. Our concern, therefore, should be centred on the ability of a child to learn in various environments rather than on learning as if that occurred only in schools (Myers 1990).

2 *Readiness for school involves more than cognitive and social readiness.* A second clarification arises from the fact that many early intervention programmes seeking to prepare children for school deal only with cognitive and social dimensions of development. Our interest is much broader, however, including programmes designed to affect nutrition and health, as well as the intellectual and social development of children. This view is particularly necessary in the Third World where health and nutrition states are often determinant, and given the interactions between psychosocial well-being and health and nutritional status, as discussed in the previous chapter.

3 *Schools as well as children need to adjust.* The idea that children should be ready for school is more common than the equally important idea that schools should be ready for children. Somehow, there seems to be an assumption that the availability and characteristics of schools are fixed and children should be adjusted to them. Schools are less often expected to adjust to the characteristics of children. However, it may be as reasonable to expect schools, for instance, to change their initial language of instruction as it is to expect a child to arrive with mastery of an 'official' language that is not the mother tongue. Or, it may be as reasonable to expect curricula to vary from region to region as it is to base the curriculum on

centrally determined, standardized material that is not recognizable or relevant to many children entering the primary school.

We will argue that readiness of children for school and the school's readiness for the child interact and should be considered together.

4 *Family and community influences are also important.* Finally, although we shall place a great deal of emphasis on the child in this chapter, readiness of the child for school involves family and community conditions and characteristics, not just characteristics of the child. Therefore, programmes directed to improving the conditions surrounding the child are as important as programmes which focus on the child.

With these clarifications in mind, we shall present evidence suggesting that:

- programmes designed to improve health, nutrition, and the psycho-social condition of children in their preschool years can affect school readiness significantly;
- better prepared children will be more likely to attend school and to perform at a higher level than less well prepared children;
- the effects can favour children who are at a social disadvantage;
- the programmes can also have a positive effect on the functioning of the primary school system by increasing both the efficiency and quality of the system; and
- the longer-term social and economic effects of early programmes as they operate through schooling can be very strong.

A FRAMEWORK FOR ANALYSIS

Guiding our analysis and discussion of the relationship between home (or the experience of the preschool child) and school is the integrative framework presented in Figure 10.1. The framework distinguishes three periods of time – from birth to the time of entry into school, the time in school, and a 'post-school' period that could begin immediately if a child never enrols, or following dropout, or in adolescence or early adulthood.

Development throughout the life span is seen as a process of interaction between a changing individual and a changing environment, with four levels of environment entering into the process. These environmental levels correspond more or less to those set out by Bronfenbrenner (1979) and emerging from the general analysis in Chapter 4. They are the same levels – family, community, institutional, and societal – that are used to define the complementary approaches to programmes of care and development set out in Chapter 5 and described with examples in Chapters 6 and 7.

Birth to school-age   Even at birth, a child is learning. The newborn brings to the learning process physical capacities (the senses, a developing central nervous system, reflexes, vocalization) and a particular temperament

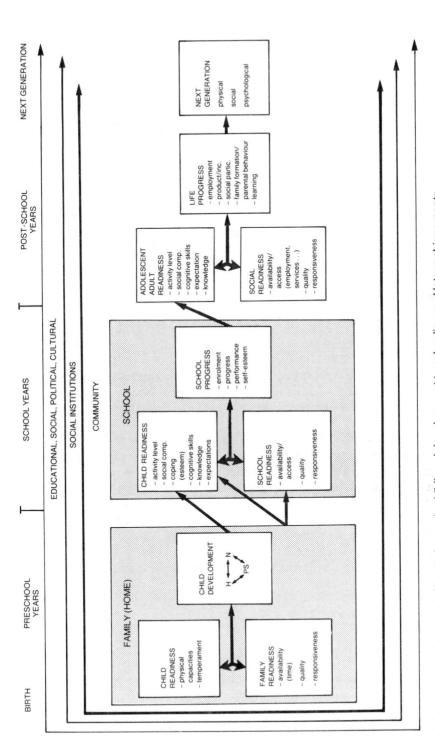

Figure 10.1 A framework for relating early childhood development to schooling and later achievements

(both individual drive and motivation and a social drive). These characteristics, which define the 'readiness' of the newborn child, are affected by what has happened during the prenatal period. The readiness of the child at this neonatal stage is indicated by such measures as birthweight and the Apgar or Brazleton scales. As the child develops during the first months and years of life, these capacities can be recognized, drawn upon and sharpened, or they can be allowed to deteriorate. The path followed will depend in large part on the family environment.

A family can be more or less well prepared to help a child develop. Family 'readiness' is in part a matter of the *availability* of different family members, the *quality* of the care they provide, and their *ability to respond* to the particular condition and capacity of each child. This readiness will be conditioned by such family characteristics as size and composition, the spacing of children, employment and income levels, and childrearing knowledge, attitudes and beliefs, and practices. These will, in turn, be influenced by the community, institutional, and larger sociocultural contexts within which families function.

In the preschool period, child readiness (which changes as the child matures) and family readiness (which changes as family characteristics change) interact, influencing each other. A child's changing state of well-being is reflected in the health and nutritional and psychosocial condition of the child at any point in time. Changing environmental variables at the levels of community, social institutions, and the sociocultural context also enter constantly into this process.

The school years   At the point of school entrance, the level of the child's development helps to define what we have called 'the readiness of children for school'. We shall return to that concept and to the interaction of the child's readiness with the readiness of schools for children as these jointly influence school enrolment, progress and performance during the primary school years. Our focus in this chapter is on that interaction and period (depicted in the central portion of Figure 10.1). First, however, we shall complete the progression that relates early development to adult achievement and beyond and which helps to set the rationale for investment during the early years.

Beyond schooling   When a child leaves school, the physical, social and mental capabilities that have been acquired (or allowed to wither) in school interact with what might be called 'the readiness of society' to receive school leavers – by the availability of employment and services, their quality, and the ability of the society to respond to the particular needs and characteristics of progressive waves of school graduates or leavers. This interaction, again within particular community, institutional and larger societal contexts, will lead to a set of outcomes over a lifetime and into the next generation.

Let us focus for the moment on the effects of primary schooling on adult characteristics and behaviours. A growing body of literature indicates that even a few years of schooling can bring important changes in skills, outlooks, and possibilities that are associated with greater economic productivity, greater solidarity and social participation, decreased fertility, and better health, nutrition, and child-care practices.

Effects on skills and outlooks   During the 1970s and 1980s a body of research began to accumulate showing that attainment of even a few years of schooling is associated with important changes in individual skills and outlooks. For example, schooled children show 'an awareness of what one knows, needs to know, and how to get needed knowledge' (Raizen and Bobrow 1974, p. 127). That is at least in part because becoming literate provides greater access to more sources of information. But schooled children also tend to be more selective in their use of information, have the ability to transfer knowledge from one situation to another, organize discrete bits of information into meaningful categories, and are more able to shift to alternative explanations (Rogoff 1980; Triandis 1980). Schooling was shown to be associated with a more 'modern' outlook (Inkeles and Smith 1974).

Effects on adult behaviour   In addition, research began to establish during the 1970s that the changes in individual skills and outlooks associated with primary schooling are related to greater economic productivity (Colclough 1980; Lockheed, Jamison, and Lau 1980; Moock 1981), to greater technological adaptiveness (Grawe 1979), to decreased fertility (e.g. Birdsall 1980), and to better health and nutrition and child-care practices (Levine 1980).

Further, studies of economic rates of return to different levels of schooling suggested that, in most places, primary schooling yielded a higher rate of return on the money spent than did secondary or university education (Psacharopoulous 1986).

Intergenerational effects   The effects of primary schooling on skills, outlooks and behaviours can be expected to extend across generations. Greater prospects of employment provide a better income base which increases not only the immediate standard of living but is related also to the participation of the next generation in schooling. Reduced fertility, linked to female education, creates better conditions for rearing the next generation, beginning with the fact that more mothers are likely to live. Also, with fewer children to care for, more attention can be given to each child. And, it is established that mothers with more schooling tend to have teaching styles more congruent with those their children will experience in school (Laosa 1982).

Together, these varied results, extracted from several different bodies of research, provide impressive evidence that the benefits to society as well as to individuals of primary schooling are substantial. But the effects of schooling on skills, outlooks, and later performance not only provide a rationale for investment in primary schools. To the extent that early child-hood programmes increase the progress and performance in primary school – and we shall show that they can have a strong effect – the invest-ment in such programmes will also bring a high return.

Against this larger picture, we turn now to the interaction between the readiness of children for school and the readiness of schools for children as these influence schooling and the outcomes of schooling.

READINESS OF CHILDREN FOR SCHOOL

A child's readiness for school is defined in terms of his/her activity level (health and nutritional status, affecting attendance, attention and concen-tration), social competencies and psychological preparedness (which affect the ability to cope with different learning environments), and cognitive abilities, including pre-literacy and pre-numeracy skills. Readiness is reflected also in the expectations the family holds for the child which relate also to the support they are ready to provide.

Health and nutrition   In the previous chapter, we discussed the syner-gistic relationship among health, nutrition, and psychosocial processes, as they jointly affect survival and development. Poor health will affect negatively the child's level and quality of activity in school, as well as school attendance patterns (Moock and Leslie 1986; Popkin and Lim-Ybanez 1982). Berg (1981) reports that in some Latin American countries children miss as much as a third of scheduled school days a year due to illness and poor health. The result may be a need to repeat a school year and/or early dropout. Thus, the child that has a continuing history of sickness is not as ready for active participation in school as a healthy child; progress and performance in school will be at risk.

Nutritional status also affects activity levels. Malnourished children (suffering protein or energy or vitamin and mineral deficiencies) are less active, less able to concentrate on learning activities and less interested in the environment than are well-nourished peers. The irritability, listlessness and distractibility of the hungry, malnourished schoolchild have been widely noted. More specifically, recent research shows clearly that there is a causal relationship between iron deficiency and school performance and that programmes to provide iron can have an effect (Pollitt and Metallinos-Katsaras 1990). Soemantri, Pollitt, and Kim (1985), working with children in an economically deprived rural area of central Java, Indonesia, have shown that a three-month iron supplementation intervention was associated with significant changes in their performance on school achievement and concentration tests (p. 1127). Similar results are now available for programmes in India (Seshadri and Gopaldas 1989) and Thailand (Pollitt *et al.* 1989).

As suggested in Chapter 9, less active infants may also be less socially attractive to caregivers, further reducing their ability to extract the responses that are essential to their well-being (Chávez and Martínez 1979). How this relationship is played out in schools is not as clear. The same principle may apply to the teacher–child relationship as to the caregiver–infant relationship. Teachers in primary school may be more inclined to work with children who are alert and demanding than with those who are listless and socially retiring. However, there is a great deal of anecdotal evidence suggesting that teachers often see active, curious young pupils as behaviour problems causing difficulties rather than presenting opportunities. In such cases, the effect of improved activity levels could be negative. Here, we see a good example of the interaction between the readiness of children for school and the readiness of schools (in this case the teachers) for children.

Intellectual and social competencies   As suggested in Table 10.1, the cognitive skills that parents (and various preschool programmes) inculcate in children are not always consonant with those skills that school will demand. For example, parents may promote primarily concrete use of language and concrete classification skills, whereas schools demand relatively more abstract and representational use of language, and classification skills based on more abstract qualities of objects (Haglund 1982). There is evidence that explicit literacy-nurturing activities are not a part of most poor children's early childhood experience in the developing countries (Pollitt 1984). To the extent that this is true, the ability to deal with the abstract and disembedded learning that is typical of some schooling will be a difficult one for these children.

Readiness is also defined by the degree of self-esteem of a young child. Children with high self-esteem are more capable of coping and adjusting to new conditions than children who are insecure and already caught up in the culture of failure.

Parental knowledge and expectations   The framework presented in Figure 10.1 suggests that a family's knowledge, attitudes or goals, and practices will have important effects on the nutrition, health and psychosocial condition of their children. Within the limits of economic possibilities and knowledge, parents take decisions about feeding and diet, about preventive and curative health care, and about the frequency and quality of psychosocial interactions they will have with their children. These decisions can lead to enhanced or impaired school readiness. These decisions will be influenced by the expectations that a parent holds for a child.

In summary, readiness of children for school (and more generally, for life beyond the home) is a product of the child's condition and family attitudes and practices, as these are influenced by the more general social and cultural surroundings.

THE READINESS OF SCHOOLS FOR CHILDREN

A brief historical note will help to put the primary school part of our discussion in perspective.

Expansion of primary schooling

One of the extraordinary achievements of the three decades prior to 1990 was the spread of primary schooling. For instance:

- In Sub-Saharan Africa, the enrolment ratio for primary school (i.e. the number of students enrolled compared with the number of children of primary school age) rose from 36 per cent to 75 per cent (of the age group that primary school is supposed to serve) in the 23 years between 1960 and 1983. For girls, the ratio rose from 24 per cent to 63 per cent (World Bank, January 1988).
- During the period from 1965 to 1985, the enrolment ratio rose from 75 to 104 per cent in 'lower middle-income' countries (GNP between US$460 and US$1570 for 1986), according to figures from the World Bank (June 1988). For girls, the increase was from 66 to 100 per cent. Bhutan, which began with the lowest enrolment ratio of all countries, increased its overall enrolment from 7 to 25 per cent and the enrolment of girls from 1 to 18 per cent. From 1960 to 1986, the enrolment ratio in India in classes 1 to 5 rose from 62 to 94 per cent (GOI 1989). Other low-income countries also showing impressive gains in the 1965 to 1985 period included:

	Total (%)	Girls (%)
Nepal	20 to 79	4 to 47
Mozambique	37 to 84	26 to 74
Tanzania	32 to 72	25 to 85
Zambia	53 to 103	46 to 96

Even allowing for some exaggeration, and recognizing that not all countries increased at this same rate, one has to admit to impressive growth of primary schooling. Why?

Changing conditions

Primary school growth was driven in the 1960s and early 1970s by favourable economic and political circumstances, combined with the increasing belief that education was a good investment for both individuals and nations. In the 1960s, the expansion of schooling had considerable political pay-off in both new nations and old states of Africa, Asia, Latin America and the Middle East. Expansion responded to a strong demand in many places, sometimes because, with the addition of a school building, a community acquired a certain prestige as well as the possibility of educating its young. Many leaders of new nations had at one time or another been teachers and believed in the value of education. They provided models as well. Moreover, the spread of schooling in new states was seen as a part of a democratizing process, essential to decolonization.

During the 1960s and early 1970s, world economic conditions were reasonably good, with relatively high growth rates helping to provide funds for investment. And, loan funds were available for educational investments (mostly school buildings) on what, at the time, seemed to be good terms. Internationally, economists were just rediscovering the value of education as an investment in human capital, providing an economic justification to go along with the perceived political and social benefits.

Even as the expansion of schooling occurred throughout the 1960s and 1970s, the conditions supporting that expansion began to deteriorate. By the early 1980s, the push from unmet demand was weakening. In a significant number of countries, communities that most wanted a primary school had it. Families whose children were not already in school usually had strong economic or moral reasons for keeping them out. Moreover, the deteriorating economic conditions associated with worldwide recession helped to moderate demand (Berstecher and Carr-Hill 1990). From a situation of satisfying demand, governments were turning to the more difficult task of creating additional demand and of reaching the unreachable.

In the 1970s and continuing into the 1980s, international economic conditions shifted, requiring many countries to cut budgets (Colclough and Lewin 1990). The problem of international debt began to influence availability of local funds and of international aid. Moreover, the initial enthusiasm by international funding agencies for education as an investment waned, at least in part because unrealistically high expectations had not been met.

Also affecting expansion, political conditions deteriorated in many Latin American and African countries. As new élites settled in, as destabilization occurred, and as the number of authoritarian governments increased, there was less push for democratization through schooling. As coverage increased, less political mileage could be gained from building schools.

As important for our purposes, much of the expansion that occurred was based on models of schooling that had served a colonial or élite population in earlier years. Moreover, ideas and school designs and materials were imported that were not in line with local needs and strengths, often as part of a programme of international assistance. Schools did not begin with the people. In addition, with growth of the schooling bureaucracy, standardization began to occur, making it ever more difficult for local adjustments to take place – in materials or scheduling or teacher training, for instance.

In brief, expansion of primary schooling was impressive during these 30 years. That expansion has brought with it an increasing gap between the organization and content of schooling and the needs and abilities which the population it is meant to serve brings to the school (Coombs 1985). During the 30-year period, conditions changed so that, throughout the 1970s and on into the early 1980s, the favourable conditions that had propitiated investments in schooling turned around. This change has slowed the growth of primary schooling (and in some areas led to a mild decline) but, more importantly, it has occurred just as many school systems were poised to confront problems of inefficiency and lagging quality in the wake of their expansion.

Lagging quality and efficiency

Although primary schooling has spread dramatically, the quality of primary schooling has not kept pace. Teachers are often poorly trained, lack motivation, and may be involved in competing activities. Educational materials are scarce. Roofs leak. The number of days a school is actually in operation may be low.

The problem of quality is present despite some concerted efforts to change content as well as coverage of schooling. For instance:

> In nearly every part of sub-Saharan Africa, texts have been adapted and new texts written so that basic skills are now taught with reference to African customs, the local environment, and the area's own history. Twenty-one of the thirty-nine countries in the region officially begin instruction in one or more African languages rather than asking children to use a European language as the medium of instruction from their first day in school.
>
> (World Bank 1988, p. 14)

The often unfavourable conditions of the school interact with cultural and socioeconomic circumstances of families to produce high rates of dropout and repetition. Continuing with the Sub-Saharan example:

> ... repeaters account for about 16 per cent of all enrolment, and because

of dropout, only 61 per cent of those who enter the first grade reach the final grade of primary school. As a result, it is estimated that the cost of each completer in the median country of Sub-Saharan Africa is 50 per cent higher than if there were no repetition and dropout.

(ibid., p. 50)

In several countries of Africa, the cost of dropout and repetition is much higher than the 50 per cent median (e.g. Guinea-Bissau = 430 per cent).

In Latin America, official statistics show repetition rates in the first grade of primary school that range up to 32 per cent (Nicaragua), with the average for the region at about 20 per cent. The repetition level is even higher if one adds dropout in the first year, most of which is temporary and really a form of repetition (UNESCO, ED-87 MINEDLAC/Ref. 2). Repetition has actually increased in the last decade, and in 1988 one of every four or five children in primary school in Latin America was a repeater (Schiefelbein 1988).

We shall argue below that improving the readiness of children for school can improve the quality and efficiency of school systems. Indeed, to put it in crass economic terms, children are probably the most important 'input' into schooling as well as its most important 'output'. To the extent that that is so, the argument for investing in early childhood programmes is strengthened.

What is meant by the readiness of schools for children?

The readiness of schools for children is defined by the *availability* of schooling (coverage and placement and days in session), by *quality* (of teachers, facilities and materials, methods), and, most importantly, by the *responsiveness* of schools to local needs and circumstances (language, adjustment of curriculum and methods to local values and circumstances, adjustment of school schedules, provision of food and health attention where needed, etc.). These readiness characteristics of schools are influenced by the actions of families and communities, and by economic and social conditions surrounding the school. They can also be influenced by policy decisions, independent of the socioeconomic conditions.

Availability   Where access to schooling is still a problem, because of lack of schools (rather than lack of demand), it is clear that school systems are not ready for children, no matter how alert and ready the children might be. With the spread of primary schooling, however, the availability of school places has become less and less of a problem.

But availability is more than simple access to school places. Even when schools have been built and children are enrolled, the availability of schooling may be low because the schools are not open on a regular basis.

Examples abound of teachers who have other jobs, who arrive on Tuesday and leave on Thursday, who are out because they are on strike, leaving the child with a drastically reduced school availability during the year.

Timing, distance and cost also affect true availability. The school that operates during harvesting and sowing seasons and sets vacations at other times curtails availability in areas where children participate in agricultural activities. Schools that are located far away or on the opposite side of streams that swell in the rainy season may prohibit children from taking advantage of what is theoretically available. Although most primary schools are 'free' in the sense that they charge no tuition or formal fees, there are many hidden costs for families (a slate, or the need to buy shoes and school clothes, for instance). If a family cannot afford schooling, then for all practical purposes the schooling is not really available.

Quality Perhaps the most important feature of school quality is the quality of the children who are in the school. The ability (or inability) of children to pay attention, their interest and motivation, and their cognitive and social abilities will set limits on what can be done in the school. Thus, the readiness of children for school should be set alongside other features of schooling that are more often included in a discussion of school quality: the quality of facilities, materials, teachers, and of the curriculum and methods used.

Regardless of what physical, cognitive, and social characteristics a child brings to school, he or she will not learn much in a class of 50 children with no textbooks, a leaky roof, and an uninspired teacher with little more than basic literacy – a situation found all too often. Not surprisingly, the research literature indicates that the quality of schooling will also have a significant effect on children's primary school progress and performance (Heyneman and Loxley 1983; Haddad 1979; Schiefelbein and Farrell 1978).

Perhaps the most important element in school quality, apart from the children, is the teacher. The ability of the teacher to take advantage of such materials that exist and to create others, to respond to children's needs, and to maintain enthusiasm in unfavourable conditions can create quality. It would be a diversion to enter into a discussion of the various factors affecting the quality of the teacher, but it is clear that the character and technical ability and motivation of the teacher constitute a key factor in the readiness of the school for the child. Another important feature of school quality is the presence of books and materials. Many children never have a book to call their own.

'Quality' is, of course, relative. What is considered to be quality schooling in one place will not constitute quality schooling in another. This reflects the need for schools to be responsive to different standards and cultures and needs.

Responsiveness to local needs and circumstances   A school may be available and reasonably well equipped and staffed by certified teachers but be unresponsive to local conditions, affecting markedly the children who enter the school. We have already mentioned potential problems that can arise from irresponsible scheduling or from programmes that function from the start in a language that is not the mother tongue of the participants. Although some excellent work has been done to adjust curricula to local circumstances (for instance, by the African Curriculum Organization, as indicated on the previous page), it is not difficult to find examples of materials that are totally foreign to the group that is using them. We have also mentioned that, in many places, schools pay little attention to health and nutrition while concentrating on the 'mental feeding' of the children.

Perhaps more difficult to achieve, however, is readiness of teachers for the children they will teach. The selection and assignment of teaching jobs often results in placement of people who are not from a local area, do not speak the local language, and are not familiar with local customs and traditions, making local adjustment difficult. Moreover, the idea of the teacher as a facilitator who uses locally available experience and materials to help children construct their own knowledge is a foreign idea to many cultures and programmes. Rather, the widespread image of the teacher is that of a custodian and dispenser of knowledge. That image applies as much to the primary school as to the university level. Teacher training tends to reflect this view which combines with a rigid, centrally controlled curriculum to inhibit adjustments to local conditions and forms of learning. Add to all of the above the poor level of pay received by most teachers, providing little incentive for teachers to take the difficult path of making needed local adjustments of curriculum and methods, and it is little wonder that teachers are often not 'ready' for the children they will receive.

ENROLMENT, PROGRESS AND PERFORMANCE

Readiness of children for schools and the readiness of schools for children interact, in our analytical framework, to influence enrolment, progress and performance of children in school.

Enrolment and participation in school is influenced by the availability of schooling (including distance and cost as well as the actual availability of a place in school) and by parental decisions. The decision to enrol a child in school (and decisions whether or not to continue) involve balancing a complex set of variables that include the non-school demands on time, the perception of the child's readiness and ability, and family aspirations as well as beliefs about the value of schooling. Aspirations and perceptions may differ for boys and girls. And parental decisions may be affected also by their perceptions of the kind and quality of the schooling the child will receive.

In addition to a decision whether or not a child should enter school, parents make decisions about the age at which enrolment should occur. Age of entrance can be significant for three reasons. First, a child could enter too soon, before achieving the competencies necessary for success. Second, the later the entrance, the more out of phase a student is and, it seems, the more likely they will be to drop out before completing primary school. In part that is because the older children are, the more valuable they are as potential contributors to family survival and livelihood, either by taking on responsibilities at home or by working outside. A third reason the age of entrance is important is that variations will create more hetero-geneous classes, making teaching more difficult. If early interventions help to lower and to regularize the age of entry, they can have a noted impact on school efficiency.

'*Progress*' in school, as used here, refers to promotion from one grade to the next. From the standpoint of the child and the family, many of the same factors that influence enrolment will influence continuation: health, perceived ability, competing demands on time, etc. But progress will also depend on available places and on promotion policies.

School systems, schools, and individual teachers vary considerably in the manner in which they select children for promotion or for retention. In some systems, children are routinely held back, even though automatic promotion has been written into the educational statutes. In some systems, the child's first year in first grade may be viewed as a preparatory year, and the second year in first grade as the 'real' year (Myers 1985), swelling both repetition rates and the feeling of failure. But no differentiation is made in the content of the two years.

Grades assigned by teachers are commonly used to promote some children, and retain others. However, a subjective element often enters into assigning grades; teachers are human and do not, therefore, take achieve-ment as the only promotion criterion. Number of days absent, skin colour, dress and social behaviour have all been found to be factors (Filp *et al.* 1983). And teachers have to consider the number of available places in the next grade when assigning grades and deciding upon promotion.

Apparently, neither parents nor teachers seem to attribute high repeti-tion rates or failure of children to the insensitivity of schools to children's needs. Teachers may point to large class sizes or lack of materials, but not to deficiencies in their training or their methods. Teachers also place blame on the home, and both teachers and parents blame the child for being lazy or lacking interest, and therefore not performing well (Toro and de Rosa 1983). Nonetheless, an association has been found between teachers' observed skills and numbers of children in a class repeating: the better the skills, the fewer the repeaters (Pozner 1983).

The *performance* of children, usually measured by some combination of tests and of marks assigned by the teachers, presumably indicates how well a child has mastered the content of the school curriculum. But the curriculum of the school may or may not have been adjusted to local circumstances so that grades may be a pale reflection of a child's general knowledge or even of her ability. Moreover, as suggested with respect to promotion, a variety of factors can influence grading, further distorting their validity as an independent assessment of mastery. Nevertheless, these measures of performance are usually the main basis for deciding on promotion and are used to label children as able or not – as successes or failures.

There are, of course, other measures of performance. For instance, teachers are often asked how well children are adjusting socially to the school and are sometimes asked to provide a grade indicating how well a student has participated, and cooperated. In the pages that follow in which early educational interventions are examined for their relationship to subsequent performance in primary school, indicators of social adjustment are less often included than measures of academic performance.

We turn now to an examination of evidence regarding the effects of various early intervention programmes on readiness for school and on primary school enrolment, progress and performance.

EFFECTS OF EARLY CHILDHOOD PROGRAMMES: A REVIEW OF THE EVIDENCE

The most broadly disseminated, systematic, and mature evidence regarding effects of early childhood programmes on primary school progress and performance comes from longitudinal evaluations of so-called 'compensatory' programmes for children, aged three to five, from 'disadvantaged' backgrounds in the United States and Europe. This evidence provides an important starting point for our discussion because studies from industrialized nations have influenced international thinking about the value of early childhood programmes. In what might be called the first round of influence, the effect was negative. Programmers drew upon early findings, with negative results, to recommend against programme support for early childhood development (e.g. Smilansky 1979). These early findings have been superseded by longer term studies suggesting a more positive (and sometimes dramatic) influence of early childhood programmes on school outcomes and on behaviour. This second round of studies sets an entirely different basis and tone for considering programme investments. It is, therefore, important to set the record straight. And, it is important to build upon the hopeful findings these more recent studies provide.

Following a brief review of evidence from the United States and Europe, the growing body of evidence from the Third World will be presented.

Early evidence from the United States

In the 1960s, a large-scale action programme called 'Headstart' was begun in the United States with the specific intention of preparing children from poor families to enter school by compensating for poor home conditions. In implementation, the programme was varied in method and content and in the adjustments to local conditions. After having participated in the programme, Headstart children were found to have significantly improved their IQ scores. However, as they were followed into primary school, this relative improvement by programme participants was not sustained; rather, it 'washed out' within the first two or three years of primary school (Cicirelli *et al.* 1969).

Also begun in the early 1960s were several small-scale experimental and quasi-experimental studies, directed to the same population as Headstart, and of a generally higher quality than the Headstart efforts. These programmes are unusual because they have been able to follow participants and a comparative group of children throughout their school careers (Berruta-Clement *et al.* 1984; Gordon and Jester 1980; Gray, Ramsey and Klaus 1982; Levenstein, O'Hara and Madden 1983; Palmer 1983; Monroe and McDonald 1981; Irvine 1982. For a summary of the characteristics of these programmes, see Lazar and Darlington 1982, or Halpern and Myers 1985). The initial emphasis in evaluation of these experimental programmes was on IQ effects, as it was in the Headstart evaluation, and results similar to the Headstart evaluation appeared. On leaving the programmes, IQ gains of one-half to one standard deviation (8 to 16 points) were found for many participating children, when compared with non-participants. However, this advantage disappeared in two to three years.

The premature conclusion drawn by many people from these early evaluations was that the compensatory early childhood programmes – experiments in improving the readiness of children for school – did not make a lasting difference and that they were not, therefore, a good investment. *This conclusion has not held up over time.*

Recent evidence from industrialized nations

As children in the experimental studies being carried out in the United States continued to move through primary school, their progress and performance was evaluated, and the content of the evaluations broadened beyond the earlier focus on IQ. Evidence of positive effects on adjustment to the demands of formal schooling began to mount. In the 1980s, a set of evaluations appeared looking at children in early or late adolescence, and showing that participation in well-implemented early childhood education programmes can have significant long-term effects on progress through the school as measured by promotion, need for special education, and high school completion (see Lazar 1989, or Halpern and Myers 1985, Table 3, for summaries of evidence). One of these studies is summarized below.

The Perry Preschool Project   Perhaps the most complete of the longitudinal studies carried out in the United States is the Perry Preschool study, providing unusually solid empirical evidence that an early intervention can have effects not only on school performance and continuation, but also on employment, earnings, and social behaviour. The participants in the Perry programme were all urban black children from low-income families in Ypsilanti, Michigan. They participated for two years, at ages three and four (except for one group that received the programme for only one school year at age four). The programme was in operation for $7\frac{1}{2}$ months each year, with classes conducted for $2\frac{1}{2}$ hours each morning, Monday through Friday. The staff–child ratio was one adult for every five or six children enrolled. Teachers made a home visit to each mother and child for $2\frac{1}{2}$ hours weekly.

In a volume titled *Changed Lives* (Berruta-Clement *et al.* 1984), results are reported of a study that followed up the Perry preschool children, and a comparative, randomly chosen group that did not participate in the programme, as of age 19. The comparison shows that programme participants were more likely than non-participants to graduate from high school (67 vs. 49 per cent) and to obtain employment (59 vs. 32 per cent). The group was also less likely to require remedial education (16 vs. 28 per cent), be in trouble with the law (31 vs. 51 per cent), or become pregnant while a teenager (64 vs. 117 per 100). At age 19, 45 per cent of the programme group were supporting themselves as compared with 25 per cent of the control group. The mean annualized welfare payments to programme group members was US$633, as compared to US$1,509 for control group members.

Clearly, the earlier findings emphasizing a 'wash-out' effect from the preschool intervention did not hold up and had to be reconsidered. The study also showed that there is utility in looking at benefits of early education programmes other than IQ gains.

Furthermore, a cost study of the Perry project was carried out that suggested the following:

1 The benefit-to-cost ratio for a preschool programme can be high. (In the Perry case, the results showed that social and individual benefits exceeded costs by a factor of 7 to 1 for one year of early childhood education accompanied by home visits. This study will be reported more completely in Chapter 15, dealing with costs.)
2 An early intervention programme that has a relatively high cost can, nevertheless, be socially beneficial and bring a high rate of return.

Headstart revisited   Is the same rethinking required with respect to the Headstart programme as its graduates have been followed over time? A number of short-term evaluations of 'typical' Headstart programmes throughout the United States have followed children into primary school. Harrell (1983) conducted a meta-analysis of 71 reports of research on such programmes, selected from a much larger number, based on adequacy of documentation. She examined effects on IQ, on developed abilities at point of entry into school (school readiness) and on achievement at the end of the early grades. She found evidence of positive Headstart effects in the three areas, with the largest effects on school readiness measures, and the smallest on achievement at the end of grades 1, 2, or 3. Harrell concludes that Headstart 'does, indeed, enhance the cognitive development of children' (p. 4). Unfortunately, however, the longer-term follow-up work that showed enduring and positive results in the case of the experimental programmes has not been undertaken.

The Child Health and Education Study   In the United Kingdom, an entire cohort of children, approximately 9,000, many of whom had participated in some form of preschool experience outside the home, were followed into school (Osborn and Milbank 1987). The study was designed to investigate whether preschool experiences had a beneficial effect on the subsequent cognitive development, educational achievement and behaviour of children. This study differs markedly from the Perry study because it did not involve a particular type of preschool intervention applied on an experimental basis; rather, it examined experiences that occurred in the natural course of events for the children studied.

Differences in educational attainment were found to be associated with participation in some form of organized preschool experience outside the home. Sometimes, the effect of the preschool experience seemed to hold even though the time of participation was relatively brief. The authors also concluded that, '... provided the child receives proper care, has interesting activities and other children to play with (which are common elements in the majority of preschool institutions) the actual type of preschool experience matters very little' (ibid., p. 239).

Explaining the results

Finding a relationship between early childhood experiences and educational attainment is one thing, explaining why that relationship appears is another. What are the explanations?

Quality?   The difference between the strong positive results found when experimental programmes in the United States were followed over many years and the weaker findings for Headstart programmes may lie in the differential quality of these initiatives. What is clear from the evaluations is that high-quality, well-implemented programmes can have an effect. This finding has three implications as one thinks about programmes in developing countries. First, it provides some assurance that effects are possible to obtain. Second, it suggests that some minimum level of quality may be needed to achieve the gains. Third, it raises (answerable) questions about financial feasibility.

Changed attitudes and perceptions from a positive experience?   One reasonable, but speculative causal explanation for effects associated with early and well-implemented interventions in the preschool years is provided by Lazar:

> Many factors influence and are influenced by school performance, including children's ability, their level of motivation, teachers' expectations and treatment, and children's self-esteem and feelings of autonomy and control. It is possible that early education gave the children just enough of a 'boost' that all these mechanisms tended to operate positively. Perhaps early education taught these children some concrete cognitive skills and also exposed them to some school-relevant non-cognitive skills such as attentiveness to teachers, ability to follow instructions, and task perseverance. When the children entered first grade they had positive attitudes towards classroom activities, were able to adapt to classroom procedures, and were able to learn and do the school work. The public school experience, in short, was also positive. The children's positive attitudes towards school were reinforced; they felt competent. In all probability their teachers identified them as competent and treated them as such. Once set in motion, success tended to breed success.
>
> (Lazar, *et al.* 1982, p. 64)

In this view, the short-term cognitive gains that were found in earlier studies take on some importance. Along with certain enhanced social skills, they may be the catalyst that evokes from children a commitment to schooling, and sets children on a positive course. Indeed, it may be that, even though early IQ gains washed out, the early gains give the parents and teachers of the young students a different view of their children's ability while helping to provide the children with a better self-image.

Parental involvement?   In the analysis of the several US early interventions, one clear finding that emerged is that programmes incorporating a home visiting component, working directly to involve parents, produced better results than a programme without such direct parent involvement (Lazar 1989).

But the question of parental involvement can be approached from another angle as well. Osborn and Milbank observed that educational attainment for the primary schoolchildren studied was strongly related to socioeconomic position and to other social and family factors, of which parental interest in the child's development was one of the most important.

> Thus, the educational benefits which in reality were due to parental interest and stimulation in the home may be spuriously attributed to the preschool institution the child attended.... Moreover, a child's educational achievement was enhanced still further if his own mother was involved in the preschool institution he attended.
>
> (pp. 238–9)

This interpretation suggests that there is self-selection to preschool programmes related to parental interest and involvement. That should not, however, be taken as a rationalization for failure to support such programmes. Rather, it underscores the need in programming for a conscious effort to reach families that are so preoccupied with the day-to-day pressures of scratching out an existence that they find it difficult to express properly an interest in their child's development.

The interpretation also points to the difficulties arising from associational analyses at a point in time. In this case, what is interpreted as a 'spurious' relationship may actually reflect the inability of the analysis to untangle causality. If a preschool is able to get a parent involved and if that action changes the parental view, then the preschool effect is not 'spurious' even though, at the time of the study, an association will be found between a positive parental interest in their child's development and academic achievement that appears to override the preschool effect. Unless individual children and families are traced and unless the attitudes of the parents were examined before their children became involved in a preschool programme, we cannot make the proper causal attribution.

Infant interventions

The prior discussion has focused on programmes for children in the three to five year old age range. Much less evidence of long-term effects is available for early childhood programmes directed towards infants. The majority of these programmes involve working with parents in the home and they tend to have a relatively greater focus on parent education in health, nutrition and home stimulation than do early education, preschool programmes.

What evidence there is of lasting effects of infant interventions in the United States (Anderson, Fox, and Lewin 1983; Halpern 1984) suggests that they do have beneficial short-term effects on parent childrearing behaviours and coping skills, and somewhat less consistently on pregnancy outcomes, infant health and development. Only a few prenatal and infant intervention programmes have followed children into their school years (e.g. Epstein and Weikart 1979). Here, the scanty evidence suggests the importance of continued attention in the early years if an effect on schooling is desired; it is not enough to intervene prenatally or in infancy, even though those interventions might bring a short-term effect.

Generalizability

But what does all of the above mean for programming in Asia, Africa and Latin America? There are, of course, many differences between the conditions of schooling, of families, and of social institutions in various Third World countries and in those of industrialized countries where the programmes and studies described above were carried out. For instance, in all Sub-Saharan countries one is more likely than in the United States to encounter, on the average, large classes, scanty instructional resources, minimally trained teachers, and an inadequate number of 'places' in each grade. These conditions are such that the newly acquired skills preschool participants bring with them to primary school may be less influential than in the US in shaping the course of children's school careers. When promotion policies are only loosely tied to children's abilities, when there is no special education to be 'avoided', and when there are resources for only 10 to 20 per cent of primary school participants to complete secondary school, the positive long-term effects on the course of children's careers found in the US may not be replicated in developing countries.

Nonetheless, it is reasonable to expect that primary school systems in the Third World can be sensitive to the kinds of skills and characteristics children bring with them. Conversely, it is reasonable to expect that children whose physical health and psychosocial development has improved will be better able to adapt to and cope with the demands of the school setting. It may even be that the severe health and nutritional and cognitive deficits that constitute a starting point for many children in the Third World open the possibility for even greater improvements there than found in the United States, and with programmes that are not of as high quality.

Because the conditions in the Third World are so different, in general, from those in industrialized nations, and because there is such large variation within the Third World itself, it would be unwise simply to generalize results from the programmes and studies we have described so far. The findings do not provide proof that similar kinds of programmes will have similar kinds of results in countries of the Third World, but they do provide hope. The causal mechanisms that seem to be at work in the United States or Europe may or may not work in the varied and distinct settings of the Third World. Results might be weaker or stronger.

Let us turn, then, to the evidence available from programmes and studies carried out in the Third World.

EVIDENCE FROM THE THIRD WORLD

Does participation in early childhood development programmes improve a child's chances of enrolling and staying in school, and, perhaps, of improving the level of performance as well? Increasingly, evidence is available from countries of the Third World that helps to answer the question. That evidence results from two kinds of studies examining two different kinds of programmes.

One group of studies originates within the nutrition and health community. The projects studied were set up as experiments involving a relatively small group of participants and relatively sophisticated experimental designs. All but one included a combination of health surveillance, nutrition supplementation, and educational intervention. With one exception, these experiments began treatment before birth. The ages at which the treatments began and the length of time of the treatments varied considerably from project to project.

A second set of studies originates in education and social science communities, and is composed largely of interventions directed towards children aged three to five or six. Improved school readiness and performance were desired outcomes of these programmes. Some of the interventions studied are small-scale demonstrations, others larger municipal, state, or national service programmes. Most include more than one component in the intervention, but the principal component is an educational intervention. In most cases, evaluations of these educational programmes are weaker methodologically because they were set up as action programmes, not as scientific experiments. Nevertheless, evaluations were done carefully and include comparisons of those who participated in the programme with a similar group that did not benefit from the programme. When taken together the results are instructive.

Nutrition-related interventions

In the 1970s, an academic interest in the relationship between malnutrition and behavioural development led to a series of studies in Latin America that have been widely quoted in the literature. At the time, emphasis was placed on protein energy malnutrition and on supplementation, with little or no attention to vitamin and/or mineral traces as they might affect growth and development. Basic information is summarized in Table 10.2 about location, sample sizes, treatment and design for each of the four intervention studies we will present.

Table 10.2 Longitudinal studies of nutrition interventions as related to schooling

Country/ intervention	Urban/ rural	Age of children	Study population	Intervention components	Comparison groups
Colombia, Bogotá (Herrera and Super 1983)	Urban marginal	Prenatal 3 months at outset followed to age 7	443 families	All groups received health care Nutrition supplementation, different ages Home visits for subgroups	Random assignment to treatment groups: 1. Supplementation nutrition – mother 2. Supplementation nutrition – child – 3 months to 3 years 3. Early stim.– birth to 3 years 4. Early stim. and nutrition Combine 2 + 3
Colombia, Cali (McKay 1982)	Urban marginal	3–7	333 children malnourished low income	Preschooled Nutrition supplementation Health surveillance/care H/N education	Random assignments to: 1. 4 years beginning age 3 2. 3 years beginning age 4 3. 2 years beginning age 5 4. 1 year beginning age 6 Also: 5. No treatment low income group with normal weight/height 6. No treatment, high income
Guatemala INCAP (Klein 1979)	Rural four villages	Prenatal 6 months at outset	671 children (450 followed longitudinally)	Nutrition supplementation (6 months to 7 years)	Two villages: high protein and high calorie supplementation Two villages: no protein, modest calorie supplementation
México (Chávez and Martínez 1983)	Rural one village	Prenatal (followed for 10 years)	34 children	Nutrition supplementation to mother during pregnancy and lactation Supplementary feeding of baby from approximately 3rd month	Control (n = 17): pregnant women who were well, normal height, and between 18–36; and selection of children born with 2.5kg or more and Apgar of 8 Intervention (n = 17): matched group, a year later

Guatemala A team of researchers at the Nutrition Institute for Central America and Panama (INCAP) found that high supplemental intake had a significant effect on birthweight, physical growth (height and weight) up to age seven, and cognitive development up to age three. The cognitive effects appeared to decrease in magnitude and generality beyond age three.

High supplementation had no significant effect on verbal performance at ages five, six, and seven, on early school progress, or on school performance. However, in three of the four participating villages, in which parental education levels were moderately higher, the amount of supplemental intake was predictive of the likelihood of school enrolment (Klein 1979; Balderston *et al.* 1981). Parents' perceptions of early intellectual ability in their children, which generally seemed to be accurate, led to earlier enrolment (for boys and girls) and to a greater likelihood of enrolment (for girls).

Although nutritional supplementation seemed to have no effect on school performance, the quality of home stimulation during the early years was strongly associated with primary school performance, especially for boys (Irwin *et al.* 1978). (Because a more select group of girls attended school, there was less variance in their achievement.) It was found in these generally poor villages that even slight differences in economic status affected family ability to cope with the costs of children's education. For the same group, Barrett and Radke-Yarrow (1985) found effects of the nutritional supplementation on the social development of children as indicated by their adjustment and behaviour in school. The results suggest, as in the earlier description of results from United States studies, that a broader view of the effects of early interventions is wise (broader than the focus on IQ or even on cognitive outcomes).

In interpreting these findings, it is well to remember that the Guatemalan intervention was continuous over a period of seven years. It did not involve a programme of parental or community education.

Colombia: Cali The Cali researchers (McKay 1982) found that all the experimental groups demonstrated significantly greater growth than low-income controls in general cognitive ability during and immediately after the treatment periods. These cognitive gains were related to the age that the treatment began (and therefore to the length of the treatment as well). Modest, albeit diminished, IQ effects were found to persist to at least age eight.

Children who received nutritional supplements but who had not yet been chosen to participate in the preschool made significant gains in their height and weight, but did not improve their cognitive abilities, relatively, until they entered the preschool programme.

Results of the follow-up of children into primary school are confounded by the fact that the children attended 93 different primary schools, many switching schools more than once. Part of the treatment group had a special programme designed for it. Many children, particularly the low-status control group children, attended private 'backyard' or 'bench' schools, being unable to enrol or stay in the public system. In these settings, children are more likely than in public settings to be 'promoted,' even though they may have the least academic ability.

With all these provisos, the researchers report that treatment group children were slightly more likely than low-income controls to be promoted through the first three grades. Thus, at the beginning of the fourth year, the average grade level for each of the groups improved, in accordance with the length of time spent in the preschool. Whereas the control group averaged 2.9 years, those who were exposed to four years of preschool averaged 3.2 years, a difference of 10 per cent.

Colombia: Bogotá   Supplementation and maternal tutoring in different combinations were associated with improved cognitive abilities in various areas at ages 18 months and 3 years, with the strongest effect found for the fully supplemented and home-visited group. Parental supplementation had a very modest (60 gram) effect on birthweight. Supplementation was also associated with improved physical growth at three years. The home visiting programme had significant positive effects on the quality of mother–infant interaction (e.g. verbal interaction, contingent responsiveness, affect) in both supplemented and unsupplemented groups. Behavioural effects were greatest for supplemented infants, who theoretically had more energy with which to respond to (or elicit) their mothers' new skills.

A school readiness test (reading readiness, maths, basic knowledge), administered to 174 children, aged 5.6 to 8.7, produced a small, but significant overall positive effect of nutritional supplementation on readiness test scores, with or without maternal tutoring. Effects were larger at low levels of father's education. There were no independent effects of maternal tutoring on test scores.

There was an important effect of maternal tutoring on age of initial primary school enrolment. Mean age was 5 years for the maternal tutoring group; 5.6 years for the maternal tutoring/nutritional supplementation group; 5.9 years for the supplementation group; 6 years for the control group. There were also significant positive effects of supplementation and tutoring, alone and combined, on first grade repetition. Children in all three intervention groups repeated at about a 4 per cent rate, in the control group at a 13 per cent rate. There were no significant overall intervention effects on teacher-assigned grades in first grade.

Reviewing the whole pattern of findings at age seven, the investigators speculate that nutritional supplementation has more general long-term effects on children (for example, on level of activity, alertness, social cooperation); whereas maternal tutoring has more selective effects (perhaps through effects on maternal–child interaction) on children's 'familiarity with a school-like learning paradigm of interaction with adults'. They reiterate that the largest effects in most domains appeared to be found among the most disadvantaged children.

Mexico: Puebla   This extraordinarily detailed follow-up study, carried out over ten years, shows clearly that supplemented children (beginning with supplementation of mothers during pregnancy), when compared with unsupplemented and, therefore, undernourished children, walked at an earlier age, exerted control over their sphincters earlier, and demonstrated language superiority from the 20th week onward. With respect to language, by the 20th month, the undernourished children were found to be on the edge of abnormality, with that result being attributed both to social factors ('Conversation between adults and children is not customary') and to organic factors.

Using direct observation, open field tests, and time sampling to quantify behaviours, the authors found that, after the age of six months, the undernourished children were much less active than the nourished (supplemented) children. This difference increased with time and was evident in the amount of time spent sleeping, in the number of steps per hour, and the time spent playing. As of the second year, there were significant differences in the amount of smiling (more) and of crying (less) of nourished versus undernourished children.

Supplemented children were not only better nourished, they also received more attention. Mothers responded more readily to their demands. Bathing and cuddling were more frequent. Fathers were more likely to participate in feeding. Beginning in the 16th week differences appeared as supplemented children were given toys, clothing and rewards for good behaviour. These findings are consistent with the interactive, synergistic model of development presented in the previous chapter.

In brief, major differences in behaviour appeared in the early months of childhood. The authors suggest that, in the sequence of events leading to these differences, the demand for care by the child is as important as the offer of care from the caregiver. Better nourished children demand more. The authors also suggest that these differences can be transitory and that later stimulation can lead to recuperation.

As children were followed into the early years of schooling, it was found that differences in mental tests between the two groups were very small, but that behavioural differences continued. School achievement during the first year of schooling was evaluated using teacher grades, performance on official and international examinations, performance on specially administered reading and writing tests, and detailed time-sampling observations of the children in the classroom. On all examinations, the supplemented children performed significantly better than unsupplemented children. Observations revealed that the supplemented children more often looked at the teacher (10 per cent vs. 3 per cent), talked or asked questions (6 per cent vs. 3 per cent), played (13 per cent vs. 4 per cent), and left their seat (7 per cent vs. 1 per cent). Conversely, the supplemented children were less likely to sleep in class (1 per cent vs. 5 per cent), or cry (1 per cent vs. 5 per cent). It is not surprising, then, that slightly more than one-third of the unsupplemented children failed the first year while there were no failures among the supplemented.

Other evidence   To the above evidence, we might add that of Moock and Leslie (1986) who found that both the probability of enrolment and grade attainment (controlling for age at enrolment) were related to nutritional status. This study was not related to a specific intervention but suggests that nutritional supplementation programmes could have an effect on enrolment and progress. Or, we could include results from the 10-year longitudinal study of 'Tierra Blanca' in Mexico (Cravioto and Arrieta 1982), which shows the negative effect on school readiness of severe malnutrition and lack of home stimulation, evident in delayed language development and handling of basic bipolar concepts (e.g. large–small).

In a compact, well-documented review titled *Beyond Survival: Children's Growth for National Development,* Maguire and Austin (1987) focus on growth promotion, and include sections on mental development, intelligence and school behaviour, school enrolment and grade completion and repetition. The authors conclude that 'Better growth is associated with better pre-school and school-age IQ. It is also associated with learning-relevant behaviour, early enrolment in school and better school achievement, all of which enhance the educational efficiency of and economic return on primary schools' (p. 16).

Increasingly, iodine, iron, zinc, vitamin A, and other micro-nutrients are recognized as having an important effect on the progress and performance of children in school (Berg and Brems 1986; Levin and Pollitt 1989). An in-depth assessment of scientific evidence on the effect of iron deficiency on cognition recently led to the following statement by a group of prominent researchers:

> Many studies have shown an association between iron-deficiency anemia and less than optimal behavior in infants and children, as demonstrated by lower scores on tests of development, learning, school achievement, etc. A problem with the interpretation of past studies has been that iron-deficiency anemia is associated with other adverse environmental and nutritional conditions. Recent studies, however, using randomized designs with appropriate controls, have shown that iron therapy in preschool and school-aged children with iron-deficiency anemia results in improvement in selective learning and school achievement tests.

(Quoted in Levin and Pollitt, p. 3)

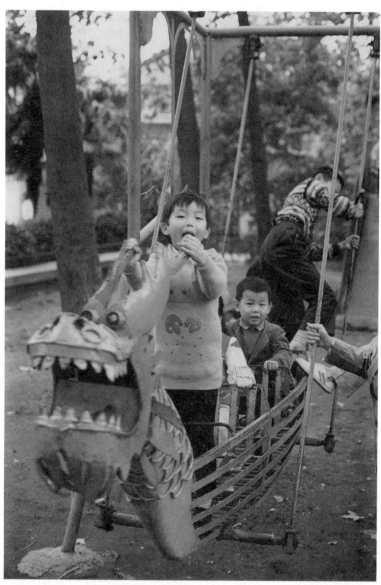
'In the playground', Nanchang, China

Early childhood education programmes

Another group of studies, focusing more directly on preschool and early education programmes, also provides evidence regarding the potential effects of early interventions on progress and performance in primary schools. Table 10.3 summarizes information describing 13 studies carried out in Asia, Latin America and the Middle East (with a heavy bias towards Latin America). These studies vary widely in their design and rigour, and in the contexts and kinds of programme interventions they examine. Several of the studies may be characterized as research projects; others as evaluations of small-scale demonstration projects; and others as evaluations of larger-scale programmes. (There is some overlapping of these categories.) One characteristic the studies share is that all have attempted to make a comparison over time between children who participated in an intervention programme and children who did not.

In the main, the designs of these 13 studies (four of which are combined in one entry in the table) are weaker methodologically than for the four experimental nutrition studies described above. For instance, only one of the early education studies assigns children randomly to comparison groups; rather, children participating in the programme being evaluated are compared with peers who are thought to be similar, except for their participation. Despite creative efforts to locate matching children for the comparison group, it is not always clear how similar the participating and non-participating groups are in fact.

In some studies, preschool-aged children, with and without participation in a specific preschool programme, are followed into the primary school. The fact that these children attend a variety of schools means that criteria used to judge promotion and progress will vary, introducing uncertainty into the comparisons. In other studies, preschool antecedents of selected primary school children are identified retrospectively in order to define the comparison groups. When working retrospectively, a possible bias is introduced by the nature of the particular primary schools chosen for study and by the possibility that some children will not have enrolled in primary school.

In spite of these limitations and some need for caution in interpreting the results, this group of studies sheds light on factors that influence children's early school careers in developing countries. And, taken as a group, the studies demonstrate clearly the potential effects of early education interventions on the age of enrolment, and on progress through the educational system.

Rather than describe each study in detail (for details, see Halpern and Myers 1985; Myers 1988, and the original documents), essentials are provided in Table 10.3 and a summary of evidence is presented in Table 10.4 regarding the effects of early intervention programmes on enrolment,

Table 10.3 Longitudinal studies of nutrition and education interventions as related to schooling

Country/ intervention	Urban/ rural	Age of children	Study population	Intervention components	Comparison groups
Turkey, comprehensive pre-school education, research project (Kağitçibaşi et al. 1987)	Urban	3–5	251 children	Maternal education using Turkish adaptation of HIPPY Preschool education vs custodial care vs home care	Children in same neighbourhoods matched on age, economic and family criteria who did not attend preschool Trained vs untrained mothers
India, Integrated Child Development Service (ICDS): Dalmau project (Chaturvedi et al. 1987)	Rural	0–6	Children ages 6–8 in primary school 214 ICDS 205 non-ICDS	Nutrition supplementation, immunization, health check-ups, health/nutrition Education, non-formal preschool education	Children in adjoining area not participating in ICDS but similar in socio-culture, geographic, anthropological features, villages within area selected randomly
India, ICDS Haryana state (Lal et al. 1986)	Rural	0–6	Primary school 1,271 ICDS 436 non-ICDS	Same as above	Children from same area who did not participate in ICDS
Morocco, literacy acquisition research (Wagner and Spratt 1987)	Urban and rural	5–7	378 children	Quranic or modern preschooling	Children in Quranic preschools compared with children in modern preschools and non preschool group Samples constructed to control for social class

Study	Setting	Age	Sample	Programme	Comparison
Latin America, 4-country study in Argentina, Bolivia, Chile, Colombia (Filp et al. 1983)	Urban and rural	4–7	2,545 children	Preschool	First grade children who had participated in preschool compared with those who had not (taken from same and other last grade classes, same schools) analysis within ses grouping
Brazil, Fortaleza preschool research (Feijo 1984)	Urban	6–7	127 children	Public kindergarten participation	Children who tried to enroll in same kindergarten but could not for lack of space, marched by gender, birth order, siblings
Perú Non-formal Programme of Initial Education (PRONOEI) (Myers et al. 1985)	Urban and rural	3–5	334 children	Non-formal preschool nutrition supplementation community improvement projects	Children in non-PRONOEI villages, with partial attempt to match on ses status
Chile, Osorno Parents and Children Project (PPH) (Richards 1985)	Rural	4–6	Children in 52 communities	Health/nutrition education Child development education community development	Children in same class who did not participate in PPH
Colombia PROMESA (Nimnicht and Posada 1986)	Rural	0–7	4 communities	Health/nutrition/child development education; early stimulation programme; community improvement projects	Children from same communities who did not participate in PROMESA
Brazil, Alagoas PROAPE (Ministerio da Saude 1983)	Urban	4–6	184 Proape 556 Casulo 320 Kinderg. 334 No pre-school	Health surveillance Nutrition supplementation Preschool	Comparisons among children from different preschool with non-preschoolers in first grade

progress and performance in school – for all 13 studies, as well as for the four nutritional studies described earlier.

Readiness of children for school

The nutritional studies showed a definite advantage in terms of children's readiness for school. Better nourished children had an advantage physically, mentally, and socially. A similar result emerges from the several studies in the education group. Each study involved a different indicator or set of indicators defining school readiness, usually focusing on cognitive development as it had been affected by the particular intervention in which the child participated.

Three examples of different programme interventions and measures will give the reader an idea of both the variations and the generally positive effect of programmes on readiness:

Turkey: Istanbul   This action research project, carried out over a four-year period (Kağitçibaşi *et al.* 1987), studied the impact on overall child development of educational preschool care combined with a programme of parental education and support. Effects of this optimal combination were compared with effects of custodial child care and home care, each taken alone and in combination with parental education. The project was carried out in five low-income areas of Istanbul with intact families, most of which were nuclear. Children were selected from existing programmes classified as custodial and educational on the basis of systematic observations and with a matched group of no-preschool children from the same neighbourhoods.

During year one of the study, baseline data were collected on child-rearing practices, patterns, and expectations and on a range of cognitive, personality, and social characteristics of the children. During years two and three, mothers of half the children in each preschool setting were provided with training, through bi-weekly home visits by trained paraprofessionals, with group discussions led by supervising professional staff in alternate weeks. Cognitive development was fostered using a Turkish adaptation of HIPPY (Home Instruction Programme for Preschool Youngsters), an enrichment programme, with materials provided for educational activities to improve language, sensory and perceptual discrimination skills, and problem-solving. Social and personality development was approached through modelling and discussions of the mother–child interaction, and by supporting mothers in developing their own feelings of competence, efficacy, and self-confidence.

Beginning with the second year (when the five-year-old group entered school), school grades were obtained at the end of each semester. In the fourth year, children were again observed and tested, and achievement data were collected.

The results of this intervention showed that children who had participated in an educational preschool programme performed significantly better than children in custodial programmes or children cared for at home on a range of measures of mental ability and cognitive skills (including IQ, as measured by the Stanford Binet; block design and the analytical triad subtests from the Weschler Intelligence Scale for Children; the Children's Embedded Figures Test; and a set of classification tasks).

Likewise, children of mothers who had participated in the parental education programme (using HIPPY) tested better than children of those who had not participated. On measures of social interaction (autonomy and dependence, aggression, self-concept and emotional difficulties), the differences were not so frequent or consistently significant. In general, however, the results showed that children from the educational preschools whose mothers had also participated in the parental education programme were more autonomous, less aggressive, and had fewer emotional difficulties than children from the home group.

In regression analyses run on the academic average of children, and on their grades in mathematics and Turkish in the fourth year of the study, the preschool environment, a comparatively high level of stimulation at home, and the mother's expectation of competence from the child were the variables most strongly and consistently related to academic achievement as reflected in school grades (ibid., pp. 65–6).

The training programme for mothers made a considerable impact on the mother's style of interaction with her child, 'leading to a style that is generally more focussed on the child, more verbal, less punitive, more cognitively stimulating, and more supportive of the child's developing autonomy' (p. 61). In addition, different outlooks and patterns of family interaction were found. 'Trained' mothers were more optimistic and likely to share in decisions and activities with their spouses.

India: ICDS   The Integrated Child Development Service has been described earlier (see Chapter 6, p. 103). Two relatively simple studies show effects of the ICDS programme on enrolment, progress, and performance of children in primary school.

1 *Chaturvedi and colleagues* (1987) randomly selected three villages from adjoining ICDS and non-ICDS areas, and studied all children aged six to eight in those villages. These two groups of children were '… well-matched according to the parental education, parental occupation, number of educated members in the household, socio-economic status, period of parental company and some other bio-social characteristics which have an association with a child's mental and social development' (p. 158).

The researchers found that children who had participated in the ICDS preschool programme scored significantly higher on the Ravens Progressive Color Matrices than those who did not. School attendance, academic performance (the average of marks on the two previous school examinations taken), and general behaviour in school (according to a rating scale used by teachers) were all significantly superior (at the 0.001 level) for ICDS participants.

2 *Lal and Wati* (1986) compared ICDS and non-ICDS children from 14 rural villages with respect to enrolment (whether students were in the right grade-for-age), dropout, and school performance as judged by the teacher. When dropout figures are examined within caste groupings, the results show that dropout was much higher by grade three for non-ICDS children than for ICDS children in the lower and middle castes, but not in the higher castes:

	ICDS	non-ICDS
lower castes	19%	35%
middle castes	5%	25%
higher castes	7%	8%

Peru: PRONOEI   In PRONOEI (Programas No-Formal de Educacion Inicial), children aged three to five are brought together for three hours, four or five mornings a week in centres. They receive education and care from a minimally trained community volunteer as well as a snack and/or noontime meal. Mothers, serving on a rotating basis, prepare the food. In some villages, this non-formal preschool programme was associated also with small income-generating projects (see also Chapter 6, p. 114, and Chapter 15, p. 407).

An evaluation (Myers *et al.* 1985) examined school readiness in terms of a criterion-referenced test, linked specifically to the behaviours that the PRONOEI non-formal preschool curriculum guide defined as desirable. The test had intellectual, motor, and social sub-scales. Results were different for the three different states in which the evaluation was carried out. In Puno, where the programme was the most extensive and where it was possible to compare children of similar backgrounds, PRONOEI children performed significantly better than non-PRONOEI children on all three of the sub-scales. This was so even though the quality of the PRONOEI programme was generally low, as judged by the teaching skills of the 'promoters', the time devoted to educational activities, the availability and use of materials, and the quality of supervision.

Although school readiness seemed to be affected positively, no effects of PRONOEI participation were found on promotion from first to second grade, or from second to third grade. Effects favouring PRONOEI participants were found on age of enrolment. A high rate of repetition in the first grade (over 50 per cent) seemed to be linked to structural conditions inherent in the local school situation, minimizing the role of individual characteristics or abilities in determining children's promotion.

Against the background of these examples, let us now look at a summary of results from the 17 interventions and evaluations set out in Table 10.4, and particularly at enrolment, progress, and performance of children in the primary school. Of the 17 studies, 10 contain comparative information about enrolment, 13 about school progress and 13 about performance.

Enrolment, progress and performance in school

School enrolment

Are children who participate in early childhood programmes more likely to enroll in primary school? Relatively little information could be found to answer this question. In one of the Indian studies (Haryana State), enrolment was higher for children who had passed through the Integrated Child Development Service programme than for those who did not. The interesting feature of this increased enrolment is that it was significant for girls, but not for boys, most of whom were already enrolled. In the Guatemalan study, the programme also showed an effect on enrolment for girls but not for boys. The early childhood programmes seemed to have an equalizing effect. The Colombian (PROMESA) study also showed a (slightly) higher enrolment level among children participating in the programme.

Is participation associated with enrolment at an earlier age? In six studies, the average age of enrolment was clearly younger for those who had been in an early childhood development programme than for those who had not. In only two cases where enrolment age was reported were there negligible differences. We do not know from the studies whether an earlier age of enrolment led to improved progress and performance. A reasonable hypothesis is that the earlier entrance regularizes flow through the system.

Progress (promotion, repetition, and dropout)

Three of the four nutrition studies showed an improvement in school progress for programme children; one failed to find a difference. Six of the 13 education studies showed a difference in promotion rates. Three showed no effect, one of which was carried out in a system with automatic promotion so no difference would be noted. Four studies did not contain information on repetition or dropout.

In some cases, the differences in promotion were rather dramatic. For instance, in the Brazilian (PROAPE) study, repetition of the first grade

Table 10.4 Impact of early childhood development programmes on school enrolment, progress and performance[1]

Country/programme	Enrolment	Progress	Performance
A. NUTRITIONAL INTERVENTIONS			
Colombia, Bogotá	Average age of enrolment 5.6 years for supplementation/home visit 6.0 years for control	Repetition: Treatment Yes 4% No 13%	Teacher assigned grades no difference (1st grade)
Colombia, Cali		Average grade level 3.2 for experimental in 4th year: 2.9 for comparison	
Guatemala	Earlier for supplemented	No effect	Academic performance: no effect/social interaction: positive effects
México (Chávez)	All enrolled	Repetition: (1st grade) Treatment Yes 0% No 35%	Significant differences found in: school exam / national exam / Detroit-Engle test / behaviour observation
B. EDUCATIONAL STUDIES			
Turkey, comprehensive preschool research project	—		Performance in grade 3 (see below)
India, (Dalmau)	Entrance by ICDS at earlier age (85% vs. 74% by age 6). Only significant for girls	Regular attendance higher for ICDS (88% vs. 74% had average of above attendance record)	1. Scholastic performance, based on teacher ratings favoured ICDS (90% vs. 76% rated average or above) 2. Behaviour: 93% vs. 81% rated average or above

Performance in grade 3

	Preschool education vs. custodial care Home care	Maternal education vs. non maternal education
1. School grades	+	+
2. Behaviour		+
3. Achievement test	+	+
4. General abilities		+

	Right age for grade:	Drop out by 3rd:	
India (Haryana State)	ICDS Yes / No Lower caste: 80% / 56% Middle caste: 75 / 56 Higher caste: 82 / 59	ICDS Yes / No 19% / 35% 5 / 25 7 / 8	1. Teacher classification: overwhelming majority of the children in top ten and 20% were those who had 2–3 years of exposure . . . to anganwadi. . . . attention span and retention power was superior
Morocco	—	No difference in promotion rates	1. Achievement test (1st grade): + For Quranic in rural areas + For modern in urban areas No difference for Quranic in urban areas 2. General abilities test
Argentina (4 country study) (C.S.)	Lower age of enrolment (all social classes, urban and rural especially low ses/rural)	Repetition (year 1): Preschool Yes / No Low ses/urban: 12% / 27% Low ses/rural: 36% / 77%	1. Reading/writing ability significantly higher for preschoolers of all ses levels
Bolivia (4 C.S.)	Negligible differences	—	1. Reading/writing ability significantly higher for preschoolers (except for urban marginal children)
Chile (4 C.S.)	Lower age of enrolment (all social classes)	No difference	1. Reading/writing ability negligible effect
Colombia (4 C.S.)	Negligible differences	Repetition (year 1): Preschool Yes / No Low ses/urban: 10% / 22%	1. Reading/writing ability negligible effect
Brazil (Fortaleza)	—	Repetition (year 1): Kindergarten Yes / No 36% / 66% (Girls benefited most)	—

Table 10.4 continued

Country/programme	Enrolment	Progress	Performance
Perú	Lower age of enrolment	No difference in 1st or 2nd grade promotion rates	
Chile	–	–	No difference in grades or on results of special math/language ability test 1st grade: Teacher rating + (71% vs. 39% rated as good) Draw-a-man + Parental assessment +
Colombia	Enrolment in 1st grade: PROMESA Yes No 100% 87%	PROMESA Yes No Reached 2nd grade 83% 77% Reached 3rd grade 73 44 Reached 4th grade 60 30	–
Brazil, Alagoas	–	PROAPE Non-PROAPE Dropout 1st grade 18% 14% Repetition 9 33 Dropout + repetition 27 47	–

Sources: see Tables 10.2 and 10.3

was only 9 per cent for the PROAPE children as compared with 33 per cent for children who did not participate in the programme. The other study from Brazil, from Fortaleza, showed a high rate of 36 per cent repetition in the first grade for children with a kindergarten experience, but an even higher rate of 66 per cent for those without such experience. (These differences for Brazil are consistent with results of other studies not reported here.)

The four studies from Colombia all show significant differences in progress through the educational system. The biggest of these is associated with a programme in the extremely impoverished area of the Choco where 60 per cent of the programme children reached the fourth grade of primary school versus only 30 per cent of the comparison group. This result is consistent with the Indian (Haryana) and Argentine studies, suggesting also that differences are most pronounced for the most disadvantaged children. In Argentina, 36 per cent of the rural children from low socioeconomic backgrounds repeated if they had a preschool experience as compared with 77 per cent for those without.

Performance

Academic performance   In two of the three nutrition studies for which information was available, no difference in academic performance was found between the programme children and the comparison group. In six of the ten education studies with available information, children from early intervention programmes performed better; in two the effect was negligible; in one there was no difference between the two groups; and, in one (Morocco), positive effects were found in a rural, but not an urban context.

Social behaviour and school adjustment   Less information was found regarding differences in social behaviour of schoolchildren as related to their participation in an intervention during the preschool years. The Guatemalan nutrition study demonstrated that programme children who received high caloric supplementation from birth to age two years had higher levels of social involvement than unsupplemented children. Both Indian studies indicated better deportment among ICDS than among non-ICDS children. The Turkish study found that adjustment was better among children whose mothers had participated in a parental training programme, but there was no difference in adjustment according to whether a child had been in a preschool centre or not.

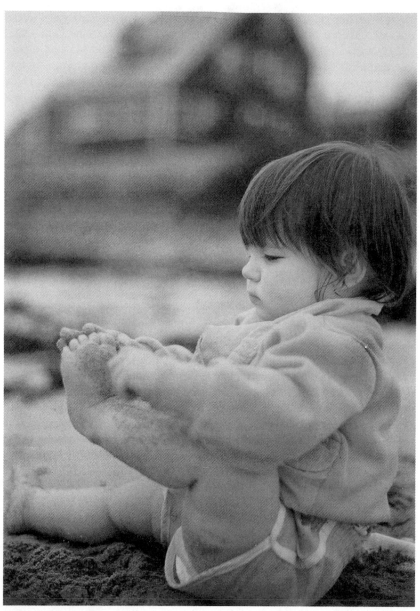

'Katie's world', Maine, US

The readiness of schools for children

Curiously, this particular body of research and evaluation information provides little insight into whether schools are ready for children or not. No analyses are available of what happens to children of similar backgrounds who go to primary schools of different quality. The unspoken assumption in more than one of the studies is that children who went to poorer quality schools would not make the same progress in spite of their involvement in the early intervention programme.

The effect of 'availability' seems to come into play in the four-country Latin American study. In Colombia and Bolivia, no differences were found between preschool and non-preschool children in their readiness at the time of entry into first grade. In these two countries, there was often a lag of one to three years between preschooling and the entry into primary school. In the Moroccan example, promotion quotas come into play. In the Peruvian study, the poor quality of the primary schools was suggested as the reason why improved readiness for school did not seem to have an effect on progress or performance.

Interestingly, it is only in the cases where school readiness did seem to improve as a result of being in an early childhood programme that the school was looked to as a possible explanation why the preschool result did not continue. But it is logical to think that, to some degree, the readiness of schools for children was operating in all cases, for good or ill. What did not occur to researchers was to examine the interaction between early interventions in the preschool years as they affect the readiness of children, and the differential availability and quality of schools.

Summary

What does all this mean? The evidence presented supports several preliminary conclusions:

1 Early intervention programmes, more often than not, have a positive effect on the probability of enrolment, on school progress (as represented by repetition and dropout rates, and by grades), and on achievement in the early years of primary school. The effect can be very large.

2 The mechanisms producing improved enrolment, progress, and performance in primary school appear to reflect some combination of earlier age of enrolment (which regularizes progress through the system), improved school readiness (related to improved health and nutritional condition, and/or to improved cognitive skills), and changes in parental expectations regarding the ability of their children and/or the importance of schooling.

3 Structural conditions and the quality of primary schooling can moderate the potential effects of improved school readiness on school progress or performance.

4 Poor children and children from social groups that have been discriminated against may benefit more than more privileged peers from early intervention programmes that are multifaceted.

5 There may be gender differences in the programme effects, helping girls to catch up to boys in circumstances where their primary school entrance lags.

6 We do not know whether effects persist over time. Only one study looked at school progress and performance beyond the third grade, and that was a cohort study that did not follow individuals. The durability of effects and the conditions under which they persist or deteriorate remain to be documented.

These conclusions are encouraging. They provide the kind of hopeful conclusions that should stimulate additional experimentation and evaluation. When placed alongside the results from the United States and Europe, they suggest that similarly positive effects of early interventions are not only possible, but that the potential for bringing about improvements is greatest where social or economic conditions prejudice entrance, continuation, and performance in primary school. When placed beside the potential cost savings of reduced repetition (see also Chapter 15), these results provide one important element in the broader rationale for investing in early childhood care and development programmes.

At the same time, it would be useful to have additional information in order to draw conclusions about the specific kinds of early childhood interventions most likely to benefit children in each of the difficult and varied circumstances found in most developing countries. Researchers and evaluators have an important task in the coming years, tracing students from different programmes over a longer period of time, examining questions of 'dosage', i.e. differences in the length of time in a programme, taking a more anthropological approach to the transition, and examining the interaction of improved readiness for school with improved readiness of schools for children. More work is needed to sort out the effects of 'empowering' parents, much as was done in the Turkish study described here.

IMPLICATIONS FOR POLICY AND PROGRAMMING

1 *An investment can bring results.* The personal and social costs of a poor entrance into school are such that improving the articulation between home and school should be a central policy goal of developing country governments and international donors, particularly in countries where repetition and dropout in the first grades of primary school are still high. Sufficient evidence exists that early childhood interventions can improve success in school; there is no need to wait for more refined and detailed studies.

2 *Combine early education with health and nutrition.* The importance of

combining health, nutrition, and educational interventions, discussed in Chapter 9, is confirmed in this chapter. It is clear from even the roughest of comparisons that greater attention will have to be given in Third World programmes to current health and nutritional needs of children than has been the case in child development programmes in the United States and Europe. That attention should go beyond simple food supplementation to include specific attention to micro-nutrient needs.

3 *Treat early education and the first years of primary together.* To improve the articulation between home, preschool and school, bringing a positive effect on schooling (and beyond to adult life and the next generation), attention needs to be given *jointly* to improving children's readiness for school and schools' readiness for children. There is need, then, for a combined approach to early childhood and the early years of primary school education.

To combine programmes requires a rethinking of the programming process. It means bridging the artificial separation between preschool and primary school children at the time of entry into school. It means getting primary school divisions of education ministries to work with preschool divisions and with pertinent parts of other ministries concerned with health and nutrition.

Combining programmes also requires a shift in attitude in which real changes in schools should be contemplated as part of their improved readiness for children, rather than thinking only or even principally that children must be adjusted to schools.

> An integrated early childhood-primary programme could serve as a vehicle for linking family and community interests and strengths to the formal schooling system; for example, fusing the values and content of the local culture into the curriculum, at first at the pre-primary then at the primary level; serving as a focus of community development energies that, once organized, could be focussed on other issues; involving teachers in the solution of community problems linked to child development but not obviously part of the formal school system's mandate; reaching parents and their children with educational services before the perceived costs of children's participation in a process with ill-defined returns becomes too high.
>
> (Halpern and Myers 1985)

Taking a combined programme view raises a series of questions – about where such a programme would be focused organizationally, about what integrative mechanisms might be used to achieve the needed coordination. If early childhood is made the responsibility exclusively of the Ministry of Education, there is a risk that the very early years will be neglected and that programmes for children aged three to six will simply become downward extensions of formal primary schooling. If that were to happen, the apparent inflexibility of primary schooling would be reinforced at the same time that programmes are created for younger children that are inappropriate to their needs.

Creating a child development/primary school unit   One organizational alternative would be to create a semi-autonomous unit within the Ministry of Education that would be charged with the responsibility for programmes covering children three to eight years of age, or even from birth or age one to eight. This unit would be a multidisciplinary unit, including individuals with health, nutrition, adult education, and community development backgrounds. The non-education personnel might be paid by ministries other than education and 'loaned', with the understanding that they would serve as a liaison to programmes in health, nutrition, etc. The actions of this group could be overseen by an inter-ministerial committee.

Possible actions   Creating such a unit might facilitate such actions as:

– The primary school curriculum might incorporate a child-to-child component in which older primary school children were not only encouraged to take child-care messages home, but were also scheduled to participate as a helper in the attached preschool for an hour or so each week, applying what they had learned, and learning from the preschool teacher. Where siblings bring their younger brothers and sisters to school with them (as happens, for instance, on a large scale in Pakistan), it would be possible to arrange child-care and early education for the preschoolers, drawing on the child-to-child strategies and/or putting the children in a separate, but adjoining, preschool/child-care class.

– Inclusion of childrearing content in literacy and post-literacy programmes.

– Greater coordination between home visiting programmes and adult education programmes of various kinds.

– 'Parental education' programmes linked to preschool and/or primary schools – through parents' committees or arranged by other organizations, providing incentives in the form of certification.

– Locating preschools and primary schools near to each other so that primary school children might bring siblings to the preschool, picking them up at the end of their school day. Such an arrangement could help to increase enrolment in primary schools (particularly for girls). This idea might require setting up as suggested above.

– Experimentation with a 'Year 0' (Schiefelbein 1988) could be tried in the primary school in which entering students are eased into primary school with a combination of play and pre-literacy/numeracy activities.

– Development of a phased bilingual education programme (as is being done in Guatemala) that would include instruction in the mother tongue in the early years.

- Where villagers expect a preschool teacher to provide children with the three Rs, the pressures on the preschool teacher to devote most of her time to such matters might be moderated by having one of the primary school teachers visit the preschool for an hour or so each week, explicitly to work with the older preschoolers on their ABCs. This might help the primary school teacher have a better idea of what children would need upon arrival at primary school. It could also help initial adjustment by the preschool children arriving at the primary school, because they would have been exposed to the teacher. In settings where the preschool teacher obtains her prestige from being a 'teacher', this idea might not work because it could undercut that prestige. Nevertheless, alternate bases for prestige could be sought and the idea could be tried out.
- Radio (and television) programmes could be created for transmission to both preschool centres and classrooms in the first one or two years of primary school. The content could include health and nutrition and play activities relevant for the age range between three and eight and could be supported by booklets with pre- and post-transmission suggestions for activities to be carried out with the children (as is being done in India). The media have the possibility of crossing bureaucratic lines.
- Joint working groups of preschool and primary school teachers could be arranged, to discuss the different expectations they have from children and to see ways in which the articulation between preschool programmes and primary school programmes might be improved through adjusted actions of both groups. (This has been tried out in Guyana.)
- Primary school teachers could be trained in how to draw more effectively on play as a learning device in the first few years of primary school. This training might be joint with preschool teachers.

There will undoubtedly be reasons why various of the above will not work in a particular location. Adjustment to local circumstances is obviously required. The intention here is simply to provide some examples of ways in which the programming process might be rethought, crossing preschool – primary school lines.

4 *Build in evaluation*   Another implication of the above review and discussion is that evaluation should be built into early childhood programmes, with extension into the early years of primary schooling. It would be wise also to accompany a rethinking and reorganization with a programme of research focused on the transitional ages.

Instruments and measures   In order to carry out evaluations it is also necessary to pay more attention than has been given in the past to indicators and instruments for measuring child development.

Readiness profiles We might also consider, in line with the way in which we have framed the issue above, creating both a child readiness profile and a school readiness profile.

A *child readiness profile* (CRP) would provide a description of children at age four or five, as they prepare to move further beyond the confines of the family, and, particularly, as they face the transition from home to school. We know that involvement and success in various life activities, including schooling, is affected by how healthy and well-nourished a child is, by how well the child handles language and basic concepts facilitating learning, by the social confidence of the child and by the expectations held for the child by others. Accordingly, a CRP might be made up of indicators of:

- morbidity
- nutritional status
- pre-literacy and pre-numeracy concepts and skills
- self-esteem
- family expectations for the child

These are suggestive. The particular indicators used in particular areas could and should be developed by an interdisciplinary team of individuals who know well the area in which the indicators would be applied. Whatever profile is developed, it would need to be validated by looking at its relationship to school performance and other indicators of positive social behaviour, determined locally. Once done, the child readiness profile could be applied periodically, on a sample basis. This would provide programmers and evaluators with an instrument to show how a given population of children is faring with respect to their readiness for school and life.

A *school readiness profile*: the indicators that might go into a school readiness profile are not so clear and might vary widely from place to place, but the profile might include indicators of:

- School availability, including locus and scheduling
- The way language is treated
- The inclusion of local materials in the curriculum
- The attitudes or expectations of teachers

5 *A need for longitudinal studies* Finally, there is a need for systematic, well-designed studies that follow children through their primary school years. We could find no equivalents in the Third World of the longitudinal studies that have had such an influence on thinking about early interventions in industrialized countries. If such studies were done it would no longer be necessary to refer, with some apologies, to research from the industrialized world when arguing the importance of investment in early interventions of various kinds. Access to such a body of research would

support the development, implementation, and evaluation of integrated programmes of early childhood development that cross bureaucratic lines and consider, in a holistic fashion, the first eight years of a child's life.

In this chapter we have examined one area in which programme integration might be sought. We turn now to another very different area, the intersecting (or competing) needs of children and women, especially as reflected in programming for child care in relation to women's work. Again, the topic will be approached with the idea that there is a need to think across intellectual and bureaucratic lines if we are to achieve the desired programme integration.

NOTE

1 This chapter draws heavily on two papers prepared for the Consultative Group on Early Childhood Care and Development: Robert Halpern and Robert Myers, 'Effects of Early Childhood Intervention on Primary School Progress and Performance in the Developing Countries', 1985; and, Robert Myers, 'Effects of Early Childhood Intervention on Primary School Progress and Performance in Developing Countries: An Update', 1985.

REFERENCES

Anderson, M., H. Fox and L. Lewin. *Reducing Infant Death and Disability: Effective Interventions and State Strategies for Implementation.* Washington DC: Lewin and Associates, 1983.

Balderston, J., A. Wilson, M. Freire and S. Simonen. *Malnourished Children of the Rural Poor.* Boston: Auburn House, 1981.

Barrett, D. and M. Radke-Yarrow. 'Effects of Nutritional Supplementation on Children's Responses to Novel, Frustrating, and Competitive Situations', *American Journal of Clinical Nutrition,* Vol. 42, No. 1 (1985), pp. 102–20.

Beirn, R., D. Kinsey and N. McGinn. 'Antecedents and Consequences of Early School Leaving', Cambridge, Mass: Harvard Graduate School of Education, Occasional Papers in Education and Development, No. 8, 1972.

Berg, A. *Malnourished People: A Policy View.* Washington: the World Bank, 1981.

Berg, A. and S. Brems. 'Micronutrient Deficiencies: Present Knowledge of Effects and Control', Technical Note 86–32B, World Bank, Population, Health and Nutritional Department, Washington DC, 1986.

Berruta-Clement, J.R., L.J. Schweinhart, W.S. Barnett, A.S. Epstein and D.T. Weikart. *Changed Lives: The Effects of the Perry Preschool Program on Youths Through Age 19.* Ypsilanti, Mich: High/Scope Educational Research Foundation, Monograph No. 8, 1984.

Berstecher, D. and R. Carr-Hill. *Primary Education and Economic Recession in the Developing World Since 1980.* A special study for the World Conference on Education for All (Thailand, 5–9 March, 1990). Paris: UNESCO, 1990.

Birdsall, N. 'Population and Poverty in the Developing World', Washington DC: the World Bank, 1980, Staff Working Paper 404.

Braithwaite, John. *Explorations in Early Childhood Education.* The Hague:

Bernard van Leer Foundation, 1983.

Bronfenbrenner, U. *The Ecology of Human Development.* Cambridge, Mass: Harvard University Press, 1979.

Chaturvedi, E., B.C. Srivastava, J.V. Singh and M. Prasad. 'Impact of Six Years Exposure to ICDS Scheme on Psycho-social Development', *Indian Pediatrics*, Vol. 24 (February 1987), pp. 153–60.

Chávez, A. and C. Martínez. *Growing Up in a Developing Community, a Bio-Ecological Study of the Development of Children from Poor Peasant Families in Mexico.* An English publication by INCAP, Guatemala, of *Nutrición y Desarrollo Infantil*, Mexico: Nueva Editorial Interamericana, S.A. de CV., 1979.

Chávez, A. and C. Martínez. 'School Performance of Supplemented and Unsupplemented Children from a Poor Rural Area', in A.E. Harper and G.K. Davis (eds), *Nutrition in Health and Disease and International Development: Symposia from the XII International Congress on Nutrition*, Vol. 77, Progress in Clinical and Biological Research, New York: Alan R. Liss, Inc., 1981.

Cicirelli, V., *The Impact of Head Start: An Evaluation of Head Start on Children's Cognitive and Affective Development.* Athens, Ohio: Westinghouse Learning Corporation, 1969.

Colclough, C. 'Primary Schooling and Economic Development: A Review of the Evidence', Washington DC: the World Bank, Staff Working Paper No 399, 1980.

Colclough, C. and K. Lewin. *Educating all the Children: The Economic Challenge for the 1990s.* A book-length manuscript prepared for the World Conference on Education for All, Thailand, 5–9 March, 1990. Brighton, University of Sussex, 1990. Mimeo.

Coombs, P. *The World Crisis in Education: The View from the Eighties.* New York: Oxford University Press, 1985.

Cravioto, J. and R. Arrieta. *Nutrición, Desarrollo Mental, Conducta y Aprendizaje*, Mexico: Sistéma Nacional para el Desarrollo Integral de la Familia, UNICEF, Mexico, 1982.

Epstein, A. and D. Weikart. 'The Ypsilanti-Carnegie Infant Education Project', Ypsilanti, Mich: High/Scope Educational Research Foundation Monograph, 1979.

Feijo, M. 'Early Childhood Education Programs and Children's Subsequent Learning: A Brazilian Case', unpublished PhD. dissertation, Stanford University, Department of Education, 1984.

Filp, J., S. Donoso, S. Cardemil, E. Dieguéz, J. Torres and E. Schiefelbein. 'Relationship between Pre-primary and Grade One Primary Education in State Schools in Chile', in K. King and R. Myers (eds) *Preventing School Failure: The Relationship Between Preschool and Primary Education.* Ottawa: the International Development Research Centre, 1983.

Gordon, I. and R. Jester. 'Middle School Performance as a Function of Early Intervention, Final Report to the Child Welfare Research and Demonstration Grants Program', Washington DC: Administration for Children, Youth and Families, 1980.

Government of India. 'Draft Report of the Working Group on Early Childhood Education and Elementary Education', New Delhi: Ministry of Human Resource Development, Department of Education, 1989. Mimeo.

Grawe, R. 'Ability in Pre-schoolers, Earnings, and Home Environment', Washington: World Bank, Working Paper No. 322, 1979.

Gray, S., B. Ramsey and R. Klaus. *From Three to Twenty – The Early Training Project.* Baltimore: University Park Press, 1982.

Haddad, W. 'Educational and Economic Effects of Promotion and Repetition Practices', Washington DC: the World Bank, Staff Working Paper No. 319.

Haglund, E. 'The Problem of the Match – Cognitive Transition Between Early Childhood and Primary School: Nigeria', *Journal of Developing Areas*, 17 (1982), pp. 77–92.

Halpern, R. and R. Myers. 'Effects of Early Childhood Intervention on Primary School Progress and Performance in the Developing Countries', a paper prepared for the United States Agency for International Development, Ypsilanti, Mich: the High/Scope Educational Research Foundation, April, 1985. Mimeo.

Harrell, A. 'The Effects of the Head Start Program on Children's Cognitive Development: Preliminary Report', Washington DC: US Department of Health and Human Services, Administration for Children, Youth and Families, 1983.

Herrera, M. and C. Super. 'School Performance and Physical Growth of Underprivileged Children: Results of the Bogotá Project at Seven Years', report to the World Bank. Cambridge, Mass: Harvard School of Public Health, 1983.

Heyneman, S. and W. Loxley. 'The Impact of Primary School Quality on Academic Achievement Across 29 High and Low Income Countries', *American Journal of Sociology*, 88 (1983), pp. 1162–94.

Inkeles, Alex and D.H. Smith. *Becoming Modern: Individual Change in Six Developing Countries*. Cambridge, Mass: Harvard University Press, 1974.

Irvine, D. 'Evaluation of the New York State Experimental Pre-Kindergarten Program', a paper presented at the annual meeting of the American Educational Research Association, New York City, 1982. Mimeo.

Irwin, M., P. Engle, C. Yarborough, R. Klein and J. Townsend. 'The Relationship of Prior Ability and Family Characteristics to School Attendance and School Achievement in Rural Guatemala', *Child Development*, 49 (1978), pp. 415–27.

Kağitçibaşi, C., D. Sunar and S. Bekman. 'Comprehensive Preschool Education Project: Final Report', Istanbul, Turkey: Boğaziçi University, November, 1987. A report prepared for the International Development Research Centre.

Klein, R. 'Malnutrition and Human Behavior: A Backward Glance at an Ongoing Longitudinal Study', in D. Levitsky (ed.), *Malnutrition, Environment and Behavior*. Ithaca: Cornell University Press, 1979, pp. 217–237.

Lal, Sunder and Raj Wati. 'Non-Formal Preschool Education – An Effort to Enhance School Enrolment', a paper presented for the National Conference on Research on ICDS, February 25–29, 1986. New Delhi: National Institute for Public Cooperation in Child Development (NIPCCD). Mimeo.

Laosa, L. 'Schooling, Occupation, Culture, and Family: The Impact of Parental Schooling on the Parent-child Relationship', *Journal of Educational Psychology*, Vol. 74, No. 6 (1982), pp. 791–827.

Lazar, I. 'Some Long Term Effects of Early Education', a paper presented to the International Conference on Early Education and Development (0-6 years), Hong Kong, July 31–August 4, 1989. Mimeo.

Lazar, I. and R. Darlington. 'Lasting Effects of Early Education: A Report from the Consortium for Longitudinal Studies', *Monographs of the Society for Research in Child Development*. No. 195, 1982.

Levenstein, P., J. O'Hara and J. Madden. 'The Mother–Child Home Program of the Verbal Interaction Project', in Consortium for Longitudinal Studies (ed.) *As the Twig is Bent – Lasting Effects of Preschool Programs*. Hillsdale, New Jersey: Lawrence Earlbaum, 1983, pp. 237–63.

Levin, H. and E. Pollitt. 'Micronutrient Deficiency Disorders', a paper prepared as part of the World Bank Sector Priorities Review, Washington DC, the World Bank, January, 1989. Draft.

Levine, R. 'Influences of Women's Schooling on Maternal Behavior in the Third World', *Comparative Education Review*, Vol 24, No. 3 (1980), Part 2, pp. 78–105.

Lockheed, M., D. Jamison and L. Lau. 'Farmer Education and Farm Efficiency: A Survey', *Economic Development and Cultural Change*, 29 (October 1980), pp. 37–76.

McKay, A. 'Longitudinal Study of the Long-term Effects of the Duration of Early Childhood Intervention on Cognitive Ability and Primary School Performance', unpublished PhD. dissertation, Northwestern University, Evanston, Illinois, 1982.

Maguire, J. and J. Austin. 'Beyond Survival: Children's Growth for National Development', *Assignment Children*, No. 2 (1987), New York: UNICEF.

Ministerio da Saude, y Instituto Nacional de Alimentação e Nutrição. 'Analição do PROAPE/Alagoas com Enfoque na Area Economica, Brasilia, MS/INAN, 1983. Mimeo.

Monroe, E. and M. McDonald. 'Follow-up Study of the 1966 Head Start Program', Home City Schools, Rome, Georgia, 1981. Mimeo.

Moock, Peter. 'Education and Technical Efficiency in Small-Farm Production', *Economic Development and Cultural Change*, 29 (July 1981), pp. 723–39.

Moock, P. and J. Leslie. 'Childhood Malnutrition and Schooling in the Terai Region of Nepal', *Journal of Development Economics*, (1986), pp. 33–52.

Myers, R. 'El niño y sus ambientes de aprendizaje', a paper prepared for a meeting on 'La transición de la familia a la escuela', Santiago, Chile, Centro de Investigación y Desarrollo Educativo, diciembre, 1990.

Myers, R. 'Effects of Early Childhood Intervention on Primary School Progress and Performance in Developing Countries: An Update, 1988'. Ypsilanti, Mich: the High/Scope Educational Research Foundation, 1988. Mimeo.

Myers, R. *et al.* 'Preschool Education as a Catalyst for Community Development', a report prepared for the US Agency for International Development, Lima, Peru, 1985. Mimeo.

Nimnicht, G. and P.E. Posada. 'The Intellectual Development of Children in Project Promesa', Medellin, Colombia, Centro Internacional de Educación y Desarrollo Humano (CINDE), Research and Evaluation Reports, No. 1, October, 1986. A report prepared for the Bernard van Leer Foundation.

Osborn, A.F. and J.E. Milbank. *The Effects of Early Education: A Report from the Child Health and Education Study.* Oxford: Clarendon Press, 1987.

Palmer, F. 'The Harlem Study: Effects by Type of Training, Age of Training and Social Class', in Consortium for Longitudinal Studies (ed.) *As the Twig is Bent – Lasting Effects of Preschool Programs.* Hillsdale, New Jersey: Lawrence Earlbaum, 1983, pp. 201–36.

Pollitt, E. 'Child Development Reference Document: (I) Risk Factors in the Mental Development of Young Children in the Developing Countries. (II) Early Childhood Intervention Programs for the Young Child in the Developing World', prepared for UNICEF, Houston, Texas Health Science Center, 1984. Mimeo.

Pollitt, E. and E. Metallinos-Katsaras. 'Iron Deficiency and Behavior: Constructs, Methods and Validity of the Findings', a chapter to be published in Wurtman and Wurtman (eds) *Nutrition and the Brain: Vol 8: Behavioral Effects of Metals, and their Biochemical Mechanisms.* New York: Raven Press, 1990, pp. 101–46.

Popkin, B. and M. Lim-Ybanez. 'Nutrition and School Achievement', *Social Science and Medicine*, 16 (1982), pp. 53–61.

Pozner, P. 'Relationship between Preschool Education and First Grade in Argentina', in K. King and R. Myers (eds) *Preventing School Failure: The Relationship between Preschool and Primary Education*. Ottawa: the International Development Research Centre, 1983, pp. 75–86.

Psacharopoulos, George. 'Returns to Education: A Further International Update and Implications', *Journal of Human Resources*, 20 (Fall 1986), pp. 583–604.

Raizen, S. and S. Bobrow. *Design for a National Evaluation of Social Competence in Head Start Children*. Santa Monica, California: the Rand Corporation, 1974.

Richards, H. *The Evaluation of Cultural Action*. London: The Macmillan Press Ltd. 1985.

Rogoff, B. 'Schooling and the development of cognitive skills', in H. Triandis and A. Heron (eds) *Handbook of Cross-cultural Psychology*, Vol. 4, Boston: Allyn-Bacon, 1980.

Schiefelbein, E. 'Siete Estrategias para Elevar la Calidad y Eficiencia del Sistéma de Educación', Santiago, Chile, Marzo de 1988. Mimeo.

Schiefelbein, E. and J. Farrell. 'Causas de la Deserción en la Enseñanza Media, *Revista de Educación*, 68 (1978), pp. 43–51.

Seshadri, S. and T. Gopaldas. 'Impact of Iron Supplementation on Cognitive Functions in Pre-School and School-aged Children: The Indian Experience', *American Journal of Clinical Nutrition*, Supplement (1989).

Smilansky, M. 'Priorities in Education: Pre-School; Evidence and Conclusions', Working Paper No. 323, Washington, the World Bank, 1979.

Soemantri, A.G., E. Pollitt and I. Kim. 'Iron Deficiency Anemia and Educational Achievement', *The American Journal of Clinical Nutrition*, Vol 42 (December 1985), pp. 1221–8.

Toro, B. and I. de Rosa. 'Papito, ¿Yo Porque Tengo que Repitir el Año?' Toronto: Ontario Institute for Studies in Education, 1983. Mimeo.

Triandis, H. 'Reflections on Trends in Cross-Cultural Research', *Journal of Cross-Cultural Psychology*, Vol. 11, No. 1 (1980), pp. 35–58.

UNESCO, Regional Office for Latin America and the Caribbean, Sub-regional Office for Central America, 'Estudio Prospectivo sobre Escolarización, Alfabetización, y Calidad de la Educación', San José, Costa Rica, 1987.

Wagner, D. and J. Spratt. 'Cognitive Consequences of Contrasting Pedagogies: The Effects of Quaranic Pre-schooling in Morocco', *Child Development*, Vol. 58 (1987), pp. 1209–19.

World Bank, *Education in Sub-Saharan Africa, Policies for Adjustment, Revitalization, and Expansion*. Washington DC: the World Bank, January, 1988.

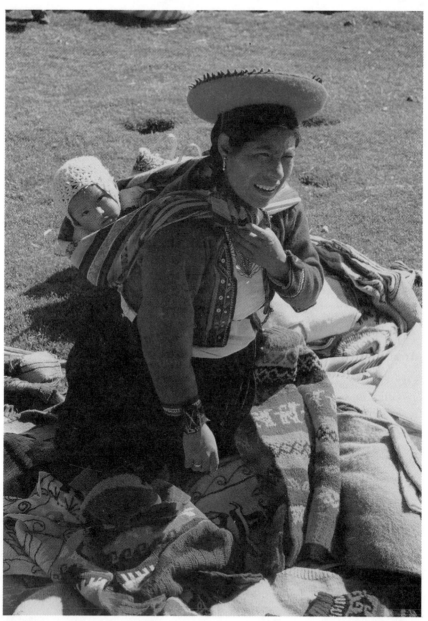

'Double duty', Chincheros, Peru

Chapter 11

Relating child care, women's work and child development[1]

Juanita Quispe edges her collapsible wooden stool a little closer in order to hear a particularly juicy bit of gossip that her friend, Olinda, has just begun to tell. She moves with care, not wanting to wake her 18-month-old daughter, asleep on her lap. Newly settled, she picks up her knitting and leans forward, only to be interrupted by a passerby who wants to know the price of the plastic combs for sale on Juanita's pushcart. After bargaining, a purchase is made and Juanita turns again to Olinda who, however, has now stopped both her talking and her spinning so she can shift her infant to a new position inside the colourful cloth keeping the baby warm and close on her back.

Each day, Juanita and Olinda, with children slung on their backs, wheel their carts to a position on a side street near the main market in Cuzco, Peru. They arrive early to get a good place and to be able to sell to people on their way to work. Before leaving home, they will have prepared food and started older children on the way to primary school. When they get home in the evening, they will have another meal to prepare and some washing to do. Typically, their work day is 16 to 18 hours, counting in the domestic labours. The children, although helpful, are all still too young to do much housework or to earn money. Their father is many kilometres away, in Lima, and only sends a small bit of money at the holidays. The meagre earnings from sales during the day barely stretch to buy needed food.

The story could continue, illustrating what happens during a typical day, or what occurs when one of the children is sick or when Olinda's estranged husband appears to abuse her or when nobody makes a purchase. Parallel scenes could be created in an African or Asian setting, and in rural as well as urban areas, showing how, within the difficult limits imposed by poverty and social convention, women have developed survival strategies, integrating their roles as mothers, homemakers, income earners, and social beings.

In concept and action, and even in time, Juanita and Olinda combine the multiple roles they must carry out to keep body and soul together. They do not separate out 'productive' from 'reproductive' roles. The way in which the two women handle their child care is intimately and directly linked to their income-earning possibilities and vice versa.

In the world of programmes, however, these roles, labelled 'reproductive' and 'productive', are often treated separately. Child-care programmes, particularly those which incorporate a child development perspective, are often created without understanding the daily life and pressures and needs and work options of caregivers. Similarly, women-in-development (WID) programmes are set in motion without considering what changes the programmes may require in child care, or what effects they may have on the welfare of children.

In this chapter, we are interested in what happens to children and to child-care routines when Juanita and Olinda, and their counterparts in poor families elsewhere, become participants in a credit or training programme, a co-op, an appropriate technology project or another effort intended to improve women's welfare (and presumably that of their children). And, we are interested in the effect on both the children and the working women when child-care programmes are created.

NEW VIEWPOINTS AND PROGRAMMES

Separate programmes for women that focus on their role as income earners or that respond to their personal needs are a relatively recent phenomenon. Prior to 1960 and the beginning of the First Development Decade, very few programmes existed in Third World countries focusing on women's needs and interests. Socialist countries, in which women were incorporated into the labour force in large numbers, constitute an exception. But, excluding a limited number of socialist countries in the Third World, benefits to women from governmental programmes or from programmes of international aid originating in the West (or provided through the United Nations) were at best indirect, often embedded within community or rural development or health programmes. Special women's ministries or divisions had not yet been created.

Slowly, however, changing economic and social conditions, changing ideas about what constitutes economic and social development, and a new consciousness among women have led governments, non-governmental organizations, and international agencies alike to include special and separate women's programmes in their portfolios. Throughout the decade of the 1960s and in the early 1970s, most WID programmes had what has been termed a welfare orientation (Buvinic, 1984). These programmes 'for' women responded almost exclusively to the needs of women in relation to the traditional roles of homemaker and childrearer. Home economics programmes, maternal and child health care, and maternal education programmes clearly fall within that category. Some 'appropriate technology' and literacy programmes could also be included. A woman's main contribution to development was still seen as occurring through her domestic or reproductive role.[2]

As long as a welfare bias was present in programming, the link between programming for women and for children was relatively easy to make. For instance, mother and child health (MCH) programmes make the link explicitly, seeking improvement in both the nutrition and health of pregnant and lactating mothers and the survival chances and welfare of children. In the MCH case, programming to benefit both mothers and children falls *within* the health sector so combining programme interests is not severely hampered by a need to cut *across* bureaucratic divisions.

As the second development decade progressed, however, changes in programme thinking began to occur. Helped along by the International Women's Year in 1975 and the Decade for Women that followed, greater emphasis was given to women in their 'productive' roles and as 'agents of change'. This contrasted with the 'reproductive' emphasis of earlier years and with the welfare view of women as passive recipients or 'targets of intervention' (Buvinic, Lycette, and McGreevey 1983).

Two closely related and relatively new strains of assistance to women evolved, one focusing on social, political, and psychological concerns, the other on the economic participation and contribution of women. The first of these new WID programming lines sought greater self-awareness, organization, and decision-making power for women – within their own families, communities and nations. This strain included programmes of women's rights and attention to such particular needs of women as protection from physical abuse. For the most part, these programmes did not stress rights or activities related to the homemaking or child-care roles of women. Indeed, this absence reflected a strong ideological and political need to de-emphasize helpmate and child-care roles which were viewed as a handicap in the search for equality and broader participation by women in all aspects of economic and social development.

A second, and dominant, strain of WID programmes placed emphasis on women's opportunities to earn income and to use it for their own purposes. Programmes to improve access by women to technology, training and education, and credit were created to support 'income-generating' projects, most involving poor women. On one hand, these projects were seen as ways of increasing and improving the contribution of women to economic development. On the other, they were seen as providing a basis for improving the power and status of women in general, as well as within their own households.

Some of these women's income-generating projects included a child-care component. However, in most cases, child-care emerged as a need once a project got under way (Evans 1985). Consistent with the emphasis on the productive role and with a shying away from maternal concerns, child care and the child typically entered the thinking of WID programmers as an afterthought. This was so even though it was relatively obvious that the lack of alternative child care would constrain women's economic choices and influence her productivity, her health, and her children's welfare.

The main function of child care, if included in women's income-generating programmes, was to give free time to women – for training and/ or work. The potential effects for *children* of substitute, or alternative care was a secondary consideration. An untested assumption was operating: that additional earnings by a mother would result naturally in improvements in child welfare because more money would be directed to that end. Accordingly, child-care programmes tended to be custodial in nature; they did not attend in an integrated way to young children's needs.

NEW ORGANIZATIONAL FORMS

As a special interest in problems facing women grew, it seemed important to many organizations not only to create separate programmes focusing explicitly on women, but also to locate them in special organizational niches. This separatist position was hotly debated, but was nevertheless reflected in the creation of women's ministries or departments or divisions within governments, within non-governmental organizations, and within international and funding agencies. In some cases, this reorganization slowed change, reinforcing a traditional view of women's roles and continuing to treat women in relation to their reproductive role. In others, a radical reorientation occurred towards programmes improving the social and economic position, and the participation of women.

With a new view that separated out productive from reproductive roles, and with the formation of bureaucratic units dedicated specifically to women's programmes, organizational structures began to emerge inhibiting programming that linked in a natural way the overlapping interests and interrelated needs of women and children. These evolving structures began to mirror those described in Chapters 9 and 10, separating health and nutrition from education, and preschool from primary school programming. Competition among units for budget, different forms of conceiving problems, separate plans, and vertical organization helped to cloud the vision of the overlapping needs of women and children, sometimes putting these two groups in competition rather than promoting a complementary and mutually beneficial view in the formulation of programmes.

THE CHANGING CONTEXT

The increasing interest in programmes 'for' and 'with' women must be seen within a context of rapid social, economic, and political change. Over the

30 years to 1990, the appearance of new technologies has affected women's work, sometimes helping to free women's time from other chores and increasing her productivity (for example, simple machines to grind grain into flour), sometimes taking away her work and removing her source of earnings. New employment opportunities for women were a mixed blessing, frequently involving drastic changes in lifestyle and/or opening employment in low-paid, exploitative jobs. For instance, the demand for women to work in low-paid, assembly-line production of clothing in many parts of the world has been accompanied by extremely poor, often life-threatening conditions. Or, new technologies in the flower industry in Colombia have employed many women, but exposure to chemicals creates an ever-present health hazard, particularly to pregnant women, accompanying low pay and long hours. With machines to help with the weeding of fields, women in some parts of India have been put out of work; what was traditionally a female job became a male job, requiring fewer people to do the work.

When these employment-related changes are set beside new and extensive forms of communication capable of reaching into remote and formerly isolated areas, expanded education, changing family systems, and extensive migration, associated with an urban explosion and other new settlement patterns, and when the effect of all these on social values is considered, the result has:

> ... been sufficient to upset a tenuous balance that women seemed to have achieved among their many roles and obligations. For women in numerous occupations, the distancing of the workplace from the home and the insoluble transportation problems of sprawling Third World cities have eliminated the possibility of combining work and child care. Work places have become larger, more bureaucratized and hostile to children. Many are extremely dangerous.... Family systems have changed and so have the local communities on which families depend for helping networks and social participation. A sharp rise in the number of female-headed households in very diverse cultural settings has perhaps been the most dramatic expression of this shift. Entirely new communities have been created such as ... the shanty communities that ring most major Third World cities. These changes ... affect men's and women's relations with their immediate human environment, their relations with each other, and their relation to their children.
>
> (Anderson 1988b, p. 2)

The worldwide recession of the 1980s has further complicated the situation by creating circumstances in which more and more women have had to enter the labour force to help make ends meet (Jolly and Cornia 1984). The recession, combined with the need to service an ever higher international debt, has forced governments to adjust their programme budgets downwards, usually to the detriment of health and education and other service programmes. These changes affect women and children dispro-portionately. They have also led governments to promote more partici-patory programmes.

What is the result of these changes? The burden on women has grown. At the same time that she is expected, or required by economic circum-stances, to increase her work load outside the home, women's domestic responsibilities remain virtually unchanged. Poor women continue to perform and manage essential tasks such as drawing water, collecting fire-wood, and caring for, nurturing, and feeding their infants and young children. It is women who bear the children and it is almost exclusively women and female children who manage the tasks of caring for them.

WOMEN'S WORK AND CHILD WELFARE: AN EVOLVING PERSPECTIVE

The difficult decisions and limited options faced by poor working women as they struggle to balance their multiple roles as mothers and economic providers have been well documented (Carloni 1984; Dwyer and Bruce 1988; Engle 1980, 1986; Nieves 1979, 1981). But the effects of these decisions, or of programmes intended to broaden options, on the well-being of both women and children are not so clear. Sorting out the effects has been hampered because ways of thinking about women's work and about child care have been slow to change. Persisting misconceptions about the work in which women engage and about child care, as care relates to the welfare of women and children, have biased analyses and misguided programmers.

Consider the following three misconceptions often underlying dis-cussions and analyses of women's work and child care:

- Women are full-time housewives who are not engaged in economically productive activity.
- Mothers are the sole caretakers of their children.
- The family is a democratic and altruistic unit maximizing welfare for all its members.

These beliefs stem from outdated Western ideas about the role of women in society and about the social and political dynamics of households. They linger, however, and they affect programmes.

Women as housewives

As the description of Juanita and Olinda at the outset of this chapter illus-trates, one cannot assume, as is often done[3], that all, or even most, women in the Third World are full-time housewives engaged exclusively in 'reproductive' activities; that is the exception rather than the norm. In fact, women are involved in a wide range of economic activities, both inside and outside the home, that contribute directly and indirectly to family income.

The absurdity of holding to a vision of women in the Third World as housewives carrying out purely domestic roles while their husbands provide the family with income is evident in the high number of female-headed households among the poor. For instance, over 40 per cent of rural households in Kenya, Botswana, Ghana, Sierra Leone, and Lesotho are headed by women (Youssef and Hamman 1985). Similarly high figures can be found in many urban slums and shanty towns. Women-headed households, as compared with those headed by men, are characterized as having less income, more and younger children, fewer secondary sources of income, and less access to productive resources. A substantial portion of the female heads of household are also in the 'prime' working age group (25–29), the period in the life cycle when the burden of household dependency is likely to be greatest (Merrick and Schmink 1983). These women must work because their families desperately need cash income (Nieves 1981; Safilios-Rothschild 1980; OEF 1979).

Viewing women as housewives engaged exclusively in domestic chores fosters the inaccurate idea that women do not work while at home (and therefore are not 'productive') or, conversely, that productive work by women must take place outside the home. A narrow definition of 'productivity' – exclusively in terms of cash income – helps to perpetuate that misconception; *paid* work more often than not does occur outside the home. This monetary definition of productivity and its link to work occurring outside the home disregards the fact that a great deal of women's work is not remunerated, occurs at home, and can be considered economically productive.

To foster a better understanding of women's work situations and the productive role of women, it is useful to set up a continuum of work situations, as presented in Table 11.1. Economists often restrict their

Table 11.1 Women's work: a continuum

Income-earning			Unpaid Family Labour		
outside home	inside home	unpaid support for income earning by others	production for family consumption	domestic chores water, wood, laundry, etc.	child care
(1)	(2)	(3)	(4)	(5)	(6)

definition of the productive role of women to the first two categories presented in the table, both of which involve earning money. However, extending the definition to include, at the very least, such non-income activities as the preparation of food for market, and home gardening, represented in categories (3) and (4), seems warranted. In most developed countries, and also among urban middle classes in the Third World, these goods or services would be purchased and the associated labour would therefore be counted as part of the productive process.

Domestic chores (5) such as collecting firewood, cooking, and washing are rarely included in a definition of economic productivity. These chores, seen as part of a woman's reproductive role, nevertheless are vital contributions to the household economy; in many societies, they too would be purchased and counted as productive.

Child care (6) is almost always considered exclusively as part of women's reproductive role. However, to the extent that child care improves the ability of a child to make a productive contribution to the family, and increases productivity in later life, it too is a productive activity. Indeed, a central argument of this book is that investment in child care and development is a productive investment, both economically and socially. That is so whether care occurs in the home and is unremunerated, or whether it occurs in a programme of child care outside the home employing paid caregivers. In the home, the costs and benefits are hidden; outside, they become part of someone's budget and are counted.

Defining productivity in terms of paid work has resulted in a significant misrepresentation of women's contribution to the household economy and an underestimation of the demands made on women's time and labour (Leslie, Lycette, and Buvinic 1988). Although national accounting systems still do not reflect the fact, it is now acknowledged that, when all working hours among family members are assigned an economic value, the contribution of women (and children) to household income can be even greater than that of men in the developing world (King and Evenson 1983; Bhatia and Singh 1987). This is so despite the fact that, whatever the location or sector, the work of women tends to be low-paying, time-intensive (often requiring long hours), labour-intensive (often requiring heavy physical labour), irregular, seasonal, and low in productivity (Anker, Buvinic, and Youssef 1982; Leslie 1988; Saradomoni 1987).

The above discussion suggests that in concept, and in fact, it is inaccurate to emphasize women's homemaking or reproductive activities, and isolate them from productive activities. To do so leads not only to an underestimation of women's productive contributions, but also to a degrading of productive contributions made in carrying out a maternal role. It contributes as well to a lack of appreciation for the 'double day' so often worked by women as they carry out their multiple roles.

The mother as sole caretaker

The idea that there is a direct trade-off, in which a child's welfare will be compromised if a woman works, depends in part on the false assumption that a mother is the only caretaker of her young children.[4] While it is true that the care and nurturing of infants and young children is primarily the responsibility of women and female children in the developing world, mothers are not the sole caretakers in most societies. Indeed, that is the exception rather than the rule (Mueller 1984; Nieves 1981; Oppong 1982; Weisner and Gallimore 1977; Engle 1989). Siblings and aunts and grand-parents and, occasionally, fathers help with child care. Neighbours and baby-sitters and child-care centre workers and home day-care mothers and preschool teachers also care for young children. A mother's direct involvement in child care depends on the availability of these 'alternative' caregivers, some of whom will do as good a job of caregiving as the mother, or better (Tucker 1989), some of whom will not do as well (Shah *et al.* 1979; Johnson 1988).

Recognizing the important role that people other than the mother play, and have always played, in taking care of children helps to unmask one objection to women's working outside the home and to creating child-care programmes – the objection that young children will not be properly attended to unless the mother provides the care. It opens the way to seeking improvements in child welfare by fashioning programmes supporting alternative caregivers, as well as mothers, in their caregiving role.

Families as democratic and altruistic units

Just as it is naive to think that the need for women to work outside the home must be harmful to children, it is naive to think that women's work will, as a result of the money earned, necessarily lead to improvements in a child's welfare or, for that matter, in her own welfare. Behind this thinking are several assumptions: 1) women will earn more than they must pay to cover any costs incurred at home by taking on a job; 2) that women will have control over spending what they earn (or that its distribution will be determined in a democratic way within the family), and 3) that the money earned and controlled by women will be used in ways that improve her child's and her own welfare.

A number of studies in recent years have shown that men and women often have different obligations and priorities for meeting family needs. Although there are variations by cultural context, research results suggest that women generally show greater and steadier allocational inputs than men for children's nutritional and health needs. Thus, mother's income seems to be a better predictor of a child's nutritional status than father's income (Cornia 1984; Kumar 1984; Popkin 1983; Safilios-Rothschild

1980; Bidinger, Nag, and Babu 1986; Johnson 1988). Additional evidence suggests that women's income routinely covers medicine and health care for children and female relatives and that women's savings are critical for medical emergencies (Leslie 1988).

However, in conditions of chronic scarcity, earning income does not guarantee control over that income or its use for improved health and nutrition. Household income is not always pooled (Guyer 1980; Jones 1983; Roldan 1982; Safilio-Rothschild 1980) and a woman may not be able to spend funds as she wishes. Then, the diversity of needs and interests among family members results in a process of negotiation – serious 'bargaining' – between male and female members. Often, the decision-making and bargaining power is unequal, favouring men, reflecting social convention as well as economic and legal inequalities between men and women (Bennett 1983).

But there is also evidence that a woman's ability to bargain and to allocate earnings can be influenced by the extent of her contribution to household income; with increased earnings, greater decision-making power. In Nepal, women's involvement in market activities increased control over their decisions (Acharya and Bennett 1982). However, when women's work is confined to the domestic and subsistence sectors, it may reduce their power *vis-à-vis* men in the household. Income earning by women may be a necessary, but not sufficient, condition for female autonomy and control over decisions. Social, cultural, and psychological dimensions are also at work (Bennett 1983; Youssef 1982; Acharya and Bennett 1982).

This brief look into the dynamics of households shows that the effect of women's work on the welfare of various family members, and particularly children, is not straightforward. Neither those who assume women's work is harmful to young children because it takes away from their attention to them, nor those who assume an income-paying job will improve the welfare of children are necessarily correct. Both women's and children's welfare is subject to mediating conditions, at the levels of family, community, and culture. One of these conditions is the availability of adequate child care.

CHILD-CARE STRATEGIES AND CHOICES

A reminder

As indicated in Chapter 3, the concept of child care is often associated with, but goes beyond 'custodial care', defined in terms of responses to a child's need for shelter, protection from accidents, clothing, feeding, and health care. A child also has psychological, social and emotional needs that must be met and these too are a part of good child care. In the best of worlds, child-care programmes and child development programmes would have the same content.

The importance assigned to each activity of child care will depend on the age of the child, the extent to which the surrounding environment puts a particular child at risk, the ability of a household to meet the needs, and the particular values of the society in which the child is growing up. Moreover, each of the needs listed can be satisfied at various levels, ranging from the minimum needed for survival to the maximum that will allow a child to realize his or her full potential.

Child-care options

There are three main ways in which child-care needs are met by working mothers, to whom most societies continue to assign the responsibility for care:

- do it yourself (work at home or take the child along)
- delegate tasks (to another caretaker, usually in the home, but organize, manage and supervise)
- delegate responsibility (by using a service or 'fostering')

In everyday life, these three child-care categories blur, with different patterns being used at different times of the year (or even during a day). During the peak agricultural season, for instance, it may not be possible for a mother to provide direct care, even though she does so during the rest of the year, so a way must be found to delegate tasks or even responsibility. Also, different caregiving functions may be associated with different caregiving options. A woman may participate directly in the nurturing of her child, but delegate the tasks of feeding and the purchase of clothing. Responsibility for care may be given to a child-care centre for part of a day but reassumed by the mother for the remainder.

Although a child-care strategy may more often involve balancing these options than choosing among them, it is nevertheless useful to distinguish among them. Each option involves a different caregiver. The first two options may occur in or outside the home, but the third is always found outside.

If a woman who must work has no one to whom she can delegate tasks and no child-care centres are available, she is forced to seek employment in jobs that will let her work at home or take the child along. Or, and this happens with too great frequency, she resorts to a fourth strategy – leaving the child alone. Although good figures for this option do not exist, there is some reason to believe that the practice is widespread (Rivera 1979; Anderson 1986; Tolbert 1990.)

Doing it yourself

Time-use and other studies indicate that, in spite of the multiple demands on poor working women, child care continues to be an important priority for them. Working women are reluctant to allocate less time to child care or to turn over child-care tasks to others as their home production or market work increases, particularly when faced with unsatisfactory alternatives (Acevedo *et al.* 1986). In order to provide as much direct care as possible, women often adjust their economic activity, and/or they reduce their 'leisure' activities.

Adjusting economic activities Perhaps the most common coping strategy used by poor women to meet multiple responsibilities is to seek a job in or near the home or work outside the home in which the child can be brought along (DaVanzo and Lee 1983; Deere 1983, Bunster 1983).[5] These activities are seldom found in the formal economic sector and tend to be labour- and time-intensive, and low in productivity. Mothers with young children may work as vendors (as in the case of Juanita and Olinda described at the outset) or take in laundry or seek other work that can be done inside the home such as making of handicrafts or piecework for others (OEF 1979; Nieves 1979; Deere 1983; Bunster 1983). This usually means that a woman's full economic potential is not realized and her earnings remain below what they would be were she to seek another job requiring a different form of child care.

Reducing so-called 'leisure' activities Another coping strategy permitting women to handle both work and child-care roles is to reduce the time spent in 'leisure' activities such as sleep and personal care (Bunster 1983; Engle 1986; Nieves 1981; OEF 1979; Popkin 1983). This strategy takes its toll on women's health. Also, if work does not permit physical proximity to a child during the day, reducing leisure time must be a part of a broader coping strategy.

Delegating tasks

In spite of her most valiant efforts, a woman who must work, whether at home or outside, cannot be expected to respond completely and at all times to the many demands of child care. Consequently, some delegating of child-care tasks is followed in almost all low-income families. Usually, although tasks are delegated, working mothers still manage to supervise the process, retaining primary responsibility for the care. The caregivers to whom tasks are most often delegated are extended family members, siblings, or neighbours and friends.

Extended family Members of the extended family have usually been the first choice of a woman who needs help in meeting her child-care needs (Anderson 1988a). (Although the role of fathers in child care and in household tasks in general is changing, fathers rarely take on child care regularly.) Grandparents or other relatives living with the family or nearby are more likely to be trusted than neighbours to give the best alternative care, simply because they are family (OEF 1979). They are preferred to siblings because they are more mature. And they need not be paid for their help. If additional family members are not at hand, women may move in to live with sisters or mothers so that domestic and income-earning responsibilities can be shared (Nieves, 1979, cites this strategy in San Salvador). In some cases, relatives are brought in to live and to care for the children (Zosa-Feranil 1982, cited in Ware 1984). Female-headed households are more likely to use this strategy than male-headed households (Safilios-Rothschild 1980).

Siblings   The use of older siblings, usually girls, to care for younger ones is a common practice (Engle 1986a, 1989; Mueller 1980; Nag and Kak 1984; Oppong 1982; Otaala *et al.* 1988; Weisner and Gallimore 1977; Werner 1983). This strategy is at once a form of child care and part of a socialization process for the siblings, many of whom are soon to be parents themselves. Often, sibling care occurs when a mother or other adult is nearby so that emergencies can be handled.

Both of these family options are available less frequently today than in the past. The number of nuclear families has increased. Migration to cities is disproportionately by young people whose older relatives stay behind in rural areas. Grandmothers may themselves be working and unavailable for substitute care. Schooling has at least partially undercut sibling care as a major form of child care, although when the need is great and no other solution is present, older children are kept out of school to help at home while mother works.

Using informal social support networks   When relatives or siblings are not available, another strategy pursued is to arrange for neighbours or close friends to care for children. Often the arrangement is very informal, with young children simply going to the home of a neighbour to play. Sometimes it is more formalized, with a neighbour receiving pay in money or kind. The use of social support networks made up of family and non-family members is an important survival strategy among the poor, not only for meeting child-care needs (Nieves 1981; Anderson 1988a; Powell *et al.* 1988), but also for a variety of goods and services used in reciprocal exchanges: information, job assistance, loans (including food, clothing, and tools), services (including housing and food), and moral support.

Delegating responsibility

When it is not possible for low-income working women to provide direct care or personally to manage tasks delegated to family or friends, children may be placed in organized programmes of child care in which the responsibility for care is, at least temporarily, given to others.[6]

Organized programmes of child care provide a way for a working mother to delegate responsibility for care while she is working. These organized programmes take many forms, ranging from the mammoth, highly organized, multifaceted child-care and preschool facilities found in Chinese cities to home day-care arrangements attending regularly to six or more neighbourhood children. The programmes may be provided within cooperatives, by factories, or by communities, and with varying degrees of participation and cost to working mothers. With the increased labour force participation of women and the decreasing availability of extended family and siblings, these organized alternative child-care programmes take on ever greater importance.

Choosing and balancing child-care options

The choice and balancing among various child-care strategies will be influenced by such diverse factors as cultural beliefs and practices, the age of the child, the composition and life-cycle stage of the household, the characteristics of available work, and the availability of organized child-care programmes.

Cultural beliefs and practices

In many cultures, women are expected to stay at home and care for the child. In others, child care is a community responsibility. The age at which it is appropriate for older children to practise sibling care is culturally linked. Second wives or mothers-in-law play special roles in child care in some societies. Spontaneous play groups of young children are a part of some societies, but not others. Fostering is common in some cultures, but virtually absent in others. These and similar practices or beliefs are seldom so fixed that they cannot be overcome when there are extenuating circumstances, but they have an influence on the choice of child-care strategies. They also influence profoundly the particular activities that are expected, regardless of who is providing the care.

Age of the child

Newborns and infants   The total dependence of babies, the intensive care they require, and the 'almost irreplaceable function of breastfeeding' (Anderson 1988; Leslie and Paolisso 1989) make it difficult and expensive to establish organized child care outside the home and without the mother. Because babies are relatively portable, it is often possible for mothers to bring babies with them to the workplace. At the work site, the mother may take full responsibility for care if the job permits, or many of the child-care functions can be delegated to another caregiver, with the mother taking time, periodically, to cuddle and breastfeed the baby.

The importance of full attention by the mother during the first weeks of a baby's life is captured in the social convention of many cultures where the mother is expected to stay at home for approximately 40 days following the birth, often in the home of the mother or mother-in-law, or with special attention by a midwife. She is then allowed to resume her home production, or other work, typically outside the formal economy. This important period has been recognized also in the laws of many countries which provide for a period of time off from work following childbirth with a guaranteed return to the job, payment during the time off, and no loss of seniority. In much of the Third World, however, maternity leaves are seldom honoured, even if they appear on the books.

Toddlers and preschoolers   As a child is weaned, becomes mobile, and is ready to talk, its needs change, affecting the choice of strategies. The growing child is less portable, needs to be watched constantly, and requires prepared food. The need for interaction with other children increases as does the importance of mastering language. These demands make it ever more difficult for a working mother, whether outside or inside the home, to handle care by herself. She must increase her dependence on others for care during working hours, or she must make drastic adjustments in her working and/or personal schedule. For poor women who must work and who have no family or other child-care support to fall back upon, this period, from approximately age one to age three, or later, can be an extraordinarily stressful period. On the other hand, if help is available, the weaned child is now more easily cared for by others, making it easier for the mother to fulfil her multiple roles.

Several reviews and studies (Leslie 1985; Engle 1986) provide evidence regarding the importance of a child's age as an intermediate variable affecting the relationship between work and a child's nutritional state. Mothers who are able to work at home or be at home during the early months of a child's life are less likely to have malnourished children. However, the reviews, and particularly Engle's work (1989) in urban Guatemala suggest that, as children grow beyond age one, the positive income effect of working outside the home may outweigh the greater child-care time mothers can provide by being at home.

Household composition and life-cycle stage

Working mothers in one-parent, nuclear or one-child families will obviously have fewer options within the family for alternate care than working mothers with a partner or relatives or older siblings present. These different family situations call for different strategies. For example, while women-headed households often rely on sibling care (Merrick and Schmink 1983; Nieves 1981; Safilios-Rothschild 1980), mothers living with men depend on friends, neighbours, and maids for child care (Rosenberg 1984, cited in Engle 1986a). The more limited the family options are, the greater the need for organized care.

A study in Caracas, Venezuela, identifies the period when the first child is born as a 'life-cycle squeeze' for many families because parents are young and have little earning power (Fundación del Niño 1979, Vol. II). The new mother may need to work to survive, but grandparents are either still in rural areas or are also young and still working. There are no older siblings to help with care. Earnings are usually meagre, even if a husband is present, because he is early in his working life. Conversely, a family in which the parents (and grandparents) are older, and which includes older siblings will be in a better position to solve its child-care needs without looking outside the family.

In larger families, another life-cycle squeeze can occur. The presence of several children can create a heavy financial burden, requiring difficult choices. Older children may have to leave school to care for younger children while the mother works or may have to enter the labour force themselves (Tienda 1980a; Galofré 1981).

Characteristics of available work

The availability of alternative child care affects work choices, but the type of work that is available will also affect the choice of child-care strategies. These two sets of options must be seen as interacting with each other.

In studies that try to sort out whether women's work is beneficial or detrimental to a child's welfare, a simplistic division is too often made between whether or not a woman works at an income-earning job. Much less attention has been given to the characteristics of the jobs available and carried out by women. Yet it seems obvious that a high-paying job will relate differently to child-care choices and produce different effects on both women and children, than a job paying well below the minimum wage, independently of whether the job is urban or rural, and whether it is in the formal or informal sector. This simplistic division helps to explain why the literature has provided us with contradictory answers about the effect of women's work on family welfare.

Let us look at several important characteristics of jobs as they relate to child care and child welfare.

Level of earnings   Behind the distinction between paid and unpaid work is the presumption that money earned can be used to purchase food, health, and child care. We have already pointed out that imbalances of decision-making and bargaining power within families can interfere with the desired use. But even when the possibility of using earned funds for general family welfare is present, the level of earnings is crucial (Leslie 1989). In most cases, the amount earned by working women is so low that purchases (of prepared food, for instance) cannot substitute for what may be given up (in home preparation of food or in breastfeeding).

The potential importance of earning levels can be illustrated by a study in India, in the state of Kerala (Kumar 1977), in which significantly lower levels of child nutrition were more apparent among children of women who were the sole earners in the family or workers in unskilled field labour, both positions of low productivity and low wages. Similarly, Soekirman (1985) in Indonesia found a significant negative effect of mother's employment on child nutritional status only if the mother worked more than 40 hours a week and earned less than the minimum wage. If a mother worked more than 40 hours and was better paid, the effect was not significant. Another study, in an urban area of Guatemala, found that the negative effect of mother's work on children's nutritional status was limited to domestic workers who worked long hours at very unskilled, poorly paid jobs (Engle, Pederson, and Smidt 1986).

Because available jobs are often so low-paying, most poor women cannot consider paying for institutionalized child care, an option that would sometimes be open if pay were higher. In the absence of organized and subsidized child-care alternatives, the most viable child-care option for working women in the Third World continues to be informal care by relatives and friends.

A kind of vicious circle may be at work here, particularly in cities, in which low-paying jobs prevent mothers from purchasing adequate child care, and the absence of adequate child care prevents mothers from seeking more stable, higher-paying employment. Provision of subsidized care that meets women's needs (including the need to acquire a technical skill) could help to break that circle, raising earnings and productivity, and benefiting both women and children.

Prestige   The prestige associated with a particular kind of work affects women's attitudes towards themselves and can affect the way in which they rear their children (Kağitçibaşi 1982), including the way in which earnings are used with respect to child survival, growth and development.

Non-monetary benefits   Most work available to poor women does not bring a guarantee of benefits such as health care or child care paid for by an employer. That seems to be the case even when women are employed in the formal sector and where laws have been passed that presumably require companies (or even employers of domestic servants) to provide benefits to

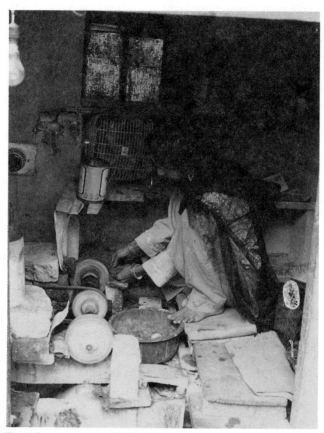

The informal sector, Old Delhi, India

their employees. One job benefit in the informal sector may simply be that a woman is able to (or is allowed to) bring her child to work with her. That was the case for Juanita and Olinda in our introduction. However, even this benefit may be denied; women working as maids in Brazil a decade ago, for instance, were often prohibited from bringing their children to work (OEF 1979).

Physical demands   A job that demands large expenditures of energy – as, for instance, harvesting and carrying crops – may leave a woman with little energy for child care and/or may have a negative effect on her health. Such a job would make it more difficult to follow a 'do it yourself' strategy of care and would push a mother towards alternative care arrangements.

Demands on time   Jobs vary widely with respect to the total number of hours, the daily scheduling, and the flexibility of the hours that can be worked. These job characteristics will affect whether a woman can realistically expect (or be expected) to be responsible for feeding, taking an infant to the health centre, administering oral rehydration, or carrying out other child-care tasks. Fitting together the time demands of a particular job with the availability of alternate child care becomes a major challenge for many poor women. It often reinforces their need to seek more flexible and less well-paid employment than they would like.

Distance from home   If a woman has to walk long distances to the field or travel long distances on public transportation to arrive at her job, taking a child with her is difficult. Even when child care is available on the job, transportation problems may make it difficult for the mother to take advantage of the service (Merrick and Schmink 1983; Anderson and Panizo 1984).

Seasonality   When work is seasonal, the several work characteristics described above seem to come together to limit child-care options and make responses to needs more difficult. Where there are wet ('hungry' or 'slack') seasons, food and cash reserves are lowest and vector-borne diseases such as malaria and guinea worm are peaking. Incidence of diarrhoea also peaks during these seasons. Where there are dry ('peak') seasons, harvesting demands are high. Pregnancies and births which occur during these times can result in maternal and infant morbidity and mortality.

Women who have to work very hard during these seasons have little time to cook, and often cook only one simple meal, or else delegate cooking altogether to young girls (Safilios-Rothschild 1980). During these times, infants needing breastfeeding or special weaning foods suffer along with lactating and pregnant women, who expend additional energy while consuming less food. The adverse conditions and/or the excessive work demands on women may lead lactating women to stop breastfeeding and prevent them from preparing special weaning foods. Health risks to children are thus increased at a time when the threat of disease is highest. (Examples from Gambia, Nigeria, Bangladesh, Korea, and Tanzania can be found in Carloni 1984; from Thailand in Palmer *et al.* 1983; from Honduras in Safilios-Rothschild, 1980; and from Bangladesh in Cornia 1984).

Children are reported to be entrusted to older siblings' care more often during the peak seasons for women's labour than at other times of the year (Carloni 1984). From Kenya there is evidence that the availability of older children to carry younger siblings when work loads for the mother were greatest decreased the incidence of diarrhoea among the young children. Moreover, when heavy work loads corresponded with the need for older children to return to school, the incidence of diarrhoea increased (Paolisso, Baksh, and Thomas 1989).

Kumar's study from Kerala (1977) showed that the child-care constraint became more pronounced during the wet, slack season when the monsoon rains bring virtually all agricultural activity to a standstill and all other household members have to work longer to alleviate the decrease in income from the primary earners. It was not uncommon to find even aged grandmothers working more often, though at very low wages, during the slack season. This meant that even they were unavailable for child care, and either the mother had to reduce her own employment, hence her income, or leave the child unattended.

From the previous discussion it is clear that there is a tension between a mother's work activities, both inside and outside the home, and her ability to provide infant/child care, even in rural traditional societies. This tension is particularly acute in resource-poor households where the effect on families of not working is highest. Among the poor, the tension is greatest:

- when children are in their first year;
- when women are the heads of the household or are in a nuclear family that relies on their earnings;
- where alternative child care by adults is not necessarily available and/ or there is heavy reliance on sibling caregivers;
- during periods of 'life-cycle squeeze';
- when work is low-paying, without benefits, far from home, and physically taxing; and
- during periods when work peaks and/or health conditions worsen.

Our discussion has also suggested that the need is increasing for organized child-care alternatives outside the home as well as for programmes that support and strengthen informal and alternative arrangements in or near the home. (For a similar position, see Maguire and Popkin (1990), whose in-depth look at the conflicting roles of women and programmes to help overcome them concludes that one key intervention is 'promoting good child care'.) To what extent is this need for good child-care programmes being met through existing programmes?

THE AVAILABILITY OF ADEQUATE CHILD CARE[7]

As suggested in Chapter 2, it is difficult to obtain full and accurate statistics describing existing forms and programmes of child care. Care by family members or friends, baby-sitting, and informal group care outside the home go unregistered. But even statistics for formal programmes, mandated or organized or supervised by or registered with national, state, and local governments, are difficult to find. The complete picture requires putting together information from a range of governmental and non-governmental organizations, each keeping separate records (e.g. Campos and Rosemberg 1988).

Household surveys provide another source of data describing child-care options and their availability. Mothers are asked what child-care arrangements they use and what their preference would be if alternatives were available (e.g. Tolbert 1990). These studies help to extend and interpret official statistics, but are not necessarily reliable. They too are likely to provide a partial picture because they fail to pick up multiple sources of care. Also, respondents' answers to questions about their needs and preferences for care are biased by a lack of knowledge about alternatives, and by a tendency to tell interviewers what they think the interviewer wants to hear.[8]

Although detailed descriptions are often lacking, the statistics and supporting studies are sufficiently clear to allow a general conclusion about the extent and quality of child-care programmes: *With the exception of a limited number of socialist countries in the Third World, publicly supported and supervised programmes of child care, explicitly set up to care for children while women work, are very limited in their coverage.*[9] For instance, according to Swaminathan (1985), only about 1 per cent of India's 33–34 million preschool aged children are formally enrolled in formal day care. Similarly, Peru is estimated to have space in regulated day care for less than 1 per cent of preschool aged children (Fort 1988). Sparse coverage of child-care programmes linked to women's work is even more pronounced in Africa, even in urban areas.

The figures just cited do not include important preschool and early childhood development programmes which were not intended first and foremost to meet the needs of working mothers. For example, through its Integrated Child Development Service alone, India now provides non-formal preschool programmes for more than 25 per cent of all children aged three to six. Peru, like India, can also point to preschool and integrated child development programmes covering more than one-fourth of all children aged three to five. But these programmes operate for only three to four hours during weekdays and children under age three rarely attend the centres; it would be stretching a point to label them child-care programmes. This problem – of combining child-care with child development programmes will be discussed below.

Why is the availability of organized alternative child care so limited?

Is need and demand low?   One explanation offered for the limited availability is that alternative care in organized programmes is really not needed; the demand is low and informal care is thought to serve adequately the existing needs. But we have already noted the declining availability of siblings and extended family members, occurring together with a growing need for alternative care, related to changes in labour force participation and family composition. Thus, although many families with working women are still able to meet the need for child care within the family or circle of friends, there seems to be a gap. One disturbing indication of the gap is the percentage of working mothers who must still resort to the drastic option of leaving children unattended for some part of the day (Anderson 1988b).

A number of studies seem to support the argument that women do not want or need organized alternative care. These studies suggest that women overwhelmingly prefer child care at home or by a trusted neighbour, rather than in a child-care centre (Rivera 1979; Engle 1980). Although the interpretation of that finding is not straightforward, it sometimes serves to rationalize decisions not to provide alternative child care outside the home. This is both inaccurate and unfortunate because the expressed preference for informal home care reflects the lack of *acceptable alternatives* more than it does simple contentment with family caregiver arrangements (Anderson 1988a).

To illustrate the point, most of the women interviewed in a six-country study of child care and women's work (OEF 1979) expressed the belief that persons other than the family are not particularly capable or motivated to provide quality care. However, the same study demonstrated that in areas where families were aware of the existence of child-care facilities offering quality care, they were anxious to have access to such services. A similar finding is reported for Mexico (Tolbert 1990). Other reports indicate that mothers not only desire such access to child-care services, but they are willing to organize and pressure officials to obtain them.[10]

A lack of demand is sometimes inferred from vacant places in existing child-care facilities. However, at least two basic reasons are given by women for this underutilization of existing facilities: 1) inconvenient location and 2) poor quality.

Location   Unfortunately, many child-care programmes are not very accessible. In the extreme cases, they are located at work sites an hour or two from the homes of the women working there. The location of child care at work sites allows children to be near mothers during the day, at least in theory. But if getting the child to the centre requires women to carry their children for long distances in conditions harmful to the child and/or if an extra transportation cost is involved, the potential advantage of nearness during the day is offset. In addition, many work sites are seen as unacceptable locations because they have environmental hazards such as pollution deemed dangerous to the children (OEF 1979; Schmink 1982; Swaminathan 1985).

There are, however, various examples of programmes that have success-fully brought child care to the work place. These include the novel Mobile Creche programme in India (see Chapter 6, p. 111) which provides on-site integrated care for children of construction workers, and a programme organized by Senegalese women to care for their children at a location near the fields during the rice-planting season (Chapter 6, p. 110).

Is the problem poor quality?   A second basic reason offered by women for the underutilization is the poor quality of child care. Many examples can be cited of programmes that are poorly staffed, poorly equipped, lack-ing play areas or proper bathroom facilities, and devoid of organized child development activity (children sit idle and aimless during the day). Often this condition is endemic.

Lack of quality is not necessarily recognized by child-care organizers as a cause for underutilization. They give too little credit to women's desires to provide their children with adequate care and to their ability to recog-nize inadequate care when they see it. For example, a study of women's child-care arrangements in the squatter settlements of Lima, Peru, showed clearly that women wanted child-care centres to be run by people in whom they had confidence – who would not physically punish children, who provided food, and who maintained a clean and well-equipped centre (Anderson 1988a).

Organizational problems   There are other reasons for underutilization as well. A look at the advantages of care by family members suggests that programmes should be *accessible, flexible, affordable,* and *accountable.* An advantage of calling on family members, traditionally, has been their availability at whatever hours they are needed, giving working mothers flexibility in their scheduling. Organized programmes of child care outside the home do not offer the same flexibility. Unfortunately, most programmes of child care have fixed and limited hours that do not neces-sarily mesh with women's working hours. This is particularly so for women in the informal sector who most need alternative care and whose days (including weekends when child-care centres may not be open) are very long.

Flexibility is also required because the need for child care can vary from day to day and season to season. The need varies with the type of work available, and with the age and health of the child. Different working mothers have very different needs. Accordingly, programmes must be prepared to meet a wide range of child-care needs if they are to be effective. A highly bureaucratized and centralized system does not easily provide this kind of flexibility.

One reason women often turn first to family is that family caregivers are not only trustworthy, but also can be supervised and are relatively accountable. In impersonalized child-care centres or in home day-care programmes, the desired trust and accountability may be lacking. This is particularly true if caregivers are not part of a national system of regulation and supervision.

Child care must be affordable. Poor families in which women must work for the family to survive cannot afford to purchase child-care services unless they are extraordinarily fortunate and obtain a relaively high-paying job, or unless no more than a token fee is involved. Grandparents and siblings do not get paid and their caregiving occurs in the home so there is no transportation cost. Many arrangements with neighbours are also costless in monetary terms although an in-kind debt may be built up. Organized programmes of care outside the home must be highly subsidized, with the main cost falling either on employers or on the public purse. If they are not affordable, places will be vacant even though a need exists.

In brief, the lack of child-care programmes is not due principally to a lack of demand or a deeply rooted preference for home care. Rather, it reflects the failure of more formal programmes to meet women's needs and expectations for programmes that are accessible, affordable, flexible, run by trusted, caring and accountable people, and of at least minimum quality.

Is low coverage a matter of high costs that organizers cannot afford or recover?   An obvious explanation why both publicly supported and supervised and mandated programmes are so few could be that such programmes involve a subsidy neither governments nor businesses have been willing (or able?) to provide. Indeed, the cost argument is often used to explain limited provision of additional child care.

> Full daycare – providing supervision, meals, health monitoring, educational and play activities, beds and quiet for rest, and loving constant attention by adults – is expensive, in absolute terms and in comparison to the investments countries might opt to make in other kinds of social services or in, say, expanding primary education. Purchasing daycare is also expensive for families. Child care can easily absorb one-fourth to

one-half of women's salaries in industrialized countries. In developing countries it must usually be heavily subsidized for it to be at all accessible to families who may be spending almost their entire incomes on food, housing, and transportation to work.

(Anderson 1988, p. 8)

There are solutions, however. For instance, a novel and workable method of raising funds to subsidize child care comes from Colombia where a 3 per cent payroll tax is levied on all employers with more than a certain number of employees. From this tax has come a huge fund for child care. The Colombian case also shows that costs can be cut drastically by adopting a neighbourhood home day-care model (Chapter 6, p. 101). It is estimated that the cost of neighbourhood day care being provided under a new programme is one-fifth of the per-child cost of the 'integrated child-care centres' placed in operation in the past (Sanz de Santamaria 1989). Cost is obviously a factor and ways must be sought to reduce costs. However, the main question to be answered, rather than 'What does it cost?' is 'Is it worth the cost?'

Part of the cost complaint is, then, really a combined problem of social convention, weak political will, and the failure to recognize that early childhood care and development is a good investment. Social convention has conveniently hidden costs under the aprons of women who spend hours daily caring for their children without pay. As we have indicated, this care does not imply a direct trade-off against work, but it often leads to the choice of low productivity jobs and to compromises in women's health and leisure. These compromises have negative effects for society at large as well as for individual women and their children.

Studies in the developed world link the availability of quality child care to increased worker productivity, noting reductions in worker tardiness, absenteeism and stress causing errors or poor performance (Galinsky 1986). Socialist countries, where women's participation in the work force is encouraged both as a means of improving their status and as a means of increasing the national product, have understood the relationship between child-care provision and worker productivity, even though the profit motive is submerged. (As part of the questioning that is occurring under recent reforms, however, there is a suggestion that too great responsibility may have been placed with institutions.)

An argument was made, as part of the rationale for investing in early childhood care and development (see Chapter 1), that early intervention programmes can reduce costs of other services and make other programmes more efficient, and this applies to child care. Good child-care programmes can reduce the need for subsequent health care, reduce repetition in primary schools, reduce social welfare costs and increase the effects of women's income-generating programmes. They also provide an entry point for other services (Evans 1985). To make good on this potential, however, requires a combined view of needs and of programming that runs up against the conceptual and organizational divisions we have seen are so prominent. In part, then, the lack of adequate child-care programmes represents a failure of programmers to integrate, or combine, child care with child development and with women's interests.

Child-centred, integrated child development programmes: a missed child-care opportunity

Unfortunately, most preschool, nursery, and other early childhood pro-grammes that could help meet the needs of poor working women are doing very little to respond to those needs. Typically, these child-centred programmes are scheduled during only three or four hours a day during weekdays. A focus within many programmes on the preparation for school has sometimes led to the neglect of other basic requirements for child care – health, for instance – which are also concerns of working women for their children. The preschool bias also favours attention beginning at age three, leaving a large gap below that age. In addition, the quality of the programmes is often poor. These 'child development' programmes are, then, subject to the same criticisms women have offered for programmes of child care.

The failure of child development programmes to combine their child-centred approach with a response to working women's needs is unsettling, given the steady expansion of such programmes in recent years. Indeed, as shown in Chapter 2, the coverage of early childhood programmes, particularly for children from age three and above, is beginning to reach significant levels in many countries. Moreover, parents attach a high value to preparing children for school and are therefore willing to place their children in such programmes, even if that causes, rather than solves, child-minding problems.

A prime example of a child-centred approach is the Integrated Child Development Service (ICDS) of India, described in Chapter 6. That programme has many features and results that must be applauded and our purpose is not to set accomplishments aside in focusing on a missing element in the programme. But the ICDS programme, while including women explicitly as a target group, is not oriented to women's child-care needs. The provision of nutrition and health and education for women are weak components in the programme and have been included more with a view towards improving the condition of the children than the women. The programme is, thus, built around the mother in her reproductive role. This may not be a bad strategy in many of the rural or tribal areas in which the programme functions because family members are present to help with care, and mothers are often at home and able to handle care while engaging in home production. In small villages, the problem of delivering and picking up the child is minor and sometimes solved by the centre worker's collecting the children to bring them to the centre. In some urban areas, however, and during peak harvest or planting seasons, the failure to respond to women's work needs can literally be fatal. As might be expected, there is pressure on the ICDS programme in some areas to take a more active role in child care, to extend hours and to improve the quality of the service. The programme is also working to improve its attention to younger children.

PROGRAMME IMPLICATIONS

Against this background, we turn now to identifying programme implications. These will be discussed in three categories. First, several general implications will be drawn. Second, ways in which women's child-care concerns can be incorporated into child development programmes will be sketched. Third, suggestions will be made regarding the integration into women's programming of child-care and development components intended to benefit women and children simultaneously.

1 *The need of working women for adequate alternative child care is not being met.*

Informal care in the home, although preferred, is not sufficient. Options exist that can provide adequate care at reasonable cost and with a more-than-reasonable return on the investment.

2 *There is no one programme solution.*

Because the circumstances and conditions of work carried out by women are so varied, no one form of child care will be able to satisfy all, or even a major portion, of child-care needs. Therefore, providing child care on a large scale should be conceived as the sum of diverse, smaller-scale programmes responding to particular needs rather than as universal coverage by one particular programme option (see Chapters 12 and 14).

3 *In many locations, strengthening traditional care is a viable and preferred option.*

In cases where alternative care involves extended family members or neighbours, these approaches can be strengthened by providing the alternative caregivers with support (for example, health and nutritional services and better physical conditions), and with training and knowledge needed to carry out their task more effectively. Strengthening these options can provide mothers with flexibility, accountability, and affordability that would be difficult to duplicate in more formal programmes.

Sibling care may be an exception; if sibling involvement in alternative care prevents school attendance, other solutions should be explored (including child-care facilities attached to primary schools).

4 *There is a need to facilitate mothers' direct care during the first year.*

Efforts should be made to see that women have the opportunity to be with their children on a full-time basis during the first critical months of life, allowing them to breastfeed and to respond to a child's need for security.

5 *In order to meet working women's needs, more formal programmes of alternative child care should be affordable, accessible, flexible, run by trusted and accountable individuals, and of at least minimum quality.*

Unless these characteristics are met, programmes created will not be used, in spite of a need on the part of women, creating a double waste rather than helping to relieve a problem.

6 *There is a need for programming that treats child care as child development and vice versa.*

The fact that child care and child development are treated separately does not make sense from either side. Programmes formulated with a child-centred goal of enhancing early development should take into consideration the child-care needs of families and respond to them. Child-care programmes should move beyond a custodial view of care to incorporate child development goals, including attention to psychological and social needs of children as well as attention to their physical needs.

7 *Women's programmes should examine programme effects on the welfare of children rather than assume that positive effects will result.*

It is clear that there are situations in which benefits associated with women's programmes will also benefit children. But it is also clear that there are situations in which this will not occur. Providing income-earning opportunities, or training, or freeing up the time of women does not by itself ensure that children will benefit. We have shown that the benefit depends on the characteristics of the particular work a woman takes on, and on the availability and quality of alternative child-care arrangements.

We turn now to examining ways in which the interests of women and families requiring alternative child care can be met within programmes of child development. We will then look at how the interests of children might be incorporated into programmes focusing on benefits to women.

Combining child development programming and women's interests

In Chapters 5, 6, and 7, we elaborated a set of complementary approaches to child development and provided examples of each strategy. These provide a starting point for discussion.

Centre-based child development programmes

Preschools   The formal preschools that exist in most countries are usually directed towards preparing children for schooling and with little thought to child-care needs of families. The hours are usually limited. Teachers are not trained to care for younger children and facilities for under-threes are seldom present. Because formal preschools are so embedded in formal bureaucratic structures, reorienting these programmes in a major way to provide the full range of child-care needs within a structure of flexible hours may be too much to expect.

Even non-formal, community-based preschools, such as those that have been described for Peru or within the Integrated Child Development Service of India, cannot easily be converted into child-care centres. In a recent experiment in India, an additional Anganwadi worker was introduced to the preschool centre and responsibility for attending to children below the age of three was added to the centre. But mothers did not bring their children and, when asked why, they said that they could provide individualized care and they did not want to have their very young child become part of a large group in which there was little possibility of direct and continuing interaction with the child (author's field notes, August 1989).

It is possible, however, to imagine some adjustments that would facilitate child care of older preschool children while family members work and be in the interests of women. For instance, in those cases where older siblings are responsible for care, placing preschools near or within primary schools, as suggested in the previous chapter, would allow siblings to bring younger brothers and sisters to the preschool prior to entering primary school and to pick them up again as they leave. This system would also allow young girls who would otherwise have to stay at home to continue in primary school. Moreover, students in the primary school could be required to spend some time helping out in the preschool, learning as they work.

Another adjustment that has been made in some places is to open preschools on non-work days and to provide courses of adult education or other activities for women while the children are cared for in the preschool centre, either by the teacher who would be paid an extra amount or on a rotating basis by the mothers.

Neighbourhood home day care   Potential advantages and disadvantages of home day care were discussed in Chapter 7. Among the potential advantages are small size, greater flexibility, a more personal relationship between the caregiver and the parent, and a home-like atmosphere. In addition, this form of care, as contrasted with centre-based care located at the workplace, can help to solidify neighbourhoods and women's groups, and lends itself to participation in the formation and supervision of programmes. Home day care can even be organized on a cooperative basis with mothers taking turns caring for children, as occurs in a Nepalese programme of women's credit. But home day care can also be exploitative of the women providing the care and can be of such poor quality (in both custodial and developmental terms) that it is not beneficial to the children. To function well, then, home day-care mothers need training and support. The Colombian example (Chapter 6, p. 101) suggests that this can be done on a relatively large scale, at low cost and with good results.

Sometimes overlooked is the fact that preschools and home day-care programmes can provide a source of earned income for women; they are potential income-generating options for women. This potential is often exploited only in middle-class communities. In low-income settings, with an emphasis on low costs, the tendency is to turn to volunteers or to provide an extremely low remuneration for the women who take on the child-care and development jobs. This is a form of exploitation of women that needs to be overcome. It feeds on the idea that women should care for children simply because they are women and that this activity should not be remunerated.

Parental education

For parental education to be carried out in a way that will best serve the interests of working women, it should not only be scheduled at times that are convenient, but should include other family members as well, recognizing that women are not (and need not be) the sole caretakers of young children. Caregiver education should, then, incorporate fathers and siblings and grandparents.

It is possible also to think of so-called education programmes directed to women as parents, with the idea that both children and women will benefit. Indeed, in the discussion of parental education in Chapter 7, we suggested that the most successful programmes will be those that bring some benefit to adults as well as to children. That benefit may be in terms of information that will improve the health and nutrition of women during pregnancy, or more generally. Or, it may be less tangible, related to the development of self-esteem or the formation of a social network or the chance for women to air problems they feel, as women. These 'by-products' of child-oriented parental education are not sufficiently encouraged.

The scheduling of parental education programmes normally occurs outside the work setting, but a novel programme of parental education was developed in Turkey where employers were persuaded to allow groups of working women to meet for an hour once a week, on company time, for a training course focusing on the cognitive development of their children (Kağıtçıbaşi 1987). These meetings proved of benefit not only to the children, but also to the women as women, helping them to change outlooks and to acquire additional authority within their own families.

Community development programmes including child-care and development components

When community development programmes begin from, or incorporate, child survival and development components, they are more likely to open up community participation by women and to include actions that will be of direct benefit to women as well as children. However, in some community-based child development programmes, women are seen simply as a source of volunteer labour, a circumstance similar to that noted above when discussing home day care. Therefore, special attention must be given in the formulation of such programmes to see that the broader interests of women are protected and fostered.

Incorporating children's interests into women-centred programmes

Women-centred programmes are no better than child-centred child development programmes at incorporating elements in their programmes that will assure mutual benefits to women and to children. Let us look at a range of programmes intended to benefit women and ask how the combined interests of both women and children might better be served.

Women's rights, social legislation and legal services

One line of programming activity to advance women's status and welfare has been to work towards changing discriminatory laws and to provide legal assistance with respect to existing laws, helping women overcome problems related to treatment in the workplace, marital disputes, property ownership, child custody and similar matters.

In some cases, this line of activity is related directly to questions of child care and women's work. For instance, laws have long existed mandating child care for women in work sites employing more than a certain number of women, ranging from 300 to 20. Although such mandated care has been on the books for many years in many countries, it has seldom been honoured. Indeed, the laws have sometimes worked against the interests of women (and children) because employers refuse to hire women or they hire one less than the legally allowed number.

In 1979, for instance, although Brazil, Peru, and the Dominican Republic had such laws, one study (OEF 1979) found no such facilities in operation in the Dominican Republic or Peru, and there were few in Brazil. Since then, however, the women's rights movement in Brazil has included this *revindicacion* on their agenda and have made progress in seeing that this right is honoured (Campos 1988). This action offers an example that could be taken up in other countries where, by way of contrast, child care has not been a concern of the women's movement or associated programmes.

Other legislative initiatives (Anderson 1988) that have been taken to help make work and child care more compatible include laws governing:
- maternity leave with guaranteed return to the job, at least some salary during the period away, and no loss in seniority;
- child sick leave, covering conditions when parental care is required within working hours;
- shortened work days or flexible scheduling of work.

Another approach to the double demand is an explicit recognition of child care as a form of productive work and the awarding of 'work points' for that work, whether it is undertaken in a formal job as a child-care attendant at a work site or as a breastfeeding mother taking time from production. This system was used in the People's Republic of China in production cooperatives, and has also been applied in cooperatives in Ethiopia (Hargot 1989).

In all of the above it is well to keep two thoughts in mind. First, the rights and benefits should contain the option of being exercised by fathers as well as mothers, where that is possible, as in sick leave or after the birth of a child. Second, and most important of all, most women (and a high proportion of men) from low-income circumstances are not employed in the formal sector so cannot easily take advantage of legal provisions. The need to survive, the self-imposed demands of their work, and the difficulty of applying laws to the informal sector require measures that look well beyond creating laws based on formal sector characteristics. One measure that is required is for greater organization among women working as maids, laundresses, and street vendors and at other jobs in the informal sector.

Consciousness raising and organization for action

During the 1970s and 1980s, an increasing number of programmes sprang up that focus on consciousness raising, fostering organization and political action. Because these efforts have usually taken on, as a first task, helping women to think beyond the maternal role, child care has not often been an early theme or concern. However, over time, the topic emerges as one of joint concern and a legitimate area for action. In a few instances, child care has provided a starting point for bringing women together and for stimulating action over a broad front. As suggested in the previous section, organization around the child-care issue (as was done in Brazil) is one means of not only ensuring better care for children but also of strengthening women's organizations.

To the extent that these programmes build confidence, strengthen support networks, reduce stress, and raise the general contentment of women, they can have an important indirect effect on the maternal as well as work roles of women. The specific topic of child care need not be discussed for there to be a benefit to children as well as women.

Income generation and related programmes

The set of programmes most closely related to our discussion in this chapter are those directed towards improving the income-earning level and capacity of women. These programmes have approached their general objective by seeking to:

- create new enterprises run by and employing women;
- free up time from domestic chores through appropriate technology;
- improve access to credit;
- upgrade women's productive skills through training; and
- strengthen support systems for women by reorienting and training individuals, providing knowledge, resources, and organizational assistance to women engaged in market activities.

1 *Income-generating programmes.*   During the First Women's Decade (1975–85), many attempts were made to establish new enterprises run by and employing women. With good intentions, many income-generating programmes built on traditional skills related to women's domestic roles – production of handicraft items or knitting or sewing, for instance. However, in too many cases these programmes were launched with inadequate attention to the real market potential of the items being produced. Adventures into 'new' fields previously dominated by men – construction and related areas, for instance – were not so frequently supported even though various projects showed the possibility of success. These newer areas required training (management or welding or other skills) and often access to credit (see below). They also involved overcoming the force of tradition, including the notion that a woman's place is always in the home, and a concern that these forms of employment would be incompatible with child-care responsibilities. Again, child care enters as an element to be taken into consideration from the outset. The need for adequate substitute care for young children of women in such programmes needs to be anticipated and assured.

2 *Appropriate technology.*   Income-generating projects and programmes can be frustrated by a series of time limitations imposed by the responsibility that societies continue to assign to women for household tasks: the debilitating 'double day'. Recognizing the need to free up time (whether of the mother or of a substitute caregiver), a set of appropriate technology projects has been promoted, the most important of which reduce time

spent in drawing water, fetching firewood, and processing food. There is little doubt that these projects have made life easier for women in many places and, in all likelihood, for their children as well.

Interestingly, however, less consideration has been given to finding or supporting ways in which working mothers can reduce time attending directly to their children, i.e. to alternative forms of child care. The failure to look towards 'alternative technologies' as well as alternative arrangements in this area is undoubtedly linked to the myth that mothers are, and should be, the sole caretakers of their children.

This lack of attention to childrearing technologies has helped the advance of one 'appropriate technology' that is seldom beneficial to the young child, the introduction of bottle-feeding. The shift away from breast-feeding, particularly in urban areas, has helped to free up time for women to work and has facilitated alternative child care. This advantage has some-times been offset by a deterioration in the nutritional status of infants. The programme implication of this is to seek ways in which women can be with their children in the earliest months and breastfeed them, to discourage bottle-feeding when it is not absolutely needed, but also to provide instruc-tion in bottle-feeding when it does occur so as to avoid the abuses of insanitary preparation and 'bottle-propping'.

The care of children involves technological choices other than the choice of breast vs. bottle-feeding. Health and nutrition choices also have implications for the time use and income-earning availability of women. Using the appropriate technologies of oral rehydration or immunization can, for instance, save child-care time. However, their use also involves time, a fact that is not always appreciated because programmes promoting these technologies have focused on the needs of children, not women, and have been planned and implemented by organizations concerned with health and nutrition, not with income-earning needs. Again, there is a need to combine programming interests. There is a need to recognize, for instance, that the administration of oral rehydration therapy is time-intensive (Leslie 1988) and will require time away from work by a mother unless there is a substitute caregiver who can properly administer the therapy.

Institutions that support organized programmes of alternative child care related to women's work also have technology choices to make. An 'appro-priate technology' approach will concentrate on neighbourhood care in homes, upgraded for the purpose, rather than on constructing separate and expensive centres. It will stress creating one's own materials rather than importing (or buying) them.

3 *Credit.*   Several innovative and much-needed credit schemes have been developed to provide women with access to credit needed in establishing or expanding their income-earning activities. Rotating credit funds and bank credit extended on the basis of group guarantees rather than linked to

individual guarantees and collateral have provided new sources of funding for innumerable small enterprises.

The programme relationship between credit and the provision of adequate child care is not obvious. However, one of the activities for which credit may be given is child care. In the Colombian home day-care programme, for instance, women are being provided with credit allowing them to make improvements in their homes so they can be used as home day care locations (Sanz de Santamaria 1989). The credit is at a favoured rate and family or community members can be paid to make the improvements, providing an income-earning opportunity in the community.

In Nepal, the formation of small groups of women to obtain credit for income-earning activities has provided the opportunity for collaboration of the group members in a programme of child care needed to help them use their funds in a productive way. The child-care initiative has been formulated with the interests of both women and children in mind. Consequently, an effort has been made to provide more than custodial care (Arnold 1989).

4 *Training.*   To permit women to enter new jobs, or to increase their productivity in their present work, training programmes have been organized covering a wide range of skills, from literacy to carpentry to driving tractors to management techniques. Although training has included upgrading of traditional skills such as sewing, in order to convert them from home production to market production activities, many, if not most, programmes have resisted such training because it is seen as reinforcing the reproductive role of women and restricting women to traditional areas carrying low prestige.

The bias in training programmes for women towards income earning unrelated to traditional domestic roles helps to explain the fact that child care has been virtually overlooked as a potential income-earning activity. Vocational training programmes established under Women-in-Development (WID) programmes do not seem to consider child care as a bona fide form of income generation. This neglect is unfortunate, not only because it misses an opportunity, but also because it places such training, when it does occur, in the hands of programmers concerned with children's, but not necessarily women's, interests. Training is minimal and usually does not include attention to needed management skills. Typically, today, the context for the training is an informal programme focused on child development leading to jobs that are 'volunteer', paying a gratuity well below the minimum salary. If programme interests could be combined, within a WID programme, or by working in cooperation, the potential benefit to both women and children is great.

5 *Strengthening support systems.*   In some WID programmes training is provided for extension workers, bank staff, community mobilizers, or others who are in a position to support women's income-earning activities.

Apparently forgotten in the list of supporting institutions are those that provide child care. Programmes to reorient the thinking of those charged with child care and child development programming would be a useful investment within some WID programmes.

Women's health

Programmes focusing on the health of working women, much like programmes of child care, seem to be an afterthought for WID programmers. As indicated earlier, most programmes of women's health have been carried out as part of maternal and child health care programmes, with attention focused on pregnant and lactating women. More general attention to women's health has lagged, having emerged only within the last two years as an important theme. Even then, at an international level, the concern became translated in some circles into 'safe motherhood'.

The Self-Employed Women's Association (SEWA) in India took on health as an issue related to income generation when it discovered that a main reason women defaulted on loans was that they lost work time due to ill health and did not therefore have the ability to pay. As a result, a health cooperative was set up responding to the health needs of working women. This scheme was successful enough to be adopted at a national level by the Indian government. Better health for women, even after they finish breast-feeding, can certainly benefit their young children as well as help pay back loans. That improvement may occur as increased earnings are translated into better conditions or as women have more energy to devote to child care. But the health of young children can also be a factor in absence from work and influence the ability to pay. It may not be surprising that SEWA is experimenting with a child-care cooperative, much as they did earlier with a women's health cooperative.

As suggested in Chapter 9 when health programmes were discussed, health (and nutrition) education programmes are often directed to women. However, such programmes are often seen simply as opportunities to instruct mothers in what to do about the physical health of their children. Our discussion of women's work and child care suggests that health education needs to be provided to a much larger audience than mothers, an audience that includes older siblings, extended family members, and other caregivers providing alternative care, both informal and institutionalized. In addition, both women and children would benefit if the health education programmes paid greater attention to the general health problems of women.

Women's education

A major strategy for bettering the condition of women has been to struggle for more and better education. A general education (as distinguished from training in particular vocational skills) can have an effect on fertility rates, birth spacing, and the care of young children, in addition to opening additional employment possibilities for women. Encouraging basic education for women, then, also encourages better care and development of children. In the long run, educational efforts may do more than any of the previous strategies discussed to benefit both women and children.

We have seen, however, in Chapter 10, that discrimination in education begins early in some cultures – in the preschool years. An attack on the problem of women's education should, therefore, include attention to the readiness of girls for primary school and to programmes of early care and development that will help overcome discriminatory barriers and gender inequalities already existing at the time of first entry into school.

The problem of an early withdrawal from school because a girl must care for a younger sibling has been mentioned previously. It is important for the girl child that ways be found to allow contined attendance at school. That means finding ways to cover the child-care responsibility that has been given to her. We have suggested locating preschools near primary schools. A shift system of schooling also increases the possibility that girls can attend, with child care on a shift system as well. There are undoubtedly other solutions and these should be sought vigorously.

Final thoughts

These several programme lines should, of course, be seen as complementary and reinforcing. All these 'women's' programmes have potential effects on children, each in a different way. But to maximize that effect and to ensure that it will be positive, it is in the best interests of those concerned with benefits to women to be consciously concerned as well and constantly to seek ways to combine these interests in their programmes to the benefit of both. More than anything else, that simply requires awareness and a willingness to overcome a blind spot that has been created by the forced distinction between the productive and reproductive roles of women.

Another blind spot continues with respect to the role of men in child care. As conditions continue to change, the role of men in assuming not only child care, but also other household tasks is likely to grow. That sharing of responsibilities can be promoted. It is likely that, in 25 years, a very different rendering of our topic will be required from the one offered here because the problem will have shifted from one of 'child care, women's work, and child development' to one of 'child care, familial roles, and family welfare'.

NOTES

1 This chapter draws heavily on: Robert Myers and Cynthia Indriso, 'Women's Work and Child Care', a paper prepared for a workshop at the Rockefeller Foundation, February 26 and 27, 1987, revised version June 1987.
2 Some confusion surrounds the notion of a 'reproductive role' because some authors link this to a woman's biological reproductivity, extended to care for the child, whereas others link it to the reproduction of societies through care and socialization of the young.
3 See, for instance, the Cornia/UNICEF model in Chapter 4.
4 This assumption is embedded in economic analyses of households that focus on how time is used.
5 These kinds of jobs are usually thought to be 'compatible' with child care whereas others, requiring substitute care, are not. This way of thinking about the relationship between work and child care feeds on the misconception that the mother is the only person who can care for the child. In fact, substitute care may make a wide range of jobs compatible with child care, including jobs that are outside the home and that do not permit the presence of a child. Moreover, proximity does not determine compatibility. A job may allow for children to be nearby and, in a sense, be cared for, but at a sacrifice to productivity on the job, and probably in the quality of care as well. In short, the concept of compatibility does not seem to be very useful for our discussion.
6 In some cultures, 'fostering' is common, in which children are sent to live with relatives or friends in another location (Dare 1983; Nieves 1981; Safilios-Rothschild 1980). We shall not discuss these arrangements, which often occur after the age of six and which tend to be made on a personal basis. Instead, we shall concentrate on organized care.
7 This section draws heavily on: Jeanine Anderson, 'Child Care and the Advancement of Women', a paper prepared for the Expert Group Meeting on Social Support Measures for the Advancement of Women, Vienna, November 14–18, 1988.
8 Household surveys now in progress as part of the International Education Achievement (IEA) project's 16-country study of child care and development should correct some of these biases. The studies request information about the multiple forms of caregiving used for children aged four.
9 The main exception among socialist countries in the Third World is China which could point to almost universal coverage in its child-care programmes prior to 1979, when the current reforms began to take hold. Now, however, something less than 25 per cent of Chinese children under six years of age are in state-run programmes of care and development for that age group. The one-child family and more flexible work schedules associated with de-collectivization have led to the reduction, with the difference reflecting a reversion to more traditional child-care solutions within the family (UNICEF, Annual Report 1987).
10 See, for instance: Swaminathan 1985 for India; Palmer, Subhadhira, and Grisanaputi 1983 for Thailand; Campos *et al.* 1988 for Brazil; and Anderson 1988a, for Peru).

REFERENCES

Acevedo, M.L., J.I. Aguilar, L.M. Brunt and M.S. Molinari. 'Child Care in Mexico City', in M. Schmink, J. Bruce, and M. Kahn (eds) *Learning about Women and Urban Services in Latin America and the Caribbean.* New York:

the Population Council, Inc., 1986, pp. 273–6.

Acharya, M. and L. Bennett. 'Women and the Subsistence Sector: Economic Participation and Household Decision-Making in Nepal', World Bank Staff Working Paper No. 526. Washington DC: the World Bank, 1982.

Anderson, J. 'Y Ahora Quién Cuida a los Niños? El Cuidado Diurno en Lima, 1981–1986'. Working papers, Working Group on Women, Low-Income Households and Urban Services (SUMBI), Lima, Peru, January 1988.

Anderson, J. 'Child Care and the Advancement of Women', a paper prepared for the Expert Group Meeting on Social Support Measures for the Advancement of Women, Vienna, November 14–18, 1988. Vienna: Centre for Social Development and Humanitarian Affairs, 1988.

Anderson, J. and N. Panizo. 'Limitaciones para el uso de los servicios urbanos por mujeres de bajos ingresos: transporte y seguridad', Working papers, Working Group on Women, Low-Income Households and Urban Services (SUMBI), Lima, 1984.

Anker, R., M. Buvinic and N. Youssef (eds) *Women's Roles and Population Trends in the Third World.* London and Sydney: Croom Helm, 1982.

Arnold, C. 'Women's Work and Child Care in Nepal: Project Entry Point', prepared for UNICEF/New York in collaboration with UNICEF/Nepal, 1989. Mimeo.

Bennett, L. 'The Role of Women in Income Production and Intra-household Allocation of Resources as a Determinant of Child Health and Nutrition', UNICEF, Geneva, December, 1983. Mimeo.

Bhatia, J.P. and D.P. Singh. 'Women's Contribution to Agricultural Economy in Hill Regions of North-West India', *Economic and Political Weekly*, Vol. 32, No. 17 (1987), pp. 7–11.

Bidinger, P.D., B. Nag and P. Babu. 'Factors Affecting Intra-Family Food Distribution in a South India Village', a report to the Ford Foundation, the Institute for Rural Health Studies, Banjara Hills, Hyderabad, India, 1986.

Bonilla, Elssy. 'Working Women in Latin America', in Inter-American Development Bank, *Economic and Social Progress in Latin America. 1990 Report.* Washington DC: Johns Hopkins University Press, for the Inter-American Development Bank, October 1990, pp. 205–56.

Bunster, X. 'Market Sellers in Lima, Peru: Talking about Work', in M. Buvinic, M. Lycette and W. McGreevey (eds) *Women and Poverty in the Third World.* Baltimore: Johns Hopkins University Press, 1983, pp. 92–103.

Buvinic, M. 'Projects for Women in the Third World: Explaining their Misbehavior'. Prepared for the Office of Women in Development, USAID, Washington DC, the International Center for Research on Women, 1984.

Buvinic, M., M. Lycette and W. McGreevey (eds). *Women and Poverty in the Third World.* Baltimore: Johns Hopkins University Press, 1983.

Cairns, G. 'Law and the Status of Women in Latin America: A Survey', Working Paper No. 13, New York, Columbia University, School of Public Health, Center for Population and Family Health, 1984.

Campos, M.M. and F. Rosemberg. *Diagnostico da Situação da Educação Preescolar na Região Metropolitana de São Paulo.* São Paulo: Fundação Carlos Chagas, 1988.

Carloni, A.S. 'The Impact of Maternal Employment and Income on the Nutritional Status of Children in Rural Areas of Developing Countries: What is Known, What is not Known, and Where the Gaps Are', a report prepared for the United Nations, FAO, Administrative Committee on Coordination, Subcommittee on Nutrition, 1984. Mimeo.

Cornia, A. 'A Survey of Cross-Sectional and Time Series Literature on Factors Affecting Child Welfare', *World Development*, Special Issue on 'The Impact of World Recession on Children', Vol. 12, No. 3 (1984), pp. 187–202.

Dare, G. and D. Adejomo. 'Traditional Fostering and its Influence on School-Related Behaviours in Nigerian Primary School Children', *International Journal of Child Development*, Vol. 15, No. 1 (1983), pp. 16–19.

DaVanzo, J. and D.L.P. Lee. 'The Compatibility of Childcare with Market and Nonmarket Activities: Preliminary Evidence from Malaysia', in M. Buvinic, M. Lycette, and W. McGreevey (eds) *Women and Poverty in the Third World*. Baltimore: Johns Hopkins University Press, 1983.

Deere, C. 'The Allocation of Familial Labor and the Formation of Peasant Household Income in the Peruvian Sierra', in M. Buvinic, M. Lycette, and W. McGreevey (eds) *Women and Poverty in the Third World*. Baltimore: Johns Hopkins University Press, 1983.

Dwyer, D. 'Women and Income in the Third World: Implications for Policy', Working Paper No. 18. New York: the Population Council, 1983.

Dwyer, D. and J. Bruce. *A Home Divided: Women and Income in the Third World*. Stanford, California: Stanford University Press, 1988.

Engle, P. 'The Intersecting Needs of Working Women and Their Young Children: A Report to the Ford Foundation', New York, the Ford Foundation, 1980. Mimeo.

Engle, P. 'The Intersecting Needs of Working Women and their Young Children: 1980 to 1985', a paper prepared for the Consultative Group on Early Childhood Care and Development, 1986. Mimeo.

Engle, P. 'Child Care Strategies of Working and Non-working Women in Rural and Urban Guatemala', in J. Leslie and M. Paolisso (eds) *Women, Work and Child Welfare in The Third World*. AAAS Selected Symposia Series. Boulder, Colorado: Westview Press, Inc., 1989, pp. 179–200.

Engle, P., M. Pederson and R. Smidt. 'The Effects of Maternal Work for Earnings on Children's Nutritional Status and School Enrolment in Rural and Urban Guatemala', Final Project Report to USAID/PPC, 1986.

Evans, J. 'Improving Program Actions to Meet the Intersecting Needs of Women and Children in Developing Countries: A Policy and Program Review', a paper produced for the Consultative Group on Early Childhood Care and Development, Ypsilanti, Michigan: the High/Scope Educational Research Foundation, 1985.

Fort, A. 'La Mujer en las Políticas de Servicios', in M. Barrig (ed.) *De Vecinas a Cuidadanas: La Mujer en el Desarrollo Urbano*. Lima, Working Group on Women, Low-Income Households, and Urban Services (SUMBI), 1988.

Fundación del Niño. 'Evaluación del Programa Hogares de Cuidado Diario'. Caracas, Venezuela, Fundación del Niño, 1979.

Galinsky, E. 'Investing in Quality Child Care. A Report for AT&T', New York: Bank Street College of Education, 1986.

Galofré, F. 'Pobreza y los Primeros Años de la Niñez. Situación en America Latina y el Caribe', in *Pobreza Crítica en La Niñez, America Latina y el Caribe*. Santiago: UNICEF, 1981.

Guyer, J. 'Household Budgets and Women's Incomes'. Working Paper No. 28. Boston, Mass: African Studies Center, Boston University, 1980.

Hargot, E. 'Case Studies of the Melba Oka and Yetnora Cooperatives in Ethiopia', a paper prepared for the Consultative Group on Early Childhood Care and Development, New York, May 1989. Mimeo.

Johnson, F.C. 'The Role of Women's Income in Determining Nutritional Status of

Preschoolers in the Dominican Republic', an unpublished dissertation, Tufts University, School of Nutrition, May 1988.

Jolly, R. and A. Cornia (eds) *The Impact of World Recession on Children.* Oxford: Pergamon Press, 1984.

Jones, C. 'The Impact of the SEMRY I Irrigation Rice Project on the Organization of Production and Consumption at the Intra-household Level', paper prepared for USAID, Washington, DC, 1983.

Kağitçibaşi, C. *The Changing Value of Children in Turkey.* Honolulu, Hawaii: East-West Population Center. Publication 60-E, 198D2.

Kağitçibaşi, C., D. Sunar and S. Bekman. 'Comprehensive Preschool Education Project, Final Report'. Prepared for the International Development Research Centre. Istanbul, Turkey: Boğaziçi University, November 1987.

King, E. and R. Evenson. 'Time Allocation and Home Production in Philippine Rural Households', in M. Buvinic, M. Lycette and W. McGreevey (eds) *Women and Poverty in the Third World.* Baltimore: Johns Hopkins University Press, 1983, pp. 35–61.

Kumar, S. 'Role of the Household Economy in Determining Child Nutrition at Low Income Levels: A Case Study in Kerala', Occasional Paper No. 95, Ithaca, New York: Cornell University, Department of Agricultural Economics, 1977.

Kumar, S. 'Differential Control over Consumption and Spending as a Function of Productive Roles'. Paper presented to the Conference on Intra-household Allocation of Resources, Gloucester, Mass., 1984.

Leslie, J. 'Women's Work and Child Nutrition in the Third World', *World Development,* Vol. 16, No. 11 (1988), pp. 1341–62.

Leslie, J. 'Women's Time: A Factor in the Use of Child Survival Technologies', *Health Policy and Planning,* Vol. 4, No. 1 (1989), pp. 1–16.

Leslie, J., M. Lycette, and M. Buvinic. 'Weathering Economic Crises: The Crucial Role of Women in Health', in D. Bell and M. Reich (eds) *Health, Nutrition, and Economic Crises: Approaches to Policy in the Third World.* Dover, Mass: Auburn House Publishing Company, 1988, pp. 307–48.

Leslie, J. and M. Paolisso. *Women, Work, and Child Welfare in the Third World.* AAAS Selected Symposia Series. Boulder, Colorado: Westview Press, Inc., 1989.

Maguire, J. and B. Popkin. 'Helping Women Improve Nutrition in the Developing World. Beating the Zero Sum Game', Washington DC, the World Bank, 1990. Technical Paper Number 114.

Merrick, T. and Schmink, M. 'Households Headed by Women and Urban Poverty in Brazil', in M. Buvinic, M. Lycette, and W. McGreevey (eds) *Women and Poverty in the Third World.* Baltimore: Johns Hopkins University Press, 1983, pp. 244-71.

Mueller, E. 'The Value and Allocation of Time in Rural Botswana', *Journal of Development Economics,* 15 (1984), pp. 329–60.

Myers, R. and C. Indriso. 'Women's Work and Childcare', a paper prepared for a workshop on 'Issues Related to Gender, Technology, and Development', February 26–27, 1987, New York, the Rockefeller Foundation, 1987. Mimeo.

Nag, M. and N. Kak. 'Demographic Transition in a Punjab Village', *Population and Development Review,* Vol. 10, No. 4 (1984), pp. 661–678.

Nieves, I. 'A Balancing Act: Strategies to Cope with Work and Motherhood in Developing Countries', a paper prepared for the International Centre for Research on Women (ICRW) Roundtable on the Interface between Poor Women's Nurturing Roles and Productive Responsibilities, Washington DC, December 10, 1981. Mimeo.

Nieves, I. 'Household Arrangements and Multiple Jobs in San Salvador', *Signs*, Vol. 5, No. 1 (1979), pp. 134–42.

Oppong, C. 'Family Structure and Women's Reproductive and Productive Roles: Some Conceptual and Methodological Issues', in R. Anker, M. Buvinic, and N. Youssef (eds) *Women's Roles and Population Trends in the Third World.* London and Sydney: Croom Helm, 1982, pp. 133–50.

Otaala, B., R. Myers, and C. Landers. 'Children Caring for Children: New Application of an Old Idea', a paper prepared for the Consultative Group on Early Childhood Care and Development, New York, 1988. Mimeo.

Overseas Education Fund (OEF). *Child Care Needs of Low Income Mothers in Less Developed Countries.* Washington DC: OEF International, 1979.

Palmer, I., Subhadhira, and Grisanaputi. 'The Northeast Rainfed Agricultural Development Project in Thailand: A Baseline Survey of Women's Roles and Household Resource Allocation for a Farming Systems Approach', in *Case Studies of the Impact of Large-Scale Development Projects on Women.* Study No. 3, New York, the Population Council, 1983.

Paolisso, M., M. Baksh and J.C. Thomas. 'Women's Agricultural Work, Child Care, and Infant Diarrhea in Rural Kenya', in J. Leslie and M. Paolisso (eds) *Women, Work and Child Welfare in The Third World.* AAAS Selected Symposia Series. Boulder, Colorado: Westview Press, Inc., 1989, pp. 217–36.

Popkin, B. 'Rural Women, Work and Child Welfare in the Philippines', in Buvinic, Lycette and McGreevey (eds), ibid. pp. 157–76.

Population Council. 'Notes', from the Seminar Series, 'The Determinants and Consequences of Female-Headed Households', New York: the Population Council, April 1989.

Powell, D., J. Leslie, G. Jackson and K. Searle. 'Women's Work, Social Support Resources and Infant Feeding Practices in Jamaica', Washington: International Council for Research on Women, December 1988.

Rivera, C. 'Labor Force Participation and Day Care Utilization by Low-Income Mothers in Bogota, Colombia', unpublished PhD dissertation, Brandeis University, May 1979.

Roldan, M. 'Intra-household Patterns of Money Allocation and Women's Subordination (A Case Study of Domestic Outworkers in Mexico City)', paper prepared for 'The Seminar on Women, Income, and Policy', 15–16 March, 1982. New York: the Population Council, 1982.

Sanz de Santamaria, A. 'Programa Social: Hogares Comunitarios de Bienestar', paper presented to the Global Seminar on Early Childhood Development, International Child Development Centre, Florence, June 12–30, 1989, Bogotá, Colombia: Instituto Colombiano de Bienestar Familiar, June 1989.

Safilios-Rothschild, C. 'The Role of the Family: A Neglected Aspect of Poverty', in *Implementing Programs of Rural Development*, World Bank Staff Working Paper No. 403. Washington DC: The World Bank, 1980.

Saradomoni, K. 'Labour, Land and Rice Production. Women's Involvement in Three States', *Economic and Political Weekly*, Vol. 32, No. 17 (1987), pp. 2–6.

Schmink, M. 'Women in the Urban Economy in Latin America', Working Paper No. 1. New York: the Population Council, 1982.

Shah, P.M., S.R. Walimbe, and V.S. Dhole. 'Wage-Earning Mothers, Mother-Substitutes and Care of Young Children in Rural Maharashtra', *Indian Pediatrics*, 16 (1979), pp. 167–73.

Soekirman. 'Women's Work and its Effect on Infants' Nutritional Status in Central Java, Indonesia', a paper presented at the 13th International Congress of Nutrition, Brighton, England, August 18–23, 1985. Mimeo.

Swaminathan, M. *Who Cares?* A Study of Child Care Facilities for Low-Income Working Women in India. New Delhi: Centre for Women's Development Studies, 1985.

Tienda, M. 'Age and Economic Dependency in Peru: A Family Life-Cycle Analysis', *Journal of Marriage and the Family*, Vol. 42 (1980), pp. 639–52.

Tienda, M. 'Dependency, Extension, and the Family Life-Cycle Squeeze in Peru', *Journal of Comparative Family Studies*, Vol. 11 (1980), pp. 413–41.

Tolbert, K. 'Availability and Need for Day-Care Services in Mexico City' a report prepared for the Ford Foundation by the Population Council, Mexico City, May 1990.

Tucker, K. 'Maternal Employment, Differentiation, and Child Health and Nutrition in Panama', in J. Leslie and M. Paolisso (eds) *Women, Work and Child Welfare in The Third World.* AAAS Selected Symposia Series. Boulder, Colorado: Westview Press, Inc., 1989, pp. 161–78.

UNICEF, State of the World's Children, 1987.

Ware, H. 'Effects of Maternal Education, Women's Roles and Child Care on Child Mortality', *Population and Development Review, A Supplement*, Vol. 10 (1984), pp. 191–214.

Weisner, T. and R. Gallimore. 'My Brother's Keeper: Child and Sibling Caretaking', *Current Anthropology*, Vol. 18, No. 2 (1977), pp. 169–90.

Werner, E.E. *Child Care: Kith, Kin and Hired Hands.* Baltimore: University Park Press, 1983. See especially Chapter 4 on sibling caregivers.

Youssef, N. 'The Inter-relationship between the Division of Labour in the Household, Women's Roles, and their Impact on Fertility', in R. Anker, M. Buvinic and N. Youssef (eds) *Women's Roles and Population Trends in the Third World.* London and Sydney: Croom Helm, 1982, pp. 173–201.

Youssef, N. and N. Hamman. 'Continuity in Women's Productive and Reproductive Roles: Implications for Food Aid and Children's Well-Being', a paper prepared for the UNICEF/WFP Workshop, 25–26 November, 1985, New York, UNICEF, 1985.

Part V

Involving people

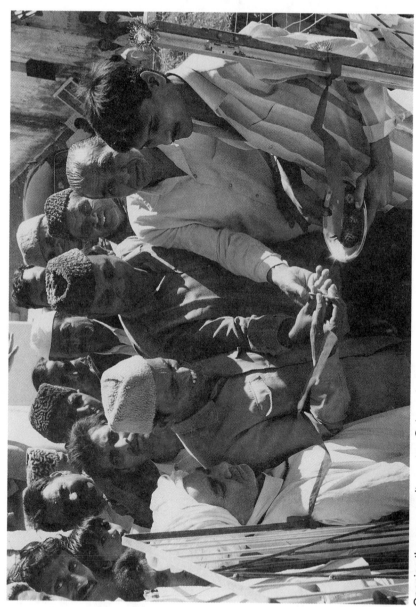

Opening the community centre, Gujarat, India

Chapter 12

Community participation: towards partnership

The people have a right and duty to participate individually and collectively in the planning and implementation of their own health care.

(Alma Alta Declaration)

One of development's 'Seven Sins' is Development without participation: Sustained development ultimately depends on enhancing people's own capacities to improve their own lives and to take more control over their own destinies.

(UNICEF, *State of the World's Children,* 1989, p. 55)

Similar quotations could be extracted from many documents issued by international and national organizations of many persuasions. Indeed, 'participation' is firmly entrenched in the rhetoric of economic and social development and its presence is not related to a particular political ideology. In different forms, participation is as much a part of neo-conservative thought (with an emphasis on democracy and decentralization and privatization) as it is a part of socialist thought with an emphasis on collectivism. It is a crucial element in popular education which, with its emphasis on praxis, owes a debt to Marxist thought. And it is part of public education, as practised in the United States, with origins closer to Rousseau.

Because the term 'participation' is so widely embraced and, seemingly, such an important element in programming, it merits closer examination. And because it is also part of the rhetoric framing this book (see Guideline 3, p. 91), we feel a need to clarify what we mean and why we think participation is such an important concept, both for child development and in the development of programmes and societies. Why is participation thought to be so important? What meanings and forms of participation can be usefully distinguished?

WHY IS PARTICIPATION SO IMPORTANT?

In human development, beginning with the newborn, active participation by individuals in constructing their own futures promotes learning and awareness, develops physical and mental capacities, and helps acquisition of self-confidence. It can bring satisfaction in accomplishment through one's own efforts and a sense of control over one's own destiny in ways that a passive, receiving, non-participatory approach to the world cannot bring. These advantages can accrue as an individual explores and interacts with the immediate physical environment – with things (watch a child experiment with and succeed in building a tower with blocks). Or, more importantly for our purposes, these benefits can result from interaction with other people. Participation with others in common tasks is part of becoming a social being, satisfying an important desire to relate to others, and helping individuals to discover the potential power of collaboration.

Community participation implies involvement together in a common enterprise by individuals who make up something called a 'community'. That participation can be in matters internal to the community and in relation to the physical environment in which community members live. But more often than not, it refers to participation by community members, collectively, in a larger project or programme that requires interaction with others outside the community. It suggests participation in the larger society of which the community is a part.

What are the presumed advantages of community participation? Some are very similar to the advantages of active participation by individuals in their own development; others go beyond. A useful listing and annotation has been provided by Alistair T. White, WHO consultant in Community Education and Participation (as quoted in Sharma 1987). The list is reproduced here, with comments and questions added.

Participation has an intrinsic value for participants, which may be difficult to measure but helps in the longer run and avoids a feeling of alienation and powerlessness. (Comment: Part of its intrinsic value may also lie in the learning that occurs naturally as part of the process.)

Participation guarantees that the felt need is involved – It might be considered that if a community agrees to participate and gives a contribution, it is sufficient to establish that the felt needs are involved in the programme. (Comment: This may depend on how extensive participation is within the community, i.e. on whether those most in need are included and what form their participation takes.)

Conscientization – Community participation results in sensitizing the community about its rights and needs. It helps close targeting of programme benefits to weaker and needed sections. It brings the masses into the picture and restores balance in the local power structure. (Comment: Again, this depends on who participates and how. Participation of 'the masses' does not occur automatically and a very special kind of participation may be needed. What about the balance between local and regional or national power?)

More will be accomplished because community's energies will be harnessed as actions are taken to provide for themselves, leading to self-reliance. (Comment: It depends on who does the 'harnessing'. Too much harnessing can lead to less rather than more effort. Is the goal really 'self-reliance'? What does that mean?)

Services can be provided at lower costs due to maximum utilization of local resources in an effective manner. (Comment: Lower costs to whom? Isn't this simply shifting the cost burden to the community from the budgets of governments or others, without really reducing costs?)

A catalyst for further development efforts – the organizational structure created once for participation within the community can be utilized for subsequent programmes or projects. (Comment: Created and utilized by whom?)

Participation leads to a sense of responsibility for the project – If a community is involved in initial stages of the planning and the implementation there is a sense of responsibility on the part of community members to see that the project is implemented effectively and is completed.

Participation ensures things are done the right way – The involvement of a community helps in adapting the project inputs according to the cultural milieu and other social traditions.

Use of indigenous knowledge and expertise – Local participation makes it possible to use indigenous resources and expertise in adapting the new technology to the advantage of local conditions and promoting the acceptance of the components of the programme. (Comment: Why put the emphasis on using the indigenous knowledge and expertise to adapt a new technology, leaving aside time-tested local ways of accomplishing the same end?)

Freedom from dependence on professionals – Community participation envisages that a community should become self-reliant in meeting all its needs at the local level. A cadre of paraprofessionals like teacher aids, volunteer workers, community workers, ANMs, if oriented and trained can make the community autonomous and reduce dependence on professionals who are few in number and costly to train. (Comment: Is the need to be free from dependence on professionals basically a cost question or are there other reasons for seeking freedom from dependence on professionals? Can a community really meet *all* its needs at a local level by creating a cadre of paraprofessionals?)

This listing of advantages helps to understand why the idea of participation is so widely accepted. But as the comments suggest, the realization of such advantages may depend to a considerable degree on who is participating (particularly on whether or not those who are most in need participate) and on the form participation takes. There are as well questions related to who controls the process or project in which participation is desired, and of the rate and rhythm and duration of participation. Let us turn now to trying to describe in a more systematic way several expressions of participation, representing several different forms that seem to be in people's minds when they use the term.

WHAT DOES IT MEAN TO PARTICIPATE?

Clearly, participation means some kind of involvement. It means 'being part of'. But this begs the question. Involvement can be token, or intense and consuming; short-lived or enduring. The something which a participant becomes part of may be smaller or larger, less or more important. The purpose of participation may be self-serving or social; concerned with transformation or with maintaining things as they are. And, there are many different forms of becoming involved: as a user, a donor, a manager, or as a planner and decision maker. Indeed, one can begin to set up a hierarchy of participation defined by origin and motive, distribution within a community, form of expression, intensity, and duration of the participation.

Let us look at several ways in which community participation is expressed and defined.

Participation through use   One form of community involvement in a project or programme occurs as people use a service or participate as learners in an education programme, or receive other programme benefits. Children who attend a preschool (and the parents who enrol them) are participants in a preschool programme. Pregnant women who visit a primary health care centre are participating in the centre.

Programme organizers and managers are often asked by cost-conscious planners and accountants how many participants they have in their project. They want to know how many individuals are using a service in order to make some judgement about per person costs. It is to the benefit of programme managers to make the number as high as possible. Replies may be based on the number of individuals a programme could potentially serve, or participation may be determined on the basis of enrolment – names on a list – with no idea of whether those enrolled actually use the service. This leads to inflated claims of the number of users, and exaggeratedly low per person costs. It distorts the idea of participation, even if one accepts this very special definition in terms of use.

Unless use is forced or mandated by law, the decision to use a service indicates a willingness to be involved. Using a service requires time and energy. And for some, that decision carries a rather high cost, requiring time away from paid work or from ever-pressing daily chores. User participation indicates that the users value the benefit they think will come from their participation as users. Conversely, not participating as a user provides one way in which individuals and communities can express their disapproval of a project and begin to pressure for change.

While recognizing that participation as a user indicates a kind of involvement in a programme, this is not the definition of participation we have in mind. Nor is it the kind of participation referred to in the opening extracts or what Alistair White was thinking about when he listed advantages. It is participation after the fact, based on acceptance of what is offered; it does not indicate active involvement in determining what is offered or in the implementation and management of a programme. It involves taking from (as beneficiaries), but not giving to, a programme. Programme responsibility remains with someone other than the user. Perhaps most important of all, participation as a user does not require working together as a community but is, rather, the sum of many individual decisions.

Participation through donation of resources   Another form of participation occurs as people contribute money or materials or time to the implementation of a project or programme. It is not unusual for community-based early childhood programmes to insist that a community participate by providing a location, by constructing a building or by helping to staff a programme. Several examples have been cited in earlier chapters in which women of a community devote time to cooking food for a snack or meal for children in an early childhood programme. A volunteer worker may run a day-care centre or a non-formal preschool or may act as a home visitor. Or, parents may be asked to help out in the centre when it is in operation.

Such donations of time and energy and materials constitute a legitimate and valued form of participation. Moreover, they reduce the costs *that are borne from outside,* by drawing on local resources. It is not difficult to understand, therefore, why governments or other organizations whose budgets are limited and tightly stretched, would seek this form of participation. By providing their own resources, communities can, in theory, establish conditions allowing influence and control over the organization and conduct of a project.

Most community contributions to externally initiated projects are made because they are a condition imposed on the community rather than because community members feel a sense of commitment to the project. This may be so even though the community has a tradition of community self-help that might be called upon if programming were approached in a different way. For the most part, this participation does not bring along any major shift in control over the programme. And often, these donations of time, energy, or material resources occur only once during the life of a programme, or are very short-lived. Once the donation has been given, participation ends. What is more, many of the contributions that are labelled 'community' contributions are really individual contributions.

For these reasons, participation in a project by donating resources usually falls short of active, committed, sustained participation. It seldom involves direct participation in decisions about the content or organization of the programme or about its functioning. Donations do not necessarily help one to feel part of a programme. Control remains outside the participants. There is no element of ownership.

Participation in programme management   Community participation can take on a different tone when the time and energy of community members is employed in managing a project or programme. The locus of control of a project – even one initiated outside the community – can shift to the community when a local management committee or a parents' committee is formed and functions effectively. Institutionalizing local management means that involvement is more likely to be continuous and over a longer period of time than is the case when participation comes through donations to programme implementation, as described above. Those who participate in the management are more likely to feel they are part of a programme.

However, projects initiated and funded from outside the community often allow little scope for decision by local managers. Rules and regulations governing the use of funds can reduce local managers to simply carrying out orders and the locus of control may not shift at all. A local group can become a channel for carrying out predetermined programme aims and methods, whether or not these correspond with local desires and conditions. Participation in management could, then, amount to donating time without much feeling of commitment or ownership.

Local management of a project or programme usually involves only a few people and they are rarely the community members who are most in need. Managers may or may not have a system of consulting other community members on a regular basis. The responsibility for management can change over time or remain in the hands of a select few. If there is no mechanism for consultation and there are no changes, and if managers are appointed from outside rather than chosen from inside the community, the degree of community participation in management will be very limited indeed. In fact, the intense and committed participation of local managers could become a basis for contention rather than for unity within a community. It could inhibit broader participation. And, it could lead to individual or personal advantage at the expense of community interests.

There is, therefore, more to community participation than handling the management of a project locally. Management must be linked to a legitimizing process of broader participation within the community and to the ability to decide and act.

Participation in setting goals, priorities, content, and in the implementation of programmes   Meaningful community participation, capable of bringing the advantages listed at the outset, requires involvement by a community in the diagnosis, design, implementation and evaluation of programmes. Only then does involvement begin to be related to real ownership and control, and carry with it the sense of being part of something that is one's own. Only then does a programme, viewed from the perspective of the community, begin to shift from being 'theirs' to being 'ours', from having been created *for* the community to having been created *by* the community (alone, or as part of a broader process with others who are viewed also as legitimate participants in the process). Only then does it bring the intrinsic benefits and the fortified community structures and other advantages that are supposed to result from a participatory approach.

But even participation in setting priorities and in plans and content can be more apparent than real, with community members simply providing information and advice, and without the power of decision or the ability to act on decisions made. Such participation may do little to 'enhance people's own capacities to improve their own lives and to take more control over their destinies', as urged in the quotation at the outset of the chapter.

With this realization, we come to the crux of the matter. *Participation, to be meaningful, should permit participants to make and act on their choices.* And community participation implies sufficient consensus and organization at the community level to be able to decide and to act together. To be able to act requires freedom and power to act, a condition that is not always present. If that is not the case, the kind of participation we have envisioned will be difficult and the advantages of participating will be limited. Thus, the focus of participatory actions, if they are to be more than superficial, shifts to creating the bases for exercising choice and action.

By viewing participation as involvement in making choices and acting on those choices, we have come a long way from seeing programme participants as the users of programmes or as donors of resources, or as managers of what others decide. We are now talking about participation by groups in the construction of their own futures through a process of analysis and action. At its best this is a continuous process of construction and reconstruction, involving all community members, that reinforces and strengthens the participatory process along the way, results in learning, and increases the basis for negotiation by the community with institutions and bureaucracies outside the community. This is the participation to which most programme rhetoric alludes and it is the participation to which we refer, but it is seldom the participation that occurs in developmental programmes.

PARTICIPATORY COMMUNITY DEVELOPMENT

To a certain degree, it is instructive to look at parallels between the active process of human development as we have described it in earlier chapters, focusing on the child, and the process of participatory community development. We have argued that the process of child development should be viewed as participatory; that the child should be recognized as (and encouraged to be) actively involved in the process, not only by bringing to it certain organic characteristics, but also by initiating, exploring, and learning through trial and error. These same principles apply to the more general process of human development, which occurs as the result of a process of constant interaction between a human being and the environment in which both the human and the environment are in '... a perpetual state of reorganization' (Sameroff and Chandler 1975, p. 235, applied to child development). This view contrasts with one in which a child, or an adult, is simply stimulated by others, or reacts, or is told what to do. It means respecting each human, children included, as an individual. It means taking a constructionist rather than a compensatory view of fostering human development.

Each person can participate in, and influence, his or her own development by exploring the surrounding environment alone, but, in the main, the process implies working (and playing) together with others, in a process of give and take. Indeed, if this did not occur, human development, which includes a social dimension, would be incomplete and distorted. For participation by a child in the development process to be meaningful, a caregiver must provide space for a child to act on its own, to explore options, to make decisions. For participation by an adult in human development to be meaningful, others with whom interaction occurs must also cede space. This means letting go of some control. (In the case of a child, however, some limits must be set to ensure that the child does not engage in activities that would be harmful to self or to others.) It also means that the people with whom interactions occur may have to modify responses, in relation to characteristics of particular individuals, and in relation to the changes over time. Friends (or caregivers in the case of the child) intervene in the individual development process by listening and reacting, providing resources when needed, motivating, recognizing accomplishments, and suggesting new ways and means of exploring and reaching goals. In so doing, caregivers as well as children, and adults who listen and support, as well as adults who talk and seek support, are also developing themselves, through their roles as co-participants in the process of development.

The process that we have described for joint participation in human development provides a good starting point for considering the participation by communities with outside institutions in projects and programmes that are intended to help a community to develop. There is some value in repeating phrases used above for human development, substituting instead community development. '(Community) development occurs as the result of a process of constant interaction between the (community) and the environment in which both the (community) and the environment are in a perpetual state of reorganization. This view contrasts with one in which a (community) is simply stimulated by others, or reacts, or is told what to do. It means respecting each (community).... It means taking a constructionist rather than a compensatory view of (community) development.'

Communities, like individual human beings, bring to the process of constructing their own futures certain cultural and social characteristics of an organic nature. A community, to develop, must also initiate, explore options, and learn by trial and error. It needs space to be able to do that. Moreover, institutions in the larger environment, with whom communities interact, must recognize that individual communities are different and that they change over time. Hence the institutions must work in different ways with different communities and be willing to vary their ways of acting as communities develop. External institutions can also participate by listening and reacting, by providing resources when needed, by suggesting new ways of doing things, and by motivating and recognizing accomplishments.

In short, there are apparent parallels between what we expect and need when dealing with human (or child) development and community development. That should not be surprising because communities are made up of humans. But there are some important differences as well which begin to appear as we reflect on the nature of communities.

WHAT IS A COMMUNITY?

In most cases when the rhetoric of community participation and development is used, a community is defined in administrative and geographic terms, encompassing all the people who are in a particular village or all people falling under the jurisdiction of a particular official, or all people living within a certain area of a city or countryside. But physical proximity and administrative organization do not provide a natural or necessarily even an appropriate basis for defining 'community'.

A community refers to a group of people who have something in common. That something is usually a common culture, including a common language and set of values and beliefs. But there is more to community. A community works together towards achieving a set of shared goals. To work together requires a sufficiently coherent social organization to be able to set common goals and to organize for common action. Shared culture facilitates organization, communication and joint action. It makes easier the process of defining and pursuing a common cause.

People who live in the same village may or may not share culture, may or may not agree upon goals, and may or may not be able to organize for common action. In a small Indian village in rural Gujarat, for instance, there is often tension between Hindus and Muslims, rooted in cultural and historical differences. Even though language is shared (Gujarati) and there is an administrative structure that is supposed to unite people, and even though there is physical closeness, the village cannot easily be called a community. Indeed, the word 'community' is used by local people to refer to the religious groupings and the word 'village' is used for the political entity incorporating both Hindus and Muslims.

In urban marginal areas, where people from very different backgrounds are often thrown together, a sense of community is often lacking completely. Furthermore, the newness and instability of inhabitants in many of these areas does not lend itself to establishing a *modus vivendi* among different groups, as can occur in a village where there are traditions, where change is seldom so abrupt and where people have more of a sense that they must live together despite differences.

What the foregoing suggests is that the first problem of community participation and development is often the problem of arriving at a level of agreement and organization that will permit a group of people who live near to each other to function in common, and that will permit participation in an activity directed towards a common goal. But how can that happen in groups that are not only far from homogeneous culturally, but where economic differences, distinctions of caste and class, and vested interests of many kinds come into play?

At least part of the answer lies in discovering common interests. When people live in the same village or neighbourhood, they are bound to face many of the same problems in their daily living. Problems of water and sanitation or of a measles epidemic or lack of employment or poor education facilities can affect all members of the village, directly or indirectly. These problems provide an opening for constructing a sense of community and for joint, participatory action among groups that might not otherwise agree or organize. These problems are also often the problems that other communities and governments and other institutions outside the community say they are interested in helping to solve. Identifying these common interests provides a basis for communities to collaborate with each other and with institutions outside the community.

The process of defining interests (or needs) and of dealing with problems at the community level can be dealt with in three main ways:

Imposed development

Problems can be identified and worked on *for* villagers by someone coming from outside the village who not only determines that there is a need for drinking water but who also drills the well – or applies a vaccine or serves as a teacher. In this case, a specific common problem may be solved, but without participation, except in the most superficial sense. And nothing will have been done to build a sense of community in the process.

Villagers may be pleased with the results of imposed development and will look in the future for actions from the beneficent institution. While seeking something more, we should not be blind to the fact that a significant effect on the living conditions within a village can be achieved with a minimum of community participation.

Self-actualized development

Or, problems can be identified and worked on *by* the community, taking initiative on its own to obtain whatever is needed for solutions, using community resources and/or resources from outside requested by and under the control of the community. In this second case, members of the community work together to identify and solve a problem, produce a solution, and build, or reinforce, a sense of community. A successful experience can strengthen community confidence and, as suggested at the outset, provide the structures to be used (in this case by the community) to work on other problems.

This second approach is easier to talk about than to realize. It tends towards the romantic. If a sense of community does not already exist that facilitates common action, or if a degree of fatalism or inertia or lack of awareness of new ways to overcome a problem inhibits action, it may be necessary to look to outsiders as participants in at least the initial stages of discovery and community building. Moreover, very few communities are able to find within themselves all the human and material resources they need; most must look to the outside for assistance in solving some of their most pressing problems.

Towards partnership

The third approach to identifying and acting upon problems faced by a community is one in which communities work together *with* institutions from the larger society to solve common problems. This approach is sometimes characterized as a partnership. A partnership cannot exist if one party always works for the other. Nor can a partnership exist if each partner works by himself or herself. In addition, partnership implies mutual respect and equality and a sharing of responsibility for both successes and failures.

Although the idea of a partnership in community development has similarities with the co-participation described for the child development process, this parallel should not be pushed too far. Villages are not children. In their early years, developing children may be given some freedom, but they also need to be protected against their own actions – touching fire or heading into a street where cars pass rapidly. But communities are run by adults and they have history and tradition. There is, therefore, no room for the 'paternal' relationship that must be maintained in parent–child interactions.

Some readers will question the idea of partnership. They will say this is a naive notion because outside institutions, and particularly government institutions, have power that communities cannot match and that they are unwilling to cede to communities. They will argue that the degree of respect and equality needed to work together in partnership cannot be achieved unless, perhaps, communities band together in broad populist movements.

These comments obviously cannot be rejected out of hand when seeking partnership with governments. The balance of power *is* unfavourable. And many governments *are* authoritarian. Even governments characterized as democratic often have such a 'top down', paternalistic approach to what they call community development that partnership seems out of the question. Moreover, it is clear from experience that the conditions necessary for working in true partnership are difficult to find in a governmental institution that is under pressure to make things happen quickly, and responds with a rhythm of work often determined by anticipated changes of government. The large scale of government operations makes certain rules and regulations and standardization necessary to maintain control over organization. These make it difficult for institutional representatives, even at a local level, to establish the kind of flexible, open, horizontal relationship that is required in a partnership. In addition, the first order of business for governments is to strengthen national spirit and vision and commitment. Too often that is seen as being equivalent with strengthening the centralized power of governments. Devolving responsibility to local communities can, therefore, be threatening.

Having said all that, however, it does not follow that working with governmental institutions is hopeless. Not all governments are equally hierarchical and set in their ways and not all efforts to change the balance of power or the outlooks of governments will be fruitless. Most governments are not monolithic and in their diversity provide openings for joint action. At local levels, the conditions may be much more favourable than at national levels. Technical agencies within governments may be able to achieve a certain level of independence and provide a different kind of basis for partnership than the rest of the bureaucracy. The question is, then, how one can move from an unbalanced form of co-participation towards partnership.

Governments are not, of course, the only institutions outside the community with which local communities can work in partnership to construct their futures. The conditions necessary for partnership are more often found in non-governmental organizations (NGOs). Such organizations may be grassroots groups that have evolved locally, or regionally. Or they may be outside organizations formed to work with communities to improve conditions. For the most part, these are smaller, less restricted by rules and more able to change themselves, less concerned with power, able to adjust to a slower rhythm, capable of reflection, and often motivated by altruistic interests. NGOs are often more stable than governments. And, typically, they are able to keep a foot firmly planted in the national culture while relating in direct and meaningful and committed ways to local communities. These NGOs can be called on, as partners and as brokers.

It would be a mistake, however, to overgeneralize about NGOs any more than it would be to treat all governments as alike. The number of NGOs has grown dramatically in the last two decades (Dichter 1988), and variations on the NGO theme are vast. In addition to the community-based and national NGOs, international NGOs are frequently present. These NGOs have grown in size and have often changed their mode of operation in recent years. Some NGOs are more oriented towards emergency support, others focus on technical assistance, others are more interested in the longer-term task of helping to build organization. Many NGOs are at least as paternalistic in their approaches to communities as some governments. Many have their own hidden agendas in working with communities. As we look towards partnership, therefore, we shall not restrict ourselves to talking about non-governmental organizations nor exclude governmental institutions.

The challenge for communities is to find appropriate partners with whom they can work towards solving specific community problems while maintaining or gaining greater control over the process of constructing their own futures. The challenge for those partners is to adopt methods and to pursue processes that not only help to solve specific problems, but are also empowering for communities, most of which are divided internally. Both groups need to recognize that local communities cannot be completely self-sufficient or self-reliant in this increasingly interdependent world. They must act to some degree within a broader social framework. The joint challenge is to locate those areas of mutual interests, within communities, and in relationship with partners, that will not only bring tangible results but will further the empowering process.

Consider the following description of a 'community-based' early childhood development project in Africa that was brought to the community by an external institution:

The major aim was certainly to mobilise the local community to take part in development activities in their area, including a day care centre

for children from 3 to 5 years of age. However, the community development officers in charge of the project seemed unclear as to how the
community was to be involved, other than by providing the food and
cooking it for the children in the day care centre. There was a delay in
erecting a building to house the centre, so it started in a local church
with the national government providing the funds for two teachers. One
mother volunteered to cook, but the community was unable to provide
the food, so the local council agreed to do so.

Very few of the parents sent their children to the day care centre,
largely because they did not appear to appreciate the importance of such
a programme for their children's growth and development. It had been
assumed by the initiators of the programme that once the centre was
opened, the children would almost automatically attend. Reasons
suggested for the lack of interest included a feeling that the project had
been started in a hurry and prematurely. Community members were
given very little time to understand the objectives and activities of the
project or to question them or offer suggestions about what they wanted.
Because the community members were treated as recipients with little or
no input into the project, they did not identify with it, and their participation and involvement has remained minimal.

> (Otaala 1989, as reported in the Bernard van Leer Foundation
> 1990, pp. 7–8)

This example illustrates in action the sometimes unhappy result when the
idea of participation is limited to donating time and materials and a
location. It also illustrates common errors committed as an external institution tries to put its project into operation. The author of the description
concluded that 'without the partnership of parents and the community,
efforts to improve early childhood care and education are unlikely to be
effective'.

What might have been done to avoid the above situation? From the
description, it is clear that community members should have been involved
from the start in the diagnosis and planning of a project, and that greater
responsibility needed to be placed within the community. The description
also suggests the need to move with less speed, allowing a process of
thought and action and evaluation to adjust what has been done (Cariola
and Rojas 1986). There was an unfulfilled need to ask and to listen (Pantin
1983).

Two kinds of knowledge

One reason community members are not asked and listened to is because
those who arrive with a programme often feel that the knowledge (or technology) they bring is superior because it has a scientific base. This is

typical of what we have called 'imposed development'. In this view, traditional wisdom tends to play a negative and obstructive role, representing outmoded ways of thinking and acting that need to be overcome. Control over knowledge is placed with scientific communities and governments who see their role as one of transmitting that knowledge to the uninitiated.

But not all valid knowledge is scientifically derived. A separate source of knowledge that drives the actions of many local communities is rooted in an unsystematic cultural accumulation of experience through trial and error over generations if not centuries. It is time-tested, rather than experimental knowledge. And there is a need to understand and to respect it as it is brought by a community to the process of formulating and carrying out a project.

Recognizing that there are two valuable sources of knowledge to be drawn upon – academic and popular – in creating and implementing programmes creates the need for a process of dialogue that will allow a kind of confrontation between the two, enriching both and promoting mutual learning. Such a dialogue is as important when dealing with problems of childrearing and child development as it is for problems in the field of agriculture (see, for instance, the work on farming systems in which agricultural scientists have recognized the virtue of locally derived wisdom about seeds and planting: Hildebrand 1978, cited in Korten and Alonso). Drawing on the two sources of knowledge is crucial for establishing a partnership in planning and action.

To work towards partnership, then, requires not only a change in conventional approaches to organization, but also a different approach to knowledge, stressing dual sources of knowledge, dialogue and mutual learning.

Dialogue and mutual learning

The ideas of dialogue and mutual learning that are essential to the partnership we seek are at the heart of a vast literature dealing with 'popular education' (Freire 1970; Gajardo 1983), 'participatory research', (Latapí 1988; Hall, Gillette and Tandon 1982; De Schutter 1986), local planning with community participation (Bosnjak 1982, 1990), 'educational communication' (Rivera 1987) and 'empowerment' (Kent 1987; Cochran 1988). A proper review of these overlapping literatures is not possible within the limits of this book, but it is here that the most convincing treatments of community participation are found, related not only to dialogue and mutual learning, but also to reflection and to action in groups that serves to empower the poor. From these various formulations come conceptual bases and specific methods that can be applied to fostering collaboration between communities and social institutions in ways that were not evident in the programme description above.

A participatory approach, in the tradition of popular education, can be contrasted with several other approaches to programming and action. The clearest of these contrasts is with a social marketing approach (Manoff 1985), captured partially in a quotation from Kent (1987):

> Consider the contrast between empowerment and social marketing. In social marketing the message is delivered in one direction, in a form like that which Paulo Freire criticized as 'banking education', a process of making information deposits into presumably empty vessels. If social marketers do undertake some sort of inquiry with their target audience, it is to learn how to design their messages and thus influence behavior more effectively. Social marketing is self-consciously manipulative, trying to induce concrete behaviors.... In empowerment, however, the agent tries to get people to create their own formulations and analyses of their problems. The decision as to what ought to be done is theirs, while in social marketing the desired behavior is predetermined by the marketer. Where the social marketer's principal medium is mass media, for the empowerment agent, the principal medium is face-to-face dialogue.

'Empowerment', as used in the above quotation, involves more than simply transferring knowledge to people. It involves creating one's own formulations and it involves face-to-face dialogue.

There is more, however. From face-to-face dialogue comes not only information and new formulations, but mutual learning and the enabling, or empowering, of groups as well as of individuals. This social and group character of empowerment, so central in the literature cited above, is being lost in current usage of the term. Unfortunately, empowerment is becoming equated, in some circles, exclusively with providing information to individuals so that they will have the power to act with respect to particular problems, say of child survival or development.

The contrast is not so clear between empowerment and social mobilization. Indeed, for some people these terms are virtually synonymous because they define social mobilization in terms of a process bringing lasting changes in participants at the grass roots that will transform conditions of living for the poor, based on their participation in the process. These lasting changes have a social, or organizational, as well as an individual dimension. To mobilize socially is to empower (Wood 1989).

But for others, social mobilization is, to oversimplify slightly, getting many people, or organizations, to do something at the same time. Social mobilization for literacy or for immunization campaigns occurs repeatedly, but seldom carries with it the same kind of longer-term changes implied in the concept of empowerment. Acting together lasts only as long as the particular action for which people are mobilized. As it is currently practised by governments and international agencies, the organizations that are mobilized for action are more likely to be scouts and the church and various parts of the government bureaucracy than community organizations. A main vehicle for the social mobilization may be a social marketing effort in which television and radio announcements play an important role, but which may include more traditional forms of communicating messages as well. Mobilization occurs around a predetermined theme.

These mobilization efforts are not 'bad'. In fact they are good because they do help to prevent deaths and to increase literacy. But they fall short because they rarely empower communities with the knowledge and organization needed to take control of their own lives.

PROGRAMME IMPLICATIONS

What are the implications of this general discussion of participation for the planning and implementation of programmes to improve child care and enhance child development? Some of the implications are obvious:

1 *Be participatory.* We should look beyond a limited view defining programme participants as individual users or beneficiaries or receivers of knowledge. Simply requesting communities to participate by donating time and materials is not sufficient. Indeed, it may backfire. To be truly participatory, programming methods should be adopted that involve community members at all stages of programming – in diagnosis, planning, implementing, and evaluation of early childhood projects. Programming for early childhood care and development should involve working in partnership, employing dialogue, drawing on both traditional wisdom and scientific knowledge, with a goal of mutual learning and of empowering communities to assume control over decisions and actions influencing their condition of life.

These points have been amply discussed earlier in the chapter. But there are a number of other implications for programming that are not simple recapitulations of earlier points. For instance:

2 *Prepare options within a broad framework.* Instead of following one narrow programme line that needs to be 'marketed' to communities, programmers need to be prepared with a set of programme options and be willing to respond to the priority needs of particular communities in different ways. The ability of any one organization to respond to all possible requests is unrealistic, hence the idea of choices that provide options within some limits, related to what an organization can do, and presumably based on experience of what people want and need.

The idea of preparing options will not be well met by some planners who feel they must have a clear idea in advance of where they are headed, or by programmers who feel they know what is best. It will not be well met by early childhood enthusiasts who feel that the best way to benefit development is by establishing a preschool or a child-care centre of a particular kind.

The idea of offering options rather than solutions operates at two levels. The first is the level of choice between an activity that is a clearly defined child development activity and an activity that works in a very general way to improve the conditions of a community, children included. For example, the choice might be between a child development activity designed to improve school readiness, and one designed to provide potable water to a village. If a community places a high priority on water, and is willing to organize itself to that end, then it is in the interest of early education specialists to support that effort while continuing to work with the community toward a partnership that will include early education. Or conversely, the idea of potable water may be attached to an initial interest in improving the integrated development of young children.

The second level at which this principle operates is at the level of choice among programmes of early childhood development. Throughout this book, we have stressed the importance of a set of complementary approaches and, within each, a variety of possible models that might be followed. The particular model (or models) that is (are) most appropriate for a particular community should be worked out with community participation.

This principle is not as limiting as it might sound. It is possible for most development-minded institutions, governmental or non-governmental, to anticipate in a general way some of the main requests that will result from a participatory diagnostic and planning process at the community level. It will be possible to prepare methods and materials that can then be adjusted through discussion in the community. Over time, the points of commonality across communities will be clearer and a revised set of options can be worked on.

The principle of preparing options is also less limiting than it seems because, in the preparation of these options, an integrating thread may well be the welfare of children. This can, and often does, serve as a starting point for the joint construction of programmes that, while benefiting children, also build community and provide benefits to adult members of the community as well. The topic captures the interest of most community members, and particularly women, who may be among the most needy community members but who may be at the margin of a participatory process. Many parents take their own physical and mental condition as (relatively) given, but will work for an improvement they feel will benefit their children. The theme cuts across cultural and other divisions in a village or neighbourhood. It is a topic that is less politically charged or threatening than many others that might be of mutual interest, such as land distribution or employment. It is less likely to be associated with a particular vested interest in a community. And it is a topic that, in the last analysis, leads to discussion of the entire gamut of conditions affecting the child; it is an integrating topic. For these reasons, one valid starting point for defining options intended to help construct community and foster participation can be the well-being of children and families.

3 *A need to decentralize.*   Institutions seeking to enhance early childhood development with participation should seek organizational adjustments that allow a truly decentralized mode of functioning, and a more realistic and responsive rhythm of work.

Decentralization can reinforce local power structures and inhibit ample participation, if done in a way that gives local tyrants greater leeway to impose their ideas. Consequently, centralized institutions must be watchful to see that participation of families in need is a part of the programming process.

4 *A new kind of professional.*   A participatory approach to planning at the local level requires a different kind of professional or technical person than is found in most organizations. This new, field-oriented institutional representative should be selected according to a set of criteria that would include empathy and familiarity with problems of the poor as well as technical expertise.

To that end, it may be necessary to develop systems of training and promotion that will allow uncertified paraprofessionals, with roots in rural villages and urban marginal areas, to qualify for technical positions within institutional bureaucracies at the local level. In addition, conventional courses for training of professionals and technicians will need to be adjusted so that, for instance, child development specialists are offered a community-based and participatory option as well as the more typical training for work in formal child-care centres and preschools, or as measurement specialists.

To attract and support these new professionals, different kinds of incentive systems will have to be developed within social institutions, providing rewards for successes in assisting communities to diagnose and organize for action, with less emphasis placed on the installation of particular kinds of programmes and on 'user counts' and the ability to disburse funds quickly.

5 *Reorganizing information systems.*   Systems of collecting and analysing information will need to be revised, from the ground up, so that the first analyses occur at community levels.

In most cases today, information is requested from local individuals and is then passed on immediately to higher levels that may or may not have the capacity for analysis. Most information is aggregated and only the general statistics are made available. Rarely is the information analysed by community or returned to the community for its own use. Thus, information gathering works against rather than for local planning, and the system lends itself to inventing information.

6 *Work with non-governmental organizations.*   There should be a greater openness on the part of both governments and international organizations to work with and support non-governmental institutions with the ability to

carry out participatory, empowering programmes of early childhood care and development. The proliferation of national and international NGOs both facilitates and complicates this recommendation, as suggested above.

The programme guidelines revisited

In Chapter 5, one of the guidelines established for successful programming was that the process should be 'participatory and community-based'. That guideline has now been elaborated and there should be little doubt about our position that community participation, seen as a form of social empowerment, should be a part of all programming efforts. But this guideline interacts with others we have set, fitting easily with some, and creating tension with others. Let us look at *participation and*:

Families at risk   The insistence that programmes focus on families and children who live in at risk conditions (Guideline 1, p. 89) places a premium on participation *by that group*, not only as users, but also in programme formulation and implementation. The challenge of making good on the rhetoric of participation is thereby increased; families and children at risk are often those who are most 'at the margin' of communities as well as of the larger society and do not normally enter into the decision-making process of communities. The example of a community-based, participatory methodology that we will describe makes a point of involving those most in need.

Comprehensiveness   Or, consider the concept of participation in relation to the idea that programmes of early childhood care and development should be part of a comprehensive, multifaceted strategy (Guideline 2, p. 89). While stressing a multifaceted strategy, we argued in Chapter 8 that it is difficult to achieve programme integration among institutions responsible for various components, given the vertical structures that are usually established to provide various services. We placed our emphasis, therefore, on convergence of services and in so doing accepted the position that whether or not a multifaceted approach is successfully realized depends, in the last analysis, on the desires and abilities of individuals, families, and communities to put the pieces together. That integration depends in part on the world view and knowledge base of individuals. But it depends also on the strength and reach and solidarity and participation that community organizations command and enjoy.

We will sketch below a method of local planning that promotes a holistic view by looking at a full range of conditions of life for children and adults in a community. Even though one area may be chosen as a starting point for action, the view is an integrated one and, over time, leads to integrated, or converging, actions.

Respecting cultural differences and beginning where people are   In the following chapter we shall return to two other guidelines – the need for flexibility related to differences in sociocultural contexts, and the need to begin where people are, building together on local ways, even while adding new information (Guidelines 4 and 5, p. 92). These are congruent with the participation guideline. Indeed, as we said, if community participation is real, programming will, by definition, be respectful of cultures. If it is not, following these two guidelines will be difficult.

Scale   By including as a programme guideline the stipulation that programmes should try to reach the largest possible number of children who are at risk (Guideline 7, p. 94), a bias against participatory programming is introduced. Growing large lends itself to programming that is impersonal, bureaucratic, standardized, ready-made, and therefore to nonparticipatory solutions and methods. In Chapter 14, we shall seek relief from this apparent tension between thinking big, and seeking participation that provides ownership and respects cultures. We shall suggest a different way of thinking about what constitutes scale and how to achieve it.

Cost-effectiveness   Finally, applying the principle of cost effectiveness (Guideline 6, p. 93) is made more complicated by the introduction of participation. First, the act of participating enters on both sides of the cost-effectiveness equation – as a desired effect, and as an action that has a cost attached, as time and energy and other resources used in the course of participating are applied to obtain specific outcomes such as enhanced child development. Second, because participation in a programme often occurs in ways that are not compensated by money, it is difficult to value. What price should be put on the time of a volunteer? How do we value contributions in kind? We shall see that the rhetoric of participation among those concerned with economic efficiency or with stretching budgets is somewhat different from the rhetoric of those who are concerned about who makes choices and about the balance of power among social groups in the process.

Examples

Colombia: Project PROMESA

In 1978, a project was begun with 100 families in four small farming and fishing villages along the Pacific Coast of Colombia, in one of the most impoverished regions of the country. Over a period of 10 years it has grown slowly to serve about 2,000 families in the area, and elements of the programme have been adapted for implementation in other parts of Colombia. A non-governmental organization, the International Center for

Education and Human Development (CINDE), acted as the external agent in the project.

In this hot, humid, isolated area, reachable only by boat or small plane, malnutrition, and infant mortality and morbidity are high, schooling attainment is low, and services are sparse. The approach taken to working on these problems was built around the healthy development of children.

> Embedded in PROMESA was a concept of community development based upon the notion that individuals must be involved in their own process of development, and that for this development to occur there must be a simultaneous process of change in the intellectual, physical, economic and sociocultural aspects of life.
>
> (CINDE 1990, p. 1)

In initial contacts with the community, CINDE staff found an interest among mothers in the intellectual development of their children. But this interest soon broadened.

> The programme began by encouraging groups of mothers, under the leadership of 'promotoras', to stimulate the physical and intellectual development of their preschool children by playing games with them. Gradually, during the meetings the mothers started to identify other problems related to topics such as health, nutrition, environmental sanitation, vocational training, income generation and cultural activities. Over time therefore, as individuals gained confidence and developed a greater understanding of their overall needs, PROMESA expanded into an integrated community development project, with the entire community participating in one or more aspects of the program.
>
> (ibid., p. 2)

A socio-intellectual component of the project involved workshops, study groups, and follow-up activities aimed at improving the quality of family interactions and life. In support of this goal, preschool and nutrition centres were organized and run by the community, with the support of local institutional agents. Physical development was approached in various ways, including the development of a primary health care system administered by the community. An economic component evolved around community groups interested in improving their income (e.g. a carpenters' cooperative) and their organizational and administrative capacities (through establishing and managing revolving funds and by organizing the marketing of their products).

> A socio-cultural component fostered the cultural identity of the groups, especially by recovering and reviewing important aspects of their past history and culture. Part of this component includes the formation of groups whose objectives are to organize and become involved in

different cultural activities, such as drama and music; local or folkloric games; and the study of native myths, legends, and natural medical practices.

From the beginning, parents have been involved in different aspects of programme planning and implementation, although this has varied from community to community according to the socio-cultural and political variables affecting the project at different moments. In fact, the parents themselves (or other community leaders) have been the main educational agents and organizers of the program. Furthermore, most of the project activities have started outside the school or other formal systems.

(ibid., pp. 3–5)

PROMESA was not without its difficult moments. However, because the external agent was an NGO, it had the flexibility to respond to a variety of needs, without being constrained by a particular sectoral approach. Funding sources also encouraged a participatory approach. It was possible to stay with the activities over a long period. CINDE facilitated the entry of several government programmes in cooperation with the community and in response to identified needs. Emphasis was placed on inter-institutional coordination from the outset, at local and regional levels.

The educational accomplishments of PROMESA children were reported in Chapter 10. Other changes, physical and organizational, have occurred slowly in the communities, but have been basic and continuing.

Although the PROMESA idea and methods have spread, the programme has been relatively contained. Applying this same method on a large scale, with the same degree of flexibility, sensitivity to cultural needs, and reliance on community members is difficult to imagine.

India: the integrated child development service

The massive ICDS programme, to which frequent reference has been made throughout the book, falls near the opposite end of the participation spectrum from the PROMESA project. Community participation is desired within the ICDS programme:

Its objectives are not limited to mere delivery of services but emphasize initiation of a process aimed at bringing social change in the life of the community by promoting awareness, changes, attitudes, beliefs and practices.

(Sharma 1987, p. 14)

Participation is, nevertheless, viewed mainly in terms of user participation and the donation of local resources. With respect to user participation, a gain has been made because the programme has been targeted to those populations most in need – in rural and tribal areas and in marginal urban areas. Even here, however, 'Most of the studies on community participation have indicated that the beneficiaries have a low awareness of the scheme, its components and the possible benefits they can get from it' (ibid.).

With respect to the local donation of time and energy, ICDS has also achieved a degree of what is sometimes called community participation. Indeed, the programme is termed a community-based programme because it involves community volunteers to manage and implement it, rather than paid functionaries. However, the Anganwadi worker charged with making the programme run is chosen by ICDS, not by the community. Moreover,

> The local coordination committees which are supposed to involve local representation in decision making and overseeing the implementation of the scheme are non-existent in most cases. Wherever committees have been set up the frequency of their meeting and taking interest in ICDS is far from what is needed. The composition of these committees is the old story of power vested with the privileged and the struggle between the haves and have nots continues. The drawing of the masses and the real beneficiaries into the process of decision making has not taken place nor has (it) been attempted.

> (ibid, pp. 14–15)

Sometimes a local community contributes in cash or kind towards supplementary nutrition or the preschool component of the programme. But these contributions are beyond the means of most. And the site of the building and other forms of contribution are closely controlled. In general, however, the service is looked upon as a 'dole'. Participation, when it occurs, is more individual than group participation. It has also been observed that project functionaries do not have adequate skills to elicit participation, despite training to that end. Incentives to involve the community are not present for either these functionaries or the grassroots worker.

As might be expected in a programme that is so large, there are exceptions to the general lack of community participation in ICDS. In some communities, women's groups have taken a very active role in overseeing operation of the local centre and in bringing parents together. In some cases, this has led to other activities at the community level. But these cases are rare.

These comments on participation should not be surprising within the Indian context. The individualistic Hindu religion, the long shadows of the caste system, traditions of Maharajas and colonial rule, and an élitist intellectual bias make community participation of the kind we have described difficult to achieve. But the lack of participation should not classify the ICDS as a failure. On the contrary, the programme has been able to point to successes in helping to reduce malnutrition, morbidity, and school repetition, even though it has not been a participatory project in the sense we have been urging. In fact, the lesson of ICDS may be that accomplishments can occur with a minimum of community participation, and that in some circumstances (even within the largest democracy in the world), the kind of community participation that involves group actions, dialogue, and empowerment is difficult to achieve on a large scale.

Other programme examples

In between the two examples presented above are many others that do not achieve the community participation of a PROMESA but are more participatory than ICDS. The reader is referred back to an example from Thailand (p. 138) in which an early education programme included accumulation of funds and management experience that allowed the external institution to withdraw from its participation in over 100 communities, leaving behind enhanced organization and a functioning programme in the hands of the community.

Or, the Kenyan experience might be described in which early childhood programmes have evolved within the context of a community-oriented movement (Njenga 1989). The harambee movement allowed the programme both to draw on and reinforce community participation.

Many cases similar to the PROMESA programme could also be cited, particularly within Latin America. For instance, mention has been made of the Chilean Parents and Children Project (see p. 140). Or, the reader can refer to a project of 'Community Children's Homes' that began in a small fishing village on the northern coast of Colombia (Amar Amar 1986), or a participatory project in Punerenas, Costa Rica (Kavanaugh 1990). Each of these projects is a small-scale project, with some extension into the surrounding area, and with participation of a non-governmental organization working in partnership with communities.

Planning and action at the local level with community and institutional participation

The final example offered in this chapter is not of a particular project, but of a participatory method facilitating the joint participation of community groups and technical staff from an external organization in the diagnosis and planning of activities at the community level. It features the confrontation of the two sources of knowledge distinguished earlier. It helps move the planning process towards partnership.

The method described in the following paragraphs (Bosnjak 1982) has been derived from field experiences in a variety of locations in Latin

America. A basic consideration underlying the methodology is that:

> The activities, goods or services that are introduced into the life of marginal groups should, as a first condition, improve the resources, knowledge and activities already existing, taking into account the value assigned to all aspects of life within a community instead of producing ruptures by means of innovations that impede a process of greater self-sufficiency.

(ibid., p. 31)

The method of local planning with community participation also assumes that:

- Marginal groups are not homogeneous and are stratified along several dimensions which have helped to maintain a condition of dependency of marginal groups on those in power.
- Although there will be differences among communities there will also appear common elements that allow definition of policies and programmes with sufficient generality to be applicable in different places. Thus, results of various local planning exercises will improve formulation and operation of regional and national policies.
- Although the community may not coincide with geographic or administrative organization, that geographic and administrative unit can offer a broad field of action that allows strengthening of existing organizations and/or promotion of new forms of association based on common interests and problems.
- The process of interaction among community members who are supposed to be the beneficiaries of a programme and institutional agents should be one of continuous dialogue and mutual learning. This requires that institutional agents have a responsibility to understand the structure of the community in order to ensure that the interests articulated are those of all community members, including and giving priority to those most in need.
- An institutional agent has a responsibility to submit his or her technical knowledge and points of view for discussion in the same way that this is expected of community members.
- Local planning is a continuous process that includes diagnosis, programming, monitoring and evaluation.
- In the joint process, information will be needed about:
    - conditions of life of various social groups in the community. These include, but will not be limited to, information about nutritional status, health, water and sanitation, work/income/expenses, housing, education, cultural expressions, communication and transportation, and degrees of participation within the existing structure of community relationships;

- factors that affect the conditions of life. These include existing patterns of action and attitudes and beliefs, organizational forms, technologies in use, both for the community and external to the community;
- community and institutional resources available for actions;
- the degree to which actions are carried out and their effectiveness.

The local planning process consists of three general steps:

1 *Diagnosis*, centred on describing the conditions of life of the community and analysing why they are that way.

2 *Project planning*. Objectives and priorities for action, in the short and long term, are set for each condition, and strategies identified to improve conditions (reinforce or modify or replace existing activities, forms of organization, resources and technologies).

3 *Project implementation*.   This includes not only carrying out actions, but also monitoring, evaluating, and adjusting along the way.

The process could develop in the following way (see Bosnjak 1982, pp. 55–7). Either the community or the institutional agent could initiate the process. In either case, the institutional agent should bring to the process at least four qualifications. First, she should have a commitment to work with the community in a participatory way. Second, she should possess technical expertise and a clear knowledge of the possibilities and limitations of the institution in working with communities. Third, the agent should know how the conditions of life of the community are described in the secondary sources of information usually kept as a part of normal bureaucratic procedure. Fourth, an understanding is necessary of the social stratification and structure of a community.

This last qualification is more difficult than the others because it requires a period of observation, informal discussion, and attendance at meetings of various organized groups in the community that are disposed to discuss the planning of a programme and their own participation in it. That means taking time, for the agent to become acquainted with the community, and vice versa. (Some would say much more is involved and that the outsider should actually live in a community for some time, participating in the everyday life of the community in order to know the community at first hand.) Consequently, the partner institution must be willing to allow time for the process to develop and must be willing to give time to its representative for that purpose. This is a labour-intensive process.

From this process of getting acquainted should come the beginnings of confidence by the community in the agent and, from the agent's side, identification of the community organizations that represent the interests of needy groups and that are willing to collaborate in the project. (If none of the existing organizations adequately represent those groups, two conditions for collaboration with other community groups might be set by the institutional agent: that the participatory process concentrate on the needs of the community members most in need, and that the process seek alternative forms for participation of the neediest at all stages.)

Once the groups that include or represent community members most in need have been identified, it is useful for those groups to begin an auto-diagnosis of the basic needs of the community, including its organization and participation. The institutional agent could offer technical assistance in that process, but the diagnosis should be undertaken by the community. This exercise has two purposes. The first is to provide a preliminary idea of the conditions of life of various groups and of the areas of greatest interest for collaborative action. To accomplish this purpose, the preliminary results of the self-diagnosis can be presented and discussed in community meetings, with comments offered by both the community and the institutional agent. (Subsequently, the diagnostic process might be carried out jointly.)

A second purpose of the preliminary self-diagnosis and discussion is to define an immediate action that might be taken to improve conditions in the community. This action ought to address a need felt by all the community (or by the neediest members), should involve some sort of institutional input that is feasible to supply quickly, and should not require feasibility or other studies before going ahead. This action should be carried out simultaneously with the continuing process of diagnosis leading to a longer-term plan. The reaction of the institution to this identified need will test the credibility, effectiveness and commitment of the institution.

With the results of the auto-diagnosis in hand, with information from secondary sources, and with growing acquaintance of the community, the institutional agent should prepare her own diagnosis. This diagnosis, like the previous one, should be presented for discussion in community meetings.

The next step involves setting objectives and priorities. From her diagnosis and the community comments, the agent should establish a list of objectives and a set of priorities for action based on a technical evaluation of the objectives. Meanwhile, the community produces its own set of objectives and priorities, based on its perception of community needs. These two sets of priorities can then be compared. If the priorities coincide, then project planning can begin; an area of mutual interest will have been identified. If they do not, the agent should explain her point of view, but be willing to postpone actions in those areas that the community does not accept.

Once the objectives and priorities have been agreed upon, the institutional agent begins the process of seeking resources within her own organization and within other public and private organizations that work within the particular areas chosen. The agent would then inform the community of the options for action that seem most appropriate from the institutional side. Meanwhile, the community begins a process of identifying the community resources that can be marshalled for the proposed actions. (In this step, community members may visit other communities in similar conditions in which similar actions have been carried out successfully.)

From this diagnosis and dialogue comes a plan for action that combines resources. As implementation occurs, the agent and community members should monitor progress and work together to overcome obstacles. Community meetings, with participation of the institutional agent, may be held to evaluate accomplishments and in light of the evaluation adjust objectives and strategies or move on to other actions.

Patience, optimism, and humility

Moving towards meaningful community participation and towards partnership in development is not an easy task. Again, the problem is not the lack of examples or of methodologies. Rather, the main problem lies in the political, institutional, and attitudinal conditions that frame programming in each particular setting. Hierarchical structures, organizational inertia, lack of empathy, established vested interests, etc. will not change quickly. But change can be helped along through programmes that strengthen organization and empower communities. And it is well to be prepared for the often unpredictable moments when change does occur, providing increased possibilities for partnership in development. To the task, one must bring patience, optimism and a degree of humility.

Meanwhile, those who would accept the challenge of pursuing improved child development through projects conceived within a framework of community participation would do well to follow the advice contained in a poem (reported in Brower and Castillo 1990, p. 11) attributed to Lao Tse in 700 BC:

> Go with the people. Live with them.
> Learn from them. Love them.
> Start with what they know.
> Build with what they have.
> But of the best leaders
> When the job is done, the task accomplished
> The people will all say,
> We have done this ourselves.

Or, if one prefers, another version (quoted in Korten 1983) of the poem would also serve, attributed to James Y.C. Yen, founder of the Rural Reconstruction Movement in China in the 1920s:

> Go with the people
> Live among the people
> Learn from the people
> Plan with the people

Work with the people
Start with what the people know
Build on what the people have
Teach by showing; learn by doing
Not a showcase but a pattern
Not odds and ends but a system
Not piecemeal but integrated approach
Not to conform but to transform
Not relief but release.

REFERENCES

Amar Amar, J.J. *Los Hogares Comunales del Niño.* Barranquilla, Colómbia: Ediciones Uninorte, 1986.

Atkin, L., T. Superveille, R. Sawyer and P. Cantón. *Paso a Paso.* México: Editorial Pax, México, Julio de 1987, Tercera Parte, pp. 382–457.

Bosnjak, V. 'Planeación y acción a nivel local con participación comunitaria', en *Proyectos locales e indicadores sociales: Implicaciones para la planificación regional y nacional.* Bogotá, Departmento Nacional de Planeación, en colaboración con UNICEF y Fundación Ford, 1982.

Bosnjak, V. *From the Margins to the Mainstream.* Manuscript in preparation, 1990.

Brower, J. and J. Castillo. 'Trabajando con Promotores', document prepared for a technical workshop in collaboration with the Centro de Investigaciones para la Infancia y la Familia (CENDIF) in Caracas, Venezuela, February 12–14, 1990. The Hague, Bernard van Leer Foundation, 1990.

Cariola, P. and A. Rojas. 'Experiencias de Educación Popular y Reflexiones para su Masificación', in UNICEF, *del Macetero al Potrero (o de lo micro a lo macro). El Aporte de la Sociedad Civil a las Políticas Sociales.* Santiago, Chile, 1986.

CINDE (International Center for Education and Human Development). 'Highlights of an Evaluation of Project Promesa', Fort Lauderdale, Florida: CINDE-USA, February, 1990. Rough draft.

Cochran, M. 'The Parental Empowerment Process: Building on Family Strengths', in John Harris (ed.) *Child Psychology: Putting Research into Practice.* London: Croom Helm, 1985.

'Community Participation: Now You See It, Now You Don't', *UNICEF News,* Issue 124 (1986). Entire issue.

De Schutter, A. *Investigación participativa: Una Opción Metodológica para la Educación de Adultos.* Pátzcuaro, México: CREFAL, 1986.

Dichter, T. 'The Changing World of Northern NGOS: Problems, Paradoxes, and Possibilities', in John Lewis (ed.) *Strengthening the Poor: What Have We Learned?* Oxford, England: Transaction Books, published for the Overseas Development Council, 1988, pp. 177–88.

Freire, P. *Pedagogy of the Oppressed.* New York: Seabury Press, 1970.

Gajardo, M. (ed.) *Teoría y Práctica de la Educación Popular.* Ottawa: the International Development Research Centre, 1983.

Hall, B., A. Gillette and R. Tandon (eds) *Creating Knowledge: A Monopoly?* New Delhi: Society for Participatory Research in Asia, 1982.

Hildebrand, P.F. 'Motivating Small Farmers to Accept Change', paper presented at the Conference on Integrated Crop and Animal Production to Optimize Resource Utilization on Small Farms in Developing Countries, the Rockefeller

Foundation Conference Center, Bellagio, Italy, October 18–23, 1978. Instituto de Ciencia y Tecnología Agricola, Guatemala, October 1978.

Kavanaugh, J. *Journey of Trust: the Participatory Design of a Citizens' Group for Social Empowerment.* Unpublished PhD. dissertation, Saybrook Institute, San Francisco, January 1990.

Kent, G. 'Empowerment for Children's Survival', Honolulu, Department of Political Science, University of Hawaii, 1987. Mimeo. Draft.

Korten, D. 'Community Organization and Rural Development. A Learning Process Approach', the Ford Foundation and the Asian Institute of Management, Makati, Metro Manila, The Philippines, April 1980.

Korten, D. 'Social Development. Putting People First', in D. Korten and F. Alonso, *Bureaucracy and the Poor. Closing the Gap.* West Hartford, Conn: Kumarian Press. Published for the Asian Institute of Management, Manila, 1983.

Latapí, P. 'Participatory Research: A New Research Paradigm?' *The Alberta Journal of Educational Research,* Vol. XXXIV, No. 3 (September 1988), pp. 310–19.

Lewis, J. (ed.). *Strengthening the Poor; What Have We Learned?* Washington DC: Overseas Development Council, 1988.

Manoff, R. *Social Marketing: New Imperative for Public Health.* New York: Praeger, 1985.

Njenga, A.W. 'The Pre-school Education and Care Programme: A Kenyan Experience', a paper prepared for the UNICEF Global Seminar on Early Childhood Development, Florence, International Child Development Centre, June 12–30, 1989. Nairobi, Kenya Institute of Education, June 1989. Mimeo.

Otaala, B. 'Alternative Approaches to Daycare in Africa: Integration of Health and Early Childhood', a paper presented to UNESCO meeting, Paris, September 4–8, 1989, as reported in the Bernard van Leer Foundation, 'The Challenge. Early Childhood Care and Education: an agenda for action', The Hague: Bernard van Leer Foundation, February 1990.

Pantin, G. *A Mole Cricket Called SERVOL.* Ypsilanti, Michigan: High/Scope Press, 1983. A study prepared for the Bernard van Leer Foundation.

Richards, H. *Evaluating Cultural Action.* London: The Macmillan Press, 1985.

Rivera, J. 'Comunicación Educativa para el Desarrollo Infantil: Conceptos y Estrategias', a document prepared for UNICEF, Regional Office for Latin America, Bogotá, August 1987. Mimeo.

Sameroff, A.J. and M.J. Chandler. 'Reproductive Risk and the Continuum of Caretaking Casualty', in F.D. Horowitz *et al.* (eds) *Review of Child Development Research, Vol. 4.* Chicago: University of Chicago Press, 1975.

Sharma, A. 'Community Participation in ICDS', *Yojana,* Vol. 31, No. 6 (April 1–15, 1987), pp. 12–16.

Whitmore, E. and P. Kerans. 'Participation, Empowerment and Welfare', *Canadian Review of Social Policy,* No. 22 (November 1988), pp. 51–60.

Wood, A.W. 'Community Mobilization', address to the Hong Kong Conference on 'Childhood in the 21st Century', July 31–August 4, 1989. The Hague, Bernard van Leer Foundation, August, 1989.

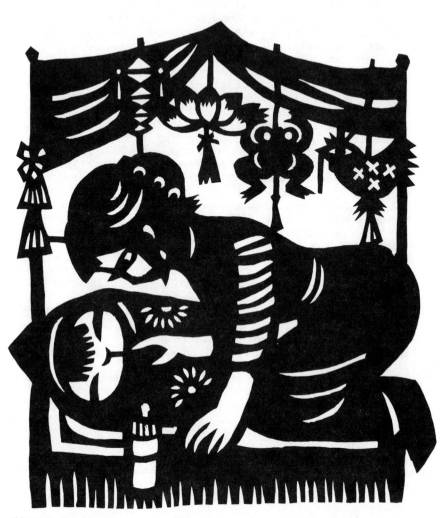

'Mother's love'
A paper cut designed by Shen Peinong for the All-China
Women's Federation

Chapter 13

Understanding cultural differences in childrearing practices and beliefs

The newborn are treated as celestial creatures entering a more humdrum existence and, at the moment of birth, are addressed with high sounding honorific phrases reserved for gods, the souls of ancestors, princes and people of a higher caste.

(Bali, Indonesia: Mead 1955)

Newborn infants are usually wrapped and placed in a basket lined with a blanket, close to the mother for a few days. Parents, relatives and neighbors usually do not openly express their enjoyment or admiration of the baby for fear that the spirits might take the baby away. Relatives usually say aloud, 'What an ugly baby he is,' in order to deceive the spirit.

(Northeast Thailand: Kotchabhakdi 1987)

Within the family, the neighbourhood or the village, all older persons were responsible for caring for the child. This is the basis, among Africans not yet cut off from their roots, of the typical strength of group feeling.

(Ki-Zerbo 1990)

Selective neglect accompanied by maternal detachment is both widespread among the poorer populations of Ladeiras but 'invisible' – generally unrecognized by those outside shantytown culture, even by professionals such as clinic doctors and teachers who come into frequent contact with severely neglected babies and young children. *Within* the shantytown, child death *a mingua* (accompanied by maternal indifference and neglect) is understood as an appropriate maternal response to a deficiency in the child. Part of learning how to mother in Alto includes learning when to 'let go'.

(Northeast Brazil: Scheper-Hughes 1985)

The number of contrasting quotations illustrating the immense variations in actual childrearing practices and beliefs could be multiplied easily, drawing on a vast and growing cross-cultural literature from anthropology, sociology and psychology. Indeed, the fact that there are major and minor cultural differences in childrearing practices will be so obvious to most people that it may not seem necessary to devote a chapter to the theme.

But the seemingly obvious does not always provide a guide to action. Programmes of child care and development in the Third World, as often as not, are designed without much thought to cultural diversities. Moreover, ideas about specific practices to be promoted frequently come from individuals who are not part of the culture or group that the programme is intended to serve. The ecological, economic, social and political conditions for urban industrial middle-class individuals who shape policy and programming differ dramatically from those of the low-income dwellers of shanty towns or from those in the impoverished agrarian settings that continue to predominate throughout most of the Third World. Accordingly, the programme goals set, and the practices suggested, may be very different from the childrearing goals set and practices carried out in daily life. Indeed, most developmental activity is aimed at influencing people to adopt institutions and technologies alien to their own culture (Myrdal 1968).

As noted in the previous chapter, programme planning and design tends also to reflect a 'scientific' way of approaching problems, based on knowledge assumed to be universally applicable. This knowledge, usually derived from a Western or northern conceptual base (see, for example, Maccoby 1980), takes precedence over experiential knowledge derived from the particular contexts in which the programmes are to function. In most programming, it is assumed that when a middle-class, scientific approach conflicts with a folkway, the folkway must be harmful and should be corrected. This judgement is made without examining how 'harm' is defined within the particular contexts for which programmes are to be recommended. It is made without an attempt to understand why such seemingly harmful practices continue. Focusing on what are considered to be harmful practices leads to a compensatory approach and to disregard for helpful local practices. In that process important knowledge and local resources that could and should be mobilized to improve development are left aside.

Contrasting with the compensatory and limited approach described above is one that respects and incorporates local wisdom by beginning with what people actually believe and practise, without judging in advance whether these beliefs and practices are harmful or helpful. We take this contrasting position for several reasons:

- Beginning where people are in their thinking and practice is crucial to developing real dialogue, mutual learning and involvement of people in programmes – as discussed in the previous chapter.
- The standards for judgement of 'helpful' and 'harmful' will vary according to the particular goals set by a society or group as they, in

turn, are conditioned by physical conditions, social organization, and beliefs. In one culture an aggressive child may be considered bad; in another, good. In one culture, low birthweight is considered to be harmful; in many cultures, it is sought as appropriate. In many cultures, allowing the death of a child is viewed as an absolute wrong whereas, in some, an individual child may be allowed to die in particular circumstances because survival of the mother or family or group is at stake. The ability of an infant to lift its head or turn over or crawl may be valued in some cultures and even used as a measure of progress, but is not valued or encouraged in others.

- Prejudging practices means prejudging people. Approaching people with the idea that their practices are wrong or immoral signals an unjustified air of superiority. When that is backed also by power, the result can go beyond imposition of ideas to creating cultural confusion and doubt, destroying vital cultural and psychological bases for living that have, for good reason, evolved over centuries.
- Traditional wisdom, even though appearing to be in conflict with 'science', may provide as good, or better, ways of meeting a particular need.

THE ROLE OF TRADITIONAL WISDOM

The value assigned above, and in previous chapters, to traditional wisdom should be put in perspective. There is always a danger of taking too romantic a view, disregarding the hardships and problems that frame existing practices, or accepting practices that prejudice a child's survival and development and that came into being under circumstances that no longer exist, making them no longer functional. There is a danger, too, in assuming that a child will always live in only one culture when most children live in two or more cultures at the same time (e.g. the dominant culture represented by a school and the popular culture of the rural home). And many children will migrate from a predominantly rural to a predominantly urban culture.

By stressing the importance of traditional wisdom, we do not mean to promote a romantic and narrow viewpoint. Our purpose is, rather, to seek for the field of child development the same kind of understanding and appreciation of the value of traditional wisdom that has been growing over the last several decades in many fields. For instance:

In the field of crop production and the management of the soil, the knowledge and experience of local farmers are unrivaled and no alternative system of food crop production has been found that is as well adjusted to the prevailing environmental conditions as that which has been practiced by the people.

(Faniran and Areola 1976, p. 403)

... traditional technologies rest on firmer local foundations than the Western technologies brought in as replacements. Whether in agriculture, crafts, food, clothing, shelter, health or transport, mounting evidence suggests that traditional technologies were optimal solutions within their societies. Their advantages included environmental soundness; very low capital costs; high labour-intensiveness; small production scales oriented towards supplying fundamental needs and use of local materials and skills.

(Brokensha, Warren and Warner, 1980)

These advantages, cited for traditional technologies within agriculture, are also applicable when thinking about early childhood care and development practices and programmes and principles.

Nor is our intent to set traditional against modern systems of care. It is, rather, to seek the good and useful in each (Negussie 1980). In medicine, for instance, it is recognized increasingly that:

The value of knowing more about traditional or folk medical systems is obvious in the potential application of knowledge derived from it to the actual health care system. ... Knowledge of traditional medicine can serve to develop new models of clinical practice. [Meanwhile], the impregnation of scientific and popular knowledge results not only in the incorporation of folk in professional or scientific medicine, but also in increasing 'medicalisation' of popular and traditional therapeutic practices.

(Pedersen and Baruffati 1989, pp. 487, 494 and 495)

If this intertwining of folkways and new ways has value for health and medicine, it should have value as well for programmes directed to enhancing psychosocial development.

CHILDREARING PRACTICES

What and how?

Childrearing practices are the generally accepted activities that respond to needs for survival and development of children in their early months and years in a way that assures the survival and maintenance (and sometimes development) of the group or culture as well as the child. For children to survive, grow and develop, they need to be nourished, to avoid disease and accident, to be nurtured, and to learn the ways of the world in order to adapt to and transform it. At this general level, one can specify practices, common to all societies, such as: feeding, sleeping, handling and carrying, bathing, preventing and attending to sickness, protecting from harm, nurturing, socializing and teaching skills.

At a more specific level, *what* is done merges with *how* it is done to define and distinguish practices that vary widely from place to place. For instance, the practice of breastfeeding contrasts with the practice of bottle-feeding. Feeding on demand contrasts with scheduled feeding. The practice of constant carrying differs dramatically from the practice of placing a child in a crib, cradle, hammock or playpen for prolonged periods. Or the practice of talking to a child about what should be done contrasts with an emphasis on non-verbal forms of communication in the socialization process.

Although it is useful to sort out particular practices, both generally and specifically, it may be more important to recognize that practices tend to group together, influencing each other – they come in clusters. These clusters are not arbitrary. They result from the fact that practices evolve together within particular settings, because a child's needs are interrelated, and because the practical choices made to satisfy one need help to determine what it is possible to do to satisfy another. For instance, the choice of breastfeeding on demand requires a kind of physical proximity to the mother at all times that scheduled bottle-feeding does not. That requirement affects carrying and sleeping practices. The physical closeness of mother to child also permits, or reinforces, a kind of nurturing that is different from that employed when there is greater physical separation.

Who cares for the child?

A discussion of childrearing practices must be concerned not only with *what* is done and *how*, but also with *who* is carrying out the practices. The range of practices that can be considered in a particular setting is influenced by who is available to carry them out. The quality of the practices and their outcomes will also be affected.

As pointed out in Chapter 11 when discussing child-care myths in relation to women's work, only rarely is the mother the only caregiver for a child, although that may be the case for the first few months of life. At one extreme, in Andean Peru, a child may still be considered to be part of the mother until it is baptized – usually during the first weeks after birth; during that period, the mother provides exclusive care. Even later, until weaning, others may only be allowed to see or talk to the baby for brief periods and then, not effusively (Ortiz and Souffez 1989). In most societies, however, multiple caregiving occurs, from very early on. In-laws, godparents, grandparents, siblings, other family and community members, and hired caregivers each play more, or less, important roles alongside the mother, depending on customs, the social organization, and the particular family composition and circumstances.

When are practices carried out?

Understanding the cultural differences in childrearing practices and beliefs requires understanding why practices occur when they do. The timing of certain practices – their initiation and duration – will be influenced by the changing developmental needs of the child, by beliefs that are embodied in rituals involving the child, and by objective conditions.

Sometimes, practices correspond to what is considered to be appropriate timing for optimal development, seen from a scientific point of view; sometimes they do not. For instance, although it is common to begin supplementary feeding at the age of four months or thereabouts, there are some cultures in which supplementation is delayed even though research tells us that delay is detrimental to the survival, growth and development of the infant (e.g. Chávez and Martínez 1982). Or, in many cultures, toilet training begins early, even though research suggests that it is not until about 15 months of age that a child is sufficiently mature physically for self-regulation to occur. Or, children are often urged to write their ABC well before the needed fine motor skills have developed and well before other pre-literacy concepts have been attained that give meaning to the exercise.

Another reason for attention to timing is that practices are sometimes related to, or keyed by, particular moments in the life of a child. These moments may be related to development of the child (e.g. the third trimester of pregnancy is a crucial period; a child's first step brings attention) and/or regulated by custom and ritual. In the Peruvian case cited above, a change in practice is linked to the ritual of baptism. Other rituals such as naming or the first haircut or circumcision will bring with them changes in practice as well. These rituals provide particularly important times when attention is focused on the child.

Not incidentally, these moments are times when parents and others involved are highly motivated to learn about what will be good for the child – within the constraints of the traditional cultural practices, and sometimes even beyond, if there is clear evidence that a change in practices will bring good results. These, together with the period of pregnancy, and the period immediately following birth, constitute what are sometimes referred to as 'touchpoints' (Brazleton 1982). Touchpoints, which may differ from place to place, are times when sensitive and sound information about child-rearing practices not only can (if applied) make a significant developmental difference, but also is more likely than at other times to be listened to and discussed and perhaps even incorporated into the childrearing repertoire.

WHY ARE PRACTICES AS THEY ARE?

To try to provide definitive answers to this question would, of course, be presumptuous. But looking at practices within a general framework that helps to understand the reasons for cultural variation is useful. We shall offer both a micro-level view that helps to explain differences at the level of individual families and caregivers and children, and a macro-level view that helps to determine, but can never fully explain, what happens in a particular setting.

The 'developmental niche'

In Chapter 4 (p. 69), the concept of a developmental niche[1] was presented in which the 1) childrearing customs, or practices, that affect development of a particular child, were depicted as directly, and reciprocally, related to 2) the physical and social conditions in which a child is born and develops, and 3) the beliefs and attitudes of the child's caregivers (Super and Harkness 1987). The immediate environment in which the child develops is set within the broader environments of the community and culture. Each part of the child's particular niche – the beliefs of the child's immediate caregivers, or the physical conditions of the home and immediate surroundings, for instance – relate, independently, to conditions in the larger environment.

This micro-level view of child development and childrearing, and its projection outward to more general physical, social and cultural conditions is useful in two ways. First, it helps to understand why there will be both regularities and differences among families in the same location. Both theory and observation would lead us to think that in relatively stable families and communities and cultures (where there has been little change in the physical conditions or social organization or beliefs over the years) childrearing practices will have accommodated to these conditions and beliefs. A homeostatic mechanism will have been at work to ensure survival – of children, families, and larger groupings. Ways of socializing children to their situation and of providing them with the skills they need to live will have evolved in accordance with the particular needs. That is, recognized practices will have been applied almost without thinking. And yet, differences in specific circumstances and in the psychology of the caregiver will lead to variations in practices.

A second way in which the model is useful is as a starting point for asking questions about what happens to childrearing practices as changes occur in physical or social conditions or in beliefs. That includes both circumstances in which an outsider arrives with a new set of practices that he or she wishes to see applied in a setting where accommodation has occurred, and circumstances in which contexts are changing rapidly (or have changed drastically) – when the harmony that existed among conditions, beliefs and practices in a particular place has been upset, or when people migrate from one context to another. It is here that the real problems associated with childrearing seem to arise and where there is the most need for action. We will return to this point after discussing briefly differences in physical and social settings, and in customs and beliefs affecting childrearing.

Physical settings

It should not be necessary to dwell on the extraordinary differences throughout the world in the climate and topography, flora and fauna, soils and subsoils, and other physical features conditioning the economic and social life of peoples. The physical setting for childrearing faced by an Eskimo family in Northern Canada contrasts dramatically with the context provided for a baby born to a family in the heart of Beijing, China, or a nomadic family in the desert of Somalia, or fishermen on the west coast of India, or a family in a tropical rain forest in Nigeria, or Peruvian or Nepalese mountain families, or.... The variation in contexts within a particular country may be equally dramatic.

It is obvious that specific childrearing practices and technologies used must be adapted to these varied settings, even though the needs they are designed to meet and the ends they serve may be similar across them. For instance, both an Eskimo (Canada) mother and a Yoruba (Nigeria) mother may carry their babies and breastfeed on demand. But for the Eskimo mother to do so requires wearing a heavy, warm, very large and loose garment that allows the baby to be carried on her back and swung around, inside the garment, at the time of feeding. A hood on the garment channels air to the baby while it is on the mother's back at the same time that it helps to keep the mother and baby warm. The Yoruba mother, faced with a tropical climate, needs only to sling the baby on her back, open to the elements. In both cases, the baby is in direct touch with the mother. In the Eskimo case, however, the baby cannot benefit from the sight of other people and of the world in general while being carried. Other means are required for providing that kind of stimulation and social interaction.

In a review of literature on this subject, John Whiting shows that '... the manner in which infants are cared for during their waking and sleeping hours is to a considerable extent constrained by the physical environment, the temperature of the coldest month of the year being the most important factor'. He also concludes that there is not sufficient evidence to indicate whether or not these variations in methods of infant care have any enduring effects (Whiting 1981).

Settlement patterns and economic and social organization

A combination of natural conditions and the technology available to deal with those conditions leads to differences in settlement patterns and in economic and social organization. The conditions for childrearing in a nomadic society differ obviously from those in a settled society. And among those who are settled, conditions will differ drastically for those who live in dispersed and in concentrated settlements. Small concentrations in rural towns provide different conditions from large concentrations in major cities.

Accompanying these differences are variations in forms of economic livelihood, the division of labour, and social organization at the level of family, community, and larger society. These include such features as divisions by caste and class, the degree of solidarity and hierarchy, family size and composition, the definition of roles for men and women, the form of governance, etc. They include extended, polygamous, nuclear, and single-parent families. It is not our purpose to try to analyse these differences cross-culturally (see, for example, Stephens 1963; Kağitçibaşi 1990), or even to try to create a full listing of relevant social differences. But to appreciate fully existing childrearing practices and to understand why they have come to be, these differences must be taken into account. Clearly, for instance, extended and polygamous families in which the kinship groupings are large, patterned and complicated will provide a different context for childrearing than either a nuclear or a single-parent family where there is isolation from other kin. When organization for work involves children as well as adults, from an early age, the context for childrearing will be different from one in which 'a child's main work is play'.

Beliefs, values, and childrearing goals

Cultures are often guided, and distinguished by, a specific set of beliefs about what happens in this world and in an unknown afterlife. The beliefs may arise from practical experiences in the particular conditions in which people live (a belief in low birthweight) or may represent attempts to deal with the unknown (a belief in the evil eye). It is possible to distinguish some rather basic differences among peoples in beliefs.

In many cultures, a newborn is considered to be a gift from god. The newborn remains in a pure state for some period. If the child dies during that early period, it returns to the spirit world, having avoided the trials and tribulations of a temporary stay on earth. This belief may have grown up around the high level of infant mortality that still exists in many places, helping to explain and accept a young child's death.

There is also in any culture a set of beliefs about how children develop. In some, it is believed necessary to teach a child to sit and walk (Super and Harkness 1986); in others it is not. In some cultures a child is believed to be fragile, in others hardy, and so forth.

Beliefs merge with values in helping to give meaning to practices by defining the kind of child (and adult) a particular society seeks to produce in the socialization process. Some cultures want children to be obedient, others foster a questioning child. Some tolerate aggressiveness; others do not. Some strengthen individualism; others a collective orientation and strong social responsibility. A more complete work dealing with child-rearing would look at each of these differences in detail, analysing the reasons for the growth of one or another set of beliefs and values in a particular society.

For example, the following set of guiding cultural values was identified in a recent study of Thai ways of childrearing (Sumon Amornvivat *et al.* 1989):

Obedience and respect for seniority	Honesty
Diligence and responsibility	Gratitude
Being economical	Self-reliance
Generosity	

It does not seem useful to label particular beliefs and values as traditional or modern. It may be useful to distinguish people in terms of whether or not they believe, for instance, in the ability to influence life's course through one's own actions. This belief, or attitude, will help to explain some practices and will affect the ability or willingness to consider changing practices.

Our purpose here is simply to call attention to and plead for greater understanding of these differences as policies and programmes are formulated.

CONTRASTING PATTERNS OF CHILDREARING

Against this general background, and in somewhat of a caricature, Table 13.1 sets out two patterns, or clusters, of childrearing practices. The practices in the first cluster approximate to what we would expect to find in a middle-class American or European home, or perhaps in an urban middle-class home in parts of the Third World. This cluster is influenced by an industrialized, technological view of the world and incorporates the results of science into childrearing. The practices of the second cluster might be found in a socially stable, but economically impoverished area in any of several parts of the Third World and are rooted in traditional wisdom.

The main point in presenting these two clusters is to illustrate the fact that different settings and value systems can be expected to produce different practices and that these practices tend to group together. Further, we shall try to show that neither set of practices should automatically be judged as superior to the other. Finally, discussion of the clusters helps to highlight how the choice of one practice (food taboos leading to a low birthweight baby) has implications for other practices to follow.

Table 13.1 A rough comparison of two clusters of selected childrearing practices

Period	Cluster 1	Cluster 2
Prenatal	Gain weight in order to have a large baby	Adhere to food taboos in order to have a small baby
Birth	Primary concern for child	Primary concern for mother
	Birth in hospital	Birth at home or in a special place
	Doctor attending	Traditional birth attendant
Perinatal	Baby given immediately to mother to hold	Delay in mother's contact with newborn
	Breastfeed within hours (colostrum given)	Wait 2/3 days to breastfeed (no colostrum given)
	Name given at birth	Naming delayed
Infant	Scheduled feeding Bottle-feeding Early weaning	On-demand feeding Breastfeeding Late weaning
	Separate sleeping	Sleep with mother
	Use crib/playpen	Hold/carry
	Walking not encouraged	Walking encouraged
	Encourage talking	Little encouragement to talk
	Light bathing	Vigorous bathing, massage
	Begin toilet training late	Begin toilet training earlier
	Emphasis on: independence individual	Emphasis on: dependence group

Prenatal and birthing practices

The practice of gaining weight in order to have a large baby contrasts with adhering to food taboos in order to have a small baby. When the results of these two practices are compared, it is clear that the latter practice often leads to a low birthweight (LBW) baby who tends also to be low in level of activity and attentiveness and who may be relatively irritable (Brazleton 1982). These characteristics are related to infant mortality and favour delayed or debilitated development. And yet, one of the more consistent findings from anthropological studies carried out in different parts of Africa, Asia and Latin America is the presence of food taboos during pregnancy (Stephens 1963). Thus, the poor nutritional status of the mother associated with LBW often results from something more than a lack of food (Negussie 1988). Why does this seemingly detrimental practice exist and continue?

One explanation suggests that the practices reflect a higher value given to survival of the species (represented in the survival of a fertile woman) than to the survival of a particular child. Saving the woman allows another child to be conceived. As the Ghanaian proverb goes, 'It is better to save the pot than to break it in attempting to save the water it contains' (quoted in Timyan 1988, p. 26). The risk to many women of having a large baby is seen, in turn, as a result of adaptations in the size and stature of women, made over the centuries in the face of food scarcities. Generations of small women reproduce themselves. Small size makes it difficult to have large babies. Difficulties may also be caused if rickets is prevalent, as was once the case over a wide area. Rickets affects the pelvic growth of young girls during the growth spurt and also makes delivery of a large baby more difficult (Negussie 1988).

Thus, while modern medicine defines low birthweight as 'at risk', some traditional societies and folk wisdom define high birthweight as 'at risk' because it increases the chances of death or of major problems for the mother (and child) at birth. According to this line of reasoning, food taboos favouring LBW have a logical basis. And, because the general stature of a population changes only slowly, it may not be appropriate in all cases to recommend larger babies. Further, in cases where increased stature and size and the elimination of rickets has occurred but food taboos and LBW continue, it is unlikely that a change in practice will occur as a result of simply providing information to women about the virtues of larger babies or about changes they should make in their eating habits during pregnancy. The traditional belief and practice will need to be confronted.

In Table 13.1, we have also contrasted the location of birth and attendance by a medical doctor rather than by a traditional birth attendant (TBA). There has been considerable emphasis placed in some countries on increasing the percentage of live births by ensuring they occur in the controlled and presumably hygienic confines of a hospital, and on increasing delivery by a qualified medical person. These practices are sometimes used as indicators of social development. However, some people would argue that the practice of isolating a woman in the antiseptic but often hostile conditions of a hospital is a barbaric custom. While recognizing the need for hygiene, this argument focuses on the need for people to be supported socially in times of stress, including birth. It also points out that a pregnant woman should not be treated as if she were sick or as a patient. Again we see the importance of incorporating a psychological and social dimension into medicine in relation to survival and development.

Perhaps ironically, there is a Western revival in the practices of giving birth at home and of admitting family members to hospitals during birth and immediately afterwards. These practices represent a recognition of the value of being supported by the family during the birthing process. But the revival incorporates hygienic practices, and complications can be handled relatively easily because a health support system is nearby. We are again faced with a question of how to rescue the positive elements of traditional wisdom while incorporating new knowledge and practices.

In this process, the traditional birth attendant is often a key person. Although much is made of 'unscientific' practices followed by some TBAs, evidence is accumulating that many TBA practices are at least as sound as those of modern medicine. In addition, the TBA typically provides a kind of social support (such as helping a woman to clean house or do other chores just before and after birth) that a medical doctor does not provide. Increasing recognition of the importance of TBAs has led to programmes providing training so that she incorporates modern medical practices into her repertoire. Similar efforts might be made to value and extend the psychosocial support she gives as well as to reinforce and improve the perinatal assistance she provides.[2]

Differences in practices during pregnancy affecting the condition of a child at birth, and differences in location and in who attends the birth are closely related to what happens immediately following the birth, in the perinatal period, to which we now turn.

Perinatal practices

Based on research on attachment that points to the importance of the earliest possible bonding between mother and child, a practice has developed in the Western hospital culture of uniting the mother and the baby as soon as the birthing process has been completed. The need for this practice has been explained by some as associated with the degree of anxiety and isolation of the mother in a hospital, creating a greater need for the immediate bonding, as compared with a situation where a woman is at home and with relatives who can attend to the baby. Current research suggests the importance of developing a strong affectionate bond in early life, without which experience it is difficult to develop a relationship of love later in life. But there is still controversy about how and to whom bonding should occur. Before making new suggestions about how that should occur, it is important to see how, in specific cultures, it does occur and under what circumstances it does not.

Another perinatal practice that differs markedly between the two clusters set out in Figure 13.1 is the practice of giving, or not giving, colostrum to the newborn. Modern medicine places a high value on colostrum, but the practice of discarding colostrum is so common throughout the world, one has the feeling that a logical reason exists for the popular practice. We have not discovered such an explanation in our brief look at the literature.

A note on attitudes towards infant mortality and survival   One result of the past and present pressure for the species to survive is to create attitudes towards the death of a young child that are not comprehensible to middle-class parents in Europe or North America or in many urban settings in the Third World. Even while babies are loved and highly valued and their death causes grief, it is possible for attitudes towards death to differ widely across cultures. Accepting death as part of the natural course of events may appear inhumane or immoral or insensitive to someone in Europe or the United States where child deaths are (now) rare, whereas it is a psychological and social necessity in conditions in which child death has been a longstanding and common occurrence.

In such circumstances, a variety of mechanisms seem to appear that help to place death in perspective. In many cultures, the death of a child is sometimes made easier by a religious belief that a child is still pure and even other-worldly in its first months or years. Death returns the child to the supernatural world without its having to live through the trials and tribulations of this world. Delaying the direct and intimate contact between child and mother is another buffering device. Delaying naming is another.

Even more difficult to understand for many middle-class urban families are those cases in which death occurs in conjunction with parental detachment or neglect, amounting to infanticide. This is most likely to occur in cases where children are born with problems or with weak constitutions in conditions where the family simply cannot provide the care needed to weaker as well as stronger children. Or, it may be directed to increasing the chances of survival of boys who are seen as a more valuable resource than girls.

These occurrences are more widespread than one would like to think, are often invisible, and are not restricted to either rural or urban areas. The extract at the outset of this chapter citing 'selective neglect', and coming from a Brazilian study of an urban *barrio* in north-east Brazil, gives one example of the acceptance of child deaths related to neglect (Scheper-Hughes 1985). In another study, in a particular area of Ecuador, it was found that girls were weaned on the average at 8 months whereas boys were weaned at 16, and the socially accepted reason was that if girls were breastfed longer they would become too aggressive. Examples of some form or other of what might be termed infanticide can be multiplied (Timyan 1988).

The reason for describing differences that may appear in the attitude towards death across cultures is not to provide an excuse for infanticide, consciously or unconsciously carried out, but simply to alert those who would solve the problem with technology that economic, social and cultural dimensions of the problem must also be dealt with.

Practices in infancy

In spite of the large number of LBW babies throughout the Third World, most children manage to arrive with their amazing capacities in functioning order. That is in part because during pregnancy, children have the first call on nourishment and it is only in extreme cases that development is permanently affected. Most LBW babies who are born in difficult circumstances can, and often do, not only survive, but catch up quickly in weight and in their activity and alertness (Brazleton 1973; Landers 1990). Many are even precocious in their early motor development, as compared with more privileged peers. Both biology and culturally concocted practices to support the biological base are at work here.

Given the historical and ecological conditions that help to explain LBW babies, and taking the position that cultures, to survive and grow, will seek ways of trying to overcome the possible complications that LBW can bring, it should not be surprising to find a set of post-natal practices that seem to be designed to help an LBW baby recover quickly, both in terms of its weight and its activity levels. Contributing to the recovery are such practices as:

- breastfeeding on demand (which increases weight, helps to cut irritability, and builds security in an infant);
- constant contact or touch which, as we have seen, facilitates growth, supporting breastfeeding on demand and helping to build security (carrying, holding, sleeping with the baby);
- stimulation, through massage and exercising;
- high levels of interaction with many people providing visual and auditory stimulation as well as early socialization.

This cluster of practices, presented in the second column of Table 13.1, fits together closely. Sleeping together and various carrying practices facilitate feeding on demand. Stimulation and interaction with various people increases activity and alertness which helps a child express its demands for food. These practices help to create an attachment to the mother which helps develop security in the child. Taken together, this set of practices helps both survival and development of infants.

In part, the higher average birthweight of European or American babies permits a very different cluster of practices, as set out in the first column of Table 13.1. But in part, the different practices reflect differences in settings and values from those that underpin cluster two. The cluster one child-rearing practices, even in infancy, are more consistent with a rapidly changing, rapidly paced urban industrial environment.

Against this background, it is instructive to reflect on what the results might be in a traditional rural culture, where poverty and hardship are still dominant and where the pace of change is still slow, of introducing such practices as:

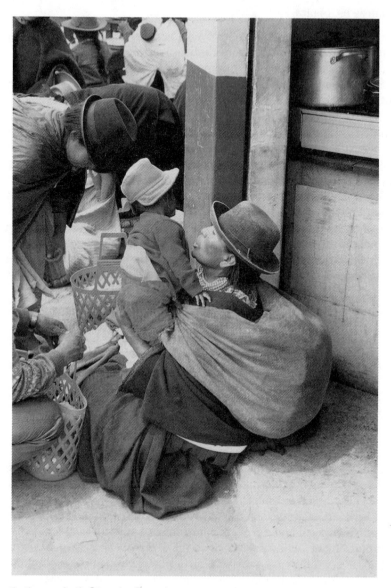

'In the market', Otavalo, Ecuador

- a change in food intake during pregnancy so as to increase birthweight (would it increase both birthweight and maternal mortality?)
- bottle-feeding (would it decrease nurturing in addition to introducing the hygiene problems that are often mentioned?)
- schooling for siblings (would it remove a primary source of child care and negatively affect women's performance in their productive role?)
- putting babies in cribs (would this cut down mother–child interaction because it substitutes for carrying?)
- scheduled feeding (while freeing mothers for a different kind of work, would it reduce the speed of recuperation from low birthweight?)

CHILDREARING IN CONDITIONS OF CHANGE

Until now, our emphasis has been on valuing and adjusting practices in relatively unchanging conditions. The programmatic implication is that one should consider very carefully the potential effects of introducing changes in childrearing practices into such situations, looking first to support the positive practices that are functioning well to fulfil children's needs in context.

But what happens when contexts change radically, or when beliefs change? The growing interest and concern with childrearing practices and with parental education is itself a reflection of the accelerating pace of social change. No culture is immune to change. Cultures can adapt to and incorporate change over time because they contain within themselves some diversity in their social structures and in their norms and values (Negussie 1988). And, as pointed out, folkways are not necessarily in conflict with newer, scientific ways, facilitating acceptance.

For the most part, however, adaptation requires time. Accordingly, the most difficult problems of adjustment occur in the conditions of the most rapid social change. That is as true for childrearing as for the other social practices to which it is related. Accordingly, these are the circumstances in which the most attention to childrearing may be needed.

There are many possible sources of abrupt or rapid change. War and natural disasters bring change. Major projects such as dams or the building of a huge sewage system or the introduction of electricity can bring drastic changes in an environment in a short time, positively affecting physical conditions but throwing existing beliefs and practices out of harmony with the new conditions. Economic shifts can bring rapid social change as, for instance, when a shift occurs from subsistence farming to a cash crop economy, undercutting existing practices without necessarily providing good replacements (i.e. making it more difficult to combine tending the fields and child care).

Another avenue of change begins with changes in beliefs. The messages of missionaries brought drastic changes in one era. The magic of the advertising media is bringing another set of drastic changes in beliefs in this era. When these forms of persuasion are linked to new technologies or practices (e.g. bottle-feeding) as well as to the creation of new values, the result can be unsettling.

Drastic change can be brought about through the introduction of new social institutions such as a school or a health centre. The arrival of the school not only affects socialization goals, but affects childrearing patterns by siphoning off siblings into the school. The substitution of school time for child-caring time can create hardships for parents. But it can also deprive the children of part of their traditional training in social responsibility and for parenthood.

Or, change can come as people move into a new setting that is very different from the one in which they were reared. The obvious example is rural to urban migration. Imagine a woman from a traditional society who has migrated to a city where she lives in precarious conditions, where she does not have an extended family, where she is expected also to work outside the home, and where her children are expected to be in school. She cannot easily breastfeed on demand after an initial period. She cannot indulge in the same carrying patterns. She cannot call on other people as sources of stimulation and interaction in the same way that she could in the rural areas. She may not be prepared to recognize and deal with the conditions of the LBW child or the inactive, malnourished child that were dealt with so naturally within the rural or traditional context and she may wonder why a child does not improve as quickly as might have occurred there. She may not be willing to consider an arrangement in which she gives up her child to strangers for a portion of a day in a child-care centre. And yet she is not in a position to cope herself. This would be all the more so if she is a single parent. The love and will may be present, but the ability to express it or the knowledge about what to do may not be present.

If we understood better the implications for childrearing practices and beliefs of these various changes, we would be able to incorporate them into the determination of populations that are at risk when deciding where to focus programmes. In general, risk would seem to be present when practices or beliefs are no longer in line with the physical and social conditions that used to support them but no longer do.

Satisfying psychosocial needs in conditions of rapid change

A child growing up in a rural community in an environment where his nutritional situation is precarious, where annual measles epidemics take their toll, where malaria and other parasitic diseases may be endemic, is correctly defined as a child physically 'at risk'. But if he is part of a family and a community which function in an integrated manner and which are intact and well-adapted to local ecological and social contexts, that child is probably not 'at risk' in his psychosocial development. Yet middle-income children living in a clean, modern home in an urban center may be well-fed, immunized and free from disease without necessarily being in a situation that is positive for psychosocial development.

(Timyan 1989, p. 10)

As the extract above suggests, improving physical conditions does not necessarily immunize a child from problems of psychosocial development. And, as shown in Table 13.2, there are many potential advantages in environments that may be labelled 'disadvantaged' economically. When change is not rapid, most of these practices are at work to foster healthy

Table 13.2 Advantages/strengths of 'disadvantaged' environments

- Close physical and emotional ties in a stable atmosphere of love and security.
- Multiple caretaking, by adults and older siblings, provides an opportunity for the child to learn from several people, balancing their strengths and weaknesses, and broadening attachments and adjustment. It also provides social support for beleaguered parents.
- Opportunity for play with peers and children of other ages, with minimal interference from adults.
- Opportunities for learning through participation in work and ritual activity (as well as play and formal education) so that learning occurs:
  - in context;
  - in naturally occurring sequences, with increasing complexity and direct and repeated monitoring; and,
  - in conjunction with building confidence, competence, and social responsibility.
- Multiple teaching and learning styles, with emphasis on modelling, observation, imitation, and self-learning through trial and error (vs. dependence on didactic learning).
- An environment providing space and many local materials that can be used in learning.
- A rich cultural heritage of toys, games, songs, riddles, stories, poems that can provide a basis for learning.
- Training in language comprehension and sensitivity to non-verbal signs, accurate reporting, and memorization skills.
- Emphasis on social solidarity and harmony and on non-material values such as respect and helping others.
- Early indulgence and strong attachments promoting emotional security.
- Stimulation associated with such customs as massage, exercise, and carrying.

Note: Obviously, not all these advantages will be present in all 'disadvantaged' settings where poverty is present. Nor is the purpose to glorify these advantages, overlooking the stressful and often debilitating aspects of living in poverty, or in constant battle with a harsh environment.

psychosocial development of the young child. When change is rapid, they may not function.

Security   For instance, the secure physical and emotional ties that came so easily in a rural area, because of the physical proximity of the mother and because of the multiple caregiving and 'indulgent' treatment of the young child, can easily be threatened in an urban environment where:

- a baby may be born in a hospital where the mother is isolated;
- nuclear families or female-headed households predominate and a social network has not been formed to provide needed support;
- the mother has to go to work outside the home and cannot bring the child along (so early weaning occurs and breastfeeding on demand is not possible for long).

When such conditions prevail, it is relatively easy to imagine that bonding and attachment will be jeopardized. This is the condition described in the disturbing study carried out in Brazil by Scheper-Hughes (1985). The study shows that where a hostile environment makes survival doubtful, social mechanisms grow that can interfere with providing love to a child, preventing rather than supporting an early attachment so that it will be easier to 'let go'. In these cases, it will be important to look for ways in which the general living conditions can be improved. But it will also be important to seek caregiving conditions that help to provide the security to the child that comes with bonding and attachment and that is related to fulfilling other basic needs of the child. This may mean helping to strengthen social networks that support a mother in ways that kin and community did in rural areas. It may mean providing alternative care for some periods during the day. It may mean reinforcing rural customs that can still be carried out in the city and that help to build security (sleeping with the child and providing massage).

Interaction and stimulation   In an urban area, it may be necessary to develop practices that substitute for the carrying practices that helped to expose children in rural areas to a rich array of people and activities, providing stimulation and a chance for interaction. If, however, mothers and other caregivers in urban areas have not been socialized to think about the need for stimulation (because the popular culture had provided natural ways for that to occur), special attention will be required to help the infant get the needed interaction.

As the child moves beyond infancy, the kind of involvement with older siblings and in groups of young children that was possible in an open rural area may not be possible in the limited space, nuclear family, school-dominated urban culture. If, as seems to be the case, a great deal of the early learning of young children in rural areas comes through their interaction with siblings and as a result of moving about a lot, observing and playing and doing simple chores (Uribe 1984), and if these options are removed in an urban area, alternative practices must be found to fulfil the need for interaction and intellectual stimulation.

Specific attention may be required to the development of language which occurred in rural areas through constant exposure to the language of siblings or grandparents or villagers. In the city, the rich cultural heritage that helped provide a basis for learning may or may not be continued. Support for the parts of that heritage (e.g. songs, riddles, etc.) that can be continued can be provided. There are, of course, many new bases for motivating the development of language, and that can be done relatively easily once an awareness of the need is present.

Socialization   In rural areas, socialization to a culture emphasizing respect and obedience and responsible behaviour is facilitated by assigning chores to children, by their learning of complex forms of greeting, and by their natural movement through an age hierarchy. In cities, running errands may be too dangerous. Helping to tend the animals is not possible. The age hierarchy is modified by changes in family composition and by peer group-ings in schools. But in all of this it is possible to imagine culturally sound and understood activities that will continue to provide a similar kind of socialization within cities and that can be supported. Chores may be continued, for instance, but the kind of chore assigned may have to be different to fit with the change in physical and social surroundings.

In the city, and with the evolution of families towards nuclear or even one-parent families, there is a tendency for a basic socialization value to shift – from one of greater dependence to one of greater independence and from one of socialization to the group to a more individualistic view. Whereas in rural areas, a child was taught to accept and adjust to the relatively unchanging environment, in the city, socialization may shift towards achieving independence of thought as well as action. Indepen-dence, or autonomy, may become more important in an urban setting in order to cope, but the need for affiliation and relatedness does not dis-appear (Kağitçibaşi 1990). Practices that help to retain the relational dimension of socialization while strengthening that of autonomy and separ-ation need to be encouraged if they continue to be considered important.

The above discussion is over-simplified. It does not do justice to the situations of absolute poverty. It does not include a discussion of children who, for all practical purposes, have no family. It does not treat problems associated with displacement and scarring brought about by war or internal oppression.

And the discussion of urban areas has involved a set of assumptions that may or may not hold. It is commonly believed that migration to urban areas isolates young adults from kin and from community support systems and that this is harmful to child development because it removes the advantages of multiple caregiving and support. This is probably so in a high percentage of cases, but it is also possible to imagine that many low-income urban families in marginal areas do manage to retain strong kinship ties, to become part of an active community within a city and to build a support system approximating that of the extended family that existed in the rural areas. In many cases, 'ruralization' of the cities (which permits continued strong kinship ties and brings with it support systems and 'community') may be stronger than the 'urbanization' of migrants to cities.

Therefore, it seems important not to accept as inevitable the hypothesized shifts in social structure and customs and beliefs that we have reflected above. A challenge of the next decade will be to do a better job of sorting out the circumstances under which these do occur and those in which they do not. More work is needed to uncover the survival strategies that are actually evolved in such conditions, in order to do a more adequate job of responding to family needs, beginning with the positive practices that exist and looking for positive deviants who have been successful in their adjustments. And, in line with the earlier review (see Chapter 4), more attention needs to be given to assisting the strengthening of social support, helping to provide a new kind of extended family where old ones are no longer operating.

IMPLICATIONS FOR PROGRAMMING

1 *Give priority to areas where rapid social change is occurring.*   Perhaps the most important implication of all for planners and implementors of programmes is that problems seem to be greatest where change is occurring most rapidly and where old methods of childrearing do not easily apply. (This observation is as valid for northern as for southern countries.) For that reason, priority should be given to such groups as urban migrants living in squatter settlements, inhabitants of areas where major changes are occurring in the environment (e.g. construction of a dam), zones where there has been a rapid shift to cash cropping, and families whose lives have been disrupted by war.

2 *Avoid a 'blueprint'.*   From our discussion, it should be painfully clear that trying to advocate uniform childrearing practices for all would be ill-advised. Although some general rules might be set down for programming, the content of programmes is going to have to differ. This implies some form of decentralization of the process. To help avoid a blueprint approach and to aid the adjustment to particular circumstances, it is important for planners to know what are the major differences in practices from place to place, who cares for the child and when in different settings.

3 *Look to and draw upon traditional wisdom and practice in programming.*   The following extract, pertaining to fertility and birth, is

equally valid for the broader spectrum of activities related to child care and development up to the age of six years (or beyond).

> It is important to identify and encourage beneficial traditional practices as they have evolved as adaptive behavior in populations that survive over time; to respect medically neutral but socially important practices such as the ritual disposing of the placenta; to discourage harmful practices such as cutting the cord with an instrument contaminated with tetanus spores, and to continue to search for meaning in practices we in the West do not understand.
>
> (MacCormack 1982, quoted in Negussie, p. 45)

Attention to the lessons of traditional wisdom is essential for developing dialogue and mutual learning. It will lead to identifying practices that are beneficial, under the control of the caregiver, low-cost and acceptable (see Table 13.2 on the advantages of 'disadvantaged' environments). It will help to identify sound reasons why change has not occurred in certain practices as well as reasons why change might not occur. It will improve the language of discussion by locating the most appropriate words and phrases denoting particular practices. It can identify the most appropriate sources of local wisdom and knowledge, as well as the actual caregivers to whom additional knowledge might be directed.

4 *Work with custodians of traditional knowledge and with those who are recognized as successful in rearing their children.* Traditional birth attendants, elderly women, and others who are the sources of wisdom about childrearing will be important sources of knowledge and important channels of transmission of new, culturally appropriate knowledge. Women who are successful in their own childrearing are natural candidates to work with other members of the community in enhancing child care and development.

5 *Look beyond parents.* We have seen that most societies are characterized by multiple caregiving rather than by caregiving restricted to the mother or parents. In some cases, caregiving responsibility extends to all community members. In others, siblings, a 'teasing uncle', a mother-in-law, a godparent, or grandparents will have important roles in assuring a child's healthy development. To the extent that programmes can involve all the relevant caregivers in ways that reinforce and improve their childrearing skills, they will be more successful programmes.

Looking beyond parents means also entertaining the possibility that forms of organized care outside the family can complement the care given within families. Characteristics of such care were discussed in Chapter 11.

6 *Present themes, not messages.* At several other points in this book, we have made reference to the need to present information about child development in terms of themes to be discussed, rather than as messages telling people what they should do. From the discussion will come locally adapted

'messages' that take into account local customs and use local language and terminology. The reason for that recommendation should now be clearer.

7 *Seek 'touchpoints'.* Different cultural traditions identify different points at which some aspect of a child's growth and development is recognized, usually in conjunction with a particular ritual (naming, a first haircut, circumcision, etc.). These, as well as the prenatal period and the period immediately following birth are times when parents and others close to the child will have much more interest in discussing issues related to the young child than at other times. Organizing discussions and providing information at these times can help to set parents more at ease and encourage them to honour and attend to the rights of their children.

8 *Understand before judging.* Finally, it seems advisable to incorporate into any programme intended to enhance early childhood care and development an effort to describe and understand existing practices without making prior judgements. Only then can desirable dialogue occur, helping to promote partnership in the improvement of practices and in the survival and development of young children.

NOTES

1   The elegant term 'niche', taken from ecology, is meant to capture the functional relationship between a living organism and its environment.
2   For detailed discussions of these and other practices during pregnancy and birth, and their implications for programming, see Pillsbury, Brownlee and Timyan 1990, and Negussie 1988.

REFERENCES

Ainsworth, M.D.S. *Infancy in Uganda: Infant Care and the Growth of Love.* Baltimore: Johns Hopkins Press, 1967.

Akinware, M.A. 'Findings in Rural Southwestern Nigeria and Implications for UNICEF Programme Planning', a paper presented at the fourth meeting of the Consultative Group on Early Childhood Care and Development, held in Ottawa, Canada, July 14–16, 1988. Lagos, Nigeria: UNICEF, July 1988. Mimeo.

Antinucci, F., B. Fiore and L. Pisani. 'Psychologie de la Petite Enfance en Afrique', in P. Coppo (ed.) *Médecine Traditionelle, Psychiatrie et Psychologie en Afrique.* Rome: Il Pensiero Scientifico Editore, 1980, pp. 131–206.

Blair, A., B. Maphathe, N. Makhetha, F. Rankhelepe and R. Thabane.'Off to a Good Start (A Study of 400 Basotho One-Year-Olds)'. Maseru: National University of Lesotho, Institute of Southern African Studies, 1986.

Brazleton, T.B. *Neonatal Behavioral Assessment Scale.* London: William Heinemann, 1973.

Brazleton, T.B. 'Early Intervention. What Does It Mean?' in H. Fitzgerald, B. Lester and M. Yogman (eds) *Theory and Research in Behavioral Pediatrics, Vol. 1.* New York: Plenum Publishing Co., 1982, pp. 1–34.

Brokensha, D., D.M. Warren and O. Warner (eds) *Indigenous Knowledge Systems and Development.* Lanham, Maryland: University Press of America, Inc., 1980.

Cayon, Edgardo. 'El Concepto de *Uriwa* entre los Quechuas', Un trabajo presentado en el Primer Congreso Nacional de Antropología, Popoyán, Colómbia,

1978. Departamento de Investigaciones Sociales, Universidad del Cauca, 1978.

Chávez, A. and C. Martínez. *Growing Up in a Developing Community*. México: Instituto Nacional de la Nutrición, 1982.

Erny, P. *L'enfant et son milieu en Afrique noire*. Paris: Editions L'Harmattan, 1987 (Re-edition of a 1971 work; also published in English by Oxford University Press of Nairobi as *The Child and His Environment in Black Africa*, Nairobi, 1981).

Faniran, A. and O. Areola. 'The Concept of Resources and Resource Utilization among Local Communities in Western State, Nigeria', *African Environment*, Vol. 2, No. 2 (1976).

Howrigan, G.A., 'Making Mothers from Adolescents: Context and Experience in Maternal Behavior in Yucatan', unpublished PhD. dissertation, Cambridge, Mass., Harvard University, Graduate School of Education, June 1984.

Kağitçibaşi, C. 'Family and Socialization in Cross-Cultural Perspective, A Model of Change', in J. Berman (ed.) *Nebraska Symposium on Motivation, 1989*. Lincoln: Nebraska University Press, 1990, pp. 135–200.

Ki-Zerbo, J. *Educate or Perish*. Abidjan: UNICEF Regional Office for West and Central Africa, 1990.

Kotchabhakdi, N.J. 'The Integration of Psycho-social Components of Early Childhood Development in a Nutrition Education Programme of Northeast Thailand', a paper prepared for the Third Meeting of the Consultative Group on Early Childhood Care and Development, Washington DC, January 12–14, 1987. New York: the Consultative Group, 1987.

Landers, C. 'Child-rearing Practices and Infant Development in South India', in N. Gunzenhauser (ed.) *Advances in Touch: New Implications in Human Development*. Skillman, N.J.: Johnson and Johnson, Inc., 1990, pp. 42–52.

Maccoby, E.E. *Social Development: Psychological Growth and the Parent–Child Relationship*. New York: Harcourt Brace Jovanovich, 1980.

Mead, M. and M. Wolfenstein (eds) *Childhood in Contemporary Cultures*. Chicago: University of Chicago Press, 1955.

Myrdal, G. *Asian Drama: An Inquiry into the Poverty of Nations*. New York: Twentieth Century Fund, 1968.

Negussie, B. *Traditional Wisdom and Modern Development, A Case Study of Traditional Peri-Natal Knowledge among Elderly Women in Southern Shewa, Ethiopia*. Stockholm: University of Stockholm, Institute of International Education, 1988.

Ortiz, A. and M. France Souffez. 'Patrones de Crianza Infantil en el Area Rural Andina', Lima: Centro Latinoamericano de Estudios Educativos, 1989.

Paolisso, M., M. Baksh and J.C. Thomas. 'Women's Agricultural Work, Child Care and Infant Diarrhea in Rural Kenya', in J. Leslie and M. Paolisso (eds) *Women, Work and Child Welfare in the Third World*. Boulder, Colorado: Westview Press, Inc., 1989, pp. 217–36.

Pedersen, D. and V. Baruffati. 'Healers, Deities, Saints and Doctors: Elements for the Analysis of Medical Systems', *Social Science Medicine*, Vol. 29, No. 4 (1989), pp. 487–96.

Pillsbury, B., A. Brownlee and J. Timyan. 'Understanding and Evaluating Traditional Practices: A Guide for Improving Maternal Care', Washington DC, International Center for Research on Women, March 1990.

Scheper-Hughes, N. 'Culture, Scarcity and Maternal Thinking. Maternal Detachment and Infant Survival in a Brazilian Shanty Town', *Ethos*, Vol. 13, No. 4 (1985), pp. 291–317.

Sears, R.R., E.E. Maccoby and H. Levin. *Patterns of Child Rearing*. Evanston, Ill: Row, Peterson, 1957.

Slothouber, A. 'Aspects of Child Rearing Practices in Liberian Society: An

Analysis', a consultant's report prepared for the UNICEF Office in Liberia, July 1986. Mimeo.

Stephens, W.N. *The Family in Cross-Cultural Perspective.* New York: Holt, Rinehart and Winston, 1963. Chapter 8 deals with childrearing.

Sumon Amornvivat, *et al. Thai Ways of Child-Rearing Practices: An Ethnographic Study.* Bangkok: Chulalongkorn University, Faculty of Education, 1989.

Super, C. 'Behavioral Development in Infancy', in R.H. Monroe, R.L. Monroe and B.B. Whiting (eds) *Handbook of Cross-Cultural Human Development.* New York: Garland Publishing Inc., 1981, pp. 181–270.

Super, C. and S. Harkness. 'The Developmental Niche: A Conceptualization at the Interface of Child and Culture', in *International Journal of Behavioral Development,* Vol. 9 (1986), pp. 545–69.

Timyan, J. 'Cultural Aspects of Psycho-social Development: An Examination of West African Childrearing Practices', a report prepared for the regional UNICEF Workshop, 'Toward a Strategy for Enhancing Early Childhood Development in the West and Central Africa Region', held January 18–22, 1988. Abidjan, Côte d'Ivoire. New York, the Consultative Group on Early Childhood Care and Development, 1988.

Tronick, E.A., S.W. Winn and G. Morelli. 'The Child-Holding Patterns of EFE (Pygmies) of Zaire', in N. Gunzenhauser (ed.) *Advances in Touch: New Implications in Human Development.* Skillman, N.J.: Johnson and Johnson Inc., 1990.

UNESCO. 'The Learning Environments of Early Childhood in Asia. Research Perspectives and Changing Programmes', Bangkok, UNESCO Principal Regional Office for Asia and the Pacific, 1988.

Uribe, M. 'Ambiente Ecológico Familiar del Niño de Puerto Merizalde', an analysis prepared for the UNICEF Office in Colombia, Cali, Julio de 1984. Mimeo.

Wagner, D.A. and H.W. Stevenson. *Cultural Perspectives on Child Development.* San Francisco: W.H. Freeman and Company, 1982.

Werner, E.E. *Cross-Cultural Child Development. A View from the Planet Earth.* Monterey, California: Brooks/Cole Publishing Company, 1979.

Whiting, B.B. (ed.) *Six Cultures: Studies of Child Rearing.* New York: John Wiley and Sons, 1963.

Whiting, B.B. and J.W.M. Whiting. *Children of Six Cultures: A Psycho-Cultural Analysis.* Cambridge, Mass: Harvard University Press, 1967.

Whiting, J.W.M. 'Environmental Constraints on Infant Care Practices', in R.H. Monroe, R.L. Monroe and B.B. Whiting (eds) *Handbook of Cross-Cultural Human Development.* New York: Garland Publishing Inc., 1981, pp. 155–79.

Zeitlin, M., F.C. Johnson and R. Houser. 'Active Maternal Feeding and Nutritional Status of 8–20 month old Low Income Mexican Children'. Mimeo n.d.

Part VI

How big and what will it cost?

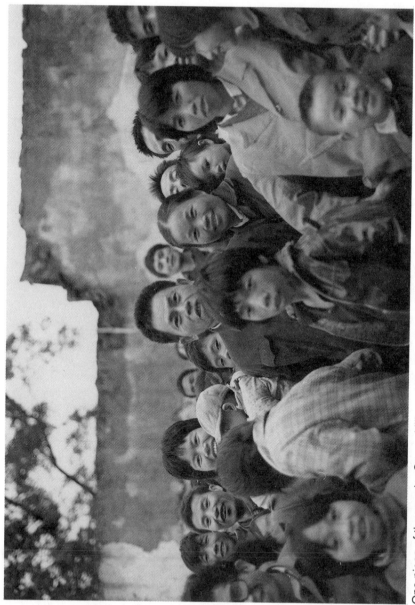

One piece of the puzzle, Guang Village, Yan Qiao Township, China

Chapter 14

Going to scale[1]

The 1980s demonstrated that many programmes related to the human goals for the 1990s lend themselves to mass application at national levels. Therefore, there is less need to concentrate on small-scale pilot projects in the 1990s as was the case in earlier decades. The challenge of the 1990s is to disseminate what has already been learned from pilot projects in earlier decades to a scale that can lead to universal coverage of most of the basic services for human development.

(UNICEF, May 1989)

How many times during the last three decades of intensive development efforts has a demonstration or pilot project provided 'the answers' to a development problem? Everyone is flushed with enthusiasm and optimism. The model that proved so successful on a small scale is expanded with the hopes of benefitting a larger portion of the population. All too often, however, impact decreases or disappears completely.

(Pyle 1984)

National governments and international development organizations are interested in reaching as many people as possible with the services or self-help programmes they promote or fund – i.e. they are interested in 'going to scale' or 'scaling up'. Indeed, scale has become one of the watchwords of the late 1980s and early 1990s.

The current interest, almost a preoccupation in some circles, with scale and how to achieve it, reflects more than an altruistic desire to make major improvements in the human condition. Operating on a larger scale is also seen as a way of using available resources more efficiently as economies of scale come into play. And political advantages are involved as well, as those in charge seek recognition and support through their extension of services.

Another reason for interest in scale is a growing frustration within organizations arising from the fact that many small-scale research, pilot, or demonstration projects have failed to get 'out of the hothouse' to have the desired large-scale influence on policies, programmes, and people. This frustration is linked, in part, to a rational view of the world in which one should be able to learn from experience and apply that learning to other settings, thereby avoiding the inefficient process of 'reinvention of the wheel'. But another part of the frustration arises from the need within organizations to show evidence of success. For governments and international organizations whose charge is a broad one, projects or programmes that fail to go to scale are often viewed as evidence of failure and wasted resources. Organizational pride, and sometimes even organizational survival, may be at stake.

Moreover, thinking big and setting large-scale targets have become part of a methodology. They are part of a process of mobilizing resources, of convincing people that the impossible (or difficult) is possible. Once a target of immunizing 80 per cent of the world's children has been set, for instance, and public agreement on this goal has been obtained by governments and international organizations, it forces actions that would otherwise not have been taken. It helps to create a self-fulfilling prophecy by putting prestige on the line, placing organizations under pressure to succeed and to do so rapidly. If the push for scale is not successful, the process of setting targets and of attempting to mobilize resources runs the risk of being interpreted as a hollow public relations ploy.

Undoubtedly, other reasons could be added, but the perceived humanitarian, economic and political benefits, the potential for mobilizing interest and resources, and organizational preoccupations with success and failure are probably sufficient to explain the present drive, expressed in the opening quotation from UNICEF, for 'mass applications' and 'a scale that can lead to universal coverage'.

But there is another side to the drive for scale. The position we shall take in this chapter is that the pressure to go to scale, while legitimate and understandable, and often beneficial, is also distracting attention from important goals and biasing the programming process. Ironically, although the motives for seeking scale are often humanitarian, a sense of humanity can easily get lost in the process of growing bigger. An emphasis on achieving the broadest coverage possible can, and often does, lead to undue emphasis on numbers which become goals in and of themselves, taking emphasis off a more fundamental concern with the human condition. Moreover, the particular way in which scale is approached favours individuals rather than groups and a centralized, standardized, directed methodology rather than participatory, empowering, community-based forms of choice and action.

This chapter has three purposes:

–   The first purpose is to analyse and elaborate and clarify the concepts of 'scale' and 'going to scale'. We shall begin with definitions because scale, as most of the other main terms used in this book, means different things to different people. We shall also examine several writings that have tried to extract lessons about the process of moving from small projects to large programmes. Then, three different ways of looking at the process will be set out and several issues related to the feasibility of going to scale will be examined.

– A second purpose is to identify a way of thinking about scale and of moving towards scale that allows a qualitative, decentralized, and participatory approach to that goal, as contrasted with the more quantitative, centralized and imposed approach that seems to predominate. By rethinking what constitutes scale and how to get there it seems possible to reconcile the seeming contradiction between achieving scale and promoting community or grassroots participation.

– Third, we shall look at the process of going to scale in relation to our particular area of interest – programming for early childhood care and development – and draw some programme implications.

SCALE AND GOING TO SCALE

What defines scale and how is it measured?

When talking about scale or size, the discussion usually begins with a particular goal in mind – of affecting the largest number of people possible in some way such as reducing infant mortality, increasing school readiness, increasing knowledge, etc. But these desired effects on people can easily be lost as the discussion proceeds and in the process of growing large. Often, the emphasis shifts to expanding a particular service (e.g. preschool education), or increasing the presence of a particular model (integrated child development centres or home day care), technology (immunization or oral rehydration packets or educational toys) or set of messages (about child survival, as presented in the UNICEF publication, *Facts for Life*).

Accordingly, the measure of what constitutes scale may differ from the original goal. Instead of measuring scale in terms of the number of people affected in a particular way (independent of the organization or model or technique), it is more likely to be indexed by increases in the size and complexity of a particular organization (e.g. the number of centres or health-care personnel in a health service), the number of examples of a particular model (e.g. the number of ICDS centres in India), or the number of people using a particular model or technique (oral rehydration packets) or receiving a set of messages (the radio audience for a group of 'spots'). The scale of a primary school system, for instance, might be indexed by referring to the number of students who reach a certain level of learning measured by an agreed upon test. But, usually, the index of scale is the number of schools or school personnel (in the system as a whole or in a particular model), or the number of students enrolled (in the system, in a model, or being taught in a particular way).

The two most typical measures of scale, then, are 1) the size of an organization and 2) 'coverage', understood as the number of people involved in a programme as users or beneficiaries of a service (or as participants in the case of self-help programmes). These are crude measures and bring with them some difficulties.

Scale as organizational size   Organizational measures of scale are essentially 'input' measures. They suggest a rather naive belief that more is better. The search for scale in these cases is tied to the premise that increases in organizational size (personnel or number of operational units) will increase the impact. At best, this may be partially true. Having more teachers or preschools may open more places and could have an effect on more children, but it is not a foregone conclusion that the service will be used or that the effect will be positive. The quality of the expanded programme could be very low and produce no result at all or even a negative effect. Still, we could say, according to an organizational definition, that a programme was 'going to scale' as more units were added. This organizational definition is not, in our view, an appropriate way to define or measure scale.

Scale as coverage   The choice of coverage as the preferred measure of size moves one step beyond equating scale with the level of material inputs into a project or programme and one step towards thinking in terms of desired outcomes. But achieving increased coverage is not the same as producing a particular result such as decreased malnutrition or improvements in mental development.

But the way in which coverage is defined varies. Coverage sometimes refers to the number of people in a particular area who, theoretically, are covered by or *have access* to a service. It sometimes refers to those who *actually use* a service. Rarely does it refer to those who *make effective use* of a service, as indicated by an outcome.

Numbers or percentages?   Coverage may be expressed in terms of absolute numbers (of potential or actual users) and arbitrary cut-off points can be assigned to classify programmes as large scale or small. In one case (APHA 1982, p. 26), the following classification was used: national or large-scale regional programmes (2,000,000–8,000,000 individuals); Medium-scale regional programmes (500,000–1,000,000); small-scale regional programmes (100,000–500,000); and small-scale programmes (under 100,000). These categories are convenient inventions, but without any particular conceptual base.

Scale is both an absolute and a relative concept. The scale of a map is expressed in relation to true size, or full scale. Scale for a programme may be defined as full scale, expressed in terms of the total number of people one would like to involve (or of all people). But scale might also be defined as a percentage of that ideal, full scale figure. That may involve looking at the percentage of geographical or administrative units covered (e.g. the Indian ICDS programme is found in 40 percent of the development districts in India) or, as is more often the case, as a percentage of individuals in the particular category to be reached (e.g. in Chile, in 1984, 13.9 per cent of the children aged 0–5 were in preschool level programmes).

Occasionally, scale is ambitiously defined in terms of full scale. However, the attempt to universalize immunization defined reaching 80 per cent of a population as a goal for going to scale. A more rigorous empirical definition of having achieved scale incorporates a distributional dimension, requiring coverage of 80 per cent of the population within each of the major administrative sub-areas of a country or sub-national region. By these standards, very few programmes can be said to have gone to scale.

Total coverage vs. coverage of a select population   We are less concerned here with the idea of *total* coverage than we are with coverage of people who are in need, or *at risk*. The programme guideline presented in Chapter 5 (p. 94) reads, 'Programmes should try to reach the largest possible number of children living in conditions that put them at risk'. In absolute terms, this seems to make the task easier by reducing the numbers of those who should be included; the population at risk may constitute 'only' 40 per cent, or even 10 per cent, of a given population. But in practice, the task is likely to be harder. Finding and working with 80 (or some other level) per cent of those at risk will be more difficult than reaching 80 per cent of the population as a whole. At risk individuals are likely to be outside the mainstream; reaching and incorporating them in a programme requires extra effort.

The population to be reached in order for a programme to be considered a full-scale programme will differ according to the particular goals and content of a programme. All children are at risk of contracting measles if they are not immunized. Therefore, the relevant population is the total population of children. But not all children are at risk of malnutrition or of suffering life-threatening bouts of diarrhoea or of delayed or debilitated mental development fostered by a lack of early childhood stimulation and interaction. A first task, then, when thinking about what constitutes scale is to identify the population which most needs the particular kind of service or self-help programme being considered. In so doing, we guard against the tendency to think that larger is automatically better.

Looking beyond the product to the process   But there is obviously more to the idea of scale than setting a target and measuring whether the target is being reached. As suggested by the title of this chapter, 'Going to Scale', we are more interested in the process of moving towards full scale, however that is defined, than we are in trying to stipulate a particular level of coverage to be reached. What are the different forms that the process can take? How are choices made about goals and methods and organization? How do different approaches vary in their pace and effect on attainment of coverage or impact as defined by increases in health or literacy or child development? How do they incorporate participation and empowerment?

Reasons for failure to go to scale

Gathering reasons why a small-scale project fails to grow into a large-scale programme can be done rather easily by asking people responsible for monitoring projects and programmes why that is so. With little effort, for instance, the following useful list of possible reasons for failure emerged from conversations by the author with a handful of field staff from several international organizations:

- Funds for the larger effort were unavailable (or were cut off).
- Political commitment was missing.
- The social organization and participation that helped make community-based pilot models work was too threatening when contemplated on a larger scale.
- The demonstration model that was successful in one region did not work in other locations.
- The organizational base was inadequate to support large-scale pro- grammes, and expansion occurred too fast for the needed changes to take place.
- Administrative methods were not in place.
- It was difficult to hold people accountable.
- Bureaucratic territoriality and malaise undercut good intentions.
- Information about the pilot projects was not available at the proper time and in the proper form to the people who counted.
- The 'mystique' associated with an original project did not transfer as the programme grew.
- The charismatic, dedicated leadership that accounted for so much of the small-scale success could not be cloned.
- Squabbling among regional groups took its toll.
- Response by the people to the programme was slow and no attempt was made to mobilize them, to gain real participation and involvement.

Readers will certainly be able to add to the list based on their own experience.

Reasons for successful scaling up

More difficult than listing potential causes for the *failure* of projects to move to scale is the task of discovering what accounts for *success*. How, for instance, have successful programmes coped with the leadership question and overcome the potential problem arising from natural limits on charismatic leadership? Have successful programmes always started on a small scale and grown large slowly? How have successful large-scale programmes organized to cope with diversity? Is it possible to identify commonalities among programmes that have successfully scaled up? Under what conditions is participation really necessary for the successful spread of a project? How is demand created?

Let us look at lessons extracted from case studies of success stories by three authors.

Lessons from five Asian success stories: Korten

David Korten (1980) has examined five extremely varied Asian programmes. Each programme began on a relatively small scale as a community-based project and grew significantly in size. From his analysis, Korten draws several conclusions about the process:

There is no blueprint.   Each project was successful because it had worked out a programme model responsive to the beneficiary needs at a particular time and place and each had built a strong organization capable of making the programme work (p. 495).

'*Successful transition from project to programme is associated with a learning process* in which villagers and programme personnel shared their knowledge and resources to create a programme which achieved a fit between needs and capacities of the beneficiaries and those of the outsiders who were providing the assistance' (p. 497). Further, 'the learning process approach calls for organisations that:(a) embrace error; (b) plan with the people; and (c) link knowledge building with action' (p. 498). Later on, three stages in this learning process will be described.

The roles of researchers, planners, and administrators were combined in a single individual or a closely knit team so that 'even as the organisations grew, the mode of operation stressed integration. Researchers worked hand-in-hand with operating personnel, and top management spent substantial time in the field keeping in contact with operations' (p. 499).

The organizational capacity developed in the pilot projects was preserved and drawn on as expansion occurred. 'The individuals who had created and sustained the fit were assigned to guide the learning experiences of others until they too gained the knowledge, commitment, and skills to make the programme work. As the programme moved into new communities, new lessons were learned, including lessons on how to maintain the fit between programme and people as the organisation expanded. New knowledge and the organisational capacity to put it to work were created simultaneously by one and the same process' (p. 499).

The lessons of success: Paul

Echoing Korten in several respects is an analysis of six successful national development programmes in Asia, Africa, and Latin America.[2] Paul's study emphasizes the importance of organizational variables but assigns importance also to political commitment and the availability of resources. Despite sectoral and national diversity, the successful programmes studied by Paul had several features in common: a marriage of planning with implementation, selectivity, organizational networking, deliberate linkages between pilot projects and national programmes, phased implementation, demand mobilizing, simple information systems, flexible selection and training, and political commitment (see Table 14.1).

According to Paul, programmes differed in: their approaches to participation, the nature of the functional and vertical integration, the degree of decentralization, and the mix of incentives used to motivate beneficiaries. For instance, Paul found that, whereas economic incentives work well for programmes with economic goals, non-economic incentives (recognition, status, a sense of challenge) are more important in social programmes.

Variations in the critical interventions from one programme to another depended on the complexity of the environment (in terms of scope, uncertainty and homogeneity) and whether single or multiple goals were sought.

The role of national governments   National governments played several particular roles with regard to successful programmes:

- Specifying broad objectives;
- Providing resources;
- Bringing programme planning and implementation together by establishing the programme agency, making the key appointments before formulating the programme, and allowing discretion to the appointed leaders in both formulation and implementation;
- Helping to monitor progress and performance;
- Providing stability, commitment, and continuity of programme leadership (continuity and commitment by leadership were more important than charisma).

Table 14.1 Features of successful large-scale programmes*

- *A marriage of planning with implementation* Programme managers were included in the formulation of programme strategies. Successful programmes avoided the tendency to import programme strategies or formulate them through internal groups without any reference to those likely to manage them. Therefore, strategy and implementation were not disjointed and were mutually adaptive.
- *Selectivity* Initial focus on a single goal or service was followed by sequential diversification.
- *Organizational networking* Even single services require complex integration of diverse inputs and skillful coordination of efforts at national, district, and community levels. That was best accomplished by relying on inter-organizational cooperation through networks rather than on hierarchical control.
- *Deliberate linkages between pilot projects and national programmes* Pilot projects were used as learning experiences.
- *Phased programme implementation* Phasing development programmes in geographic or functional terms allows adaptation to the uncertainty, diversity, and scope of the environment and to the lack of techno-managerial resources. It also serves as a means by which programmes can successfully build on experience.
- *Mobilizing demand* was an important feature of programming.
- *Simple information systems* with fast feedback were developed and used.
- *Flexible selection and training processes* were used.
- *Political commitment* was evident in a degree of flexibility and in the organizational autonomy given to programme leaders by the government.

Source: Samuel Paul, *Managing Development Programs: The Lessons of Success.* Boulder, Colorado: Westview Press Inc., 1982.

An analysis of seven Indian experiences: Pyle

In his manuscript, 'Life after Project', David Pyle (1984) examines seven successful pilot projects carried out in the Indian state of Maharashtra. According to Pyle, approaching the problem of scale with an emphasis on inputs and cost effectiveness is inadequate. The assumption that increasing inputs and solving technical problems will be sufficient to bring about the desired results is faulty. More important, he suggests, are the organizational and political dimensions of projects.

Focusing on the process of implementation, Pyle draws an ideal type from the seven small-scale projects. Comparing the small project ideal with the characteristics of large-scale programmes, he finds organizational deviations with respect to objectives, the populations served, the orientation towards results, teamwork, training and supervision, selection and incentives, administrative control and informational procedures (see Table 14.2).

Pyle adds a political analysis to his organizational review by examining commitment, accountability, how programmes relate to the structure of interest groups, and the degree of self-sufficiency sought. *Commitment* should be evident in policy statements, budget allocations, motivations and the willingness to make needed structural reforms. However, this last indicator of commitment is seldom present. Needed structural reforms run counter to many vested interests. The commitment to decentralization, for instance, requires an unusually strong and secure central government.

Table 14.2 A comparison of project and programme characteristics

Project characteristics	*Programme characteristics*
1 Specific, time-bounded *objectives*.	1 Vague, ambitious objectives without time boundaries.
2 *Targeting* the most vulnerable.	2 Lack of targeting.
3 A *results orientation*; evaluations concerned with process and impact.	3 Concern with inputs, reducing the attention to education, maintenance and follow-up.
4 *Teamwork*.	4 Hierarchical relations in which paraprofessional contributions are discounted.
5 *Training as an ongoing process*, with emphasis on developing self-esteem and a social orientation.	5 Training is one-shot and overloaded, particularly with technical material.
6 *Selection based on motivation and values*, not on test results.	6 Selection on test results or other 'objective' criteria (e.g. education levels).
7 *Non-monetary incentives*; individual initiative is rewarded.	7 Monetary incentives. Initiative is discouraged.
8 *Supervision* of reasonable scope, based on clearly defined responsibilities. Supervisors function as trainers.	8 Supervision is thin, plagued by logistical problems. Responsibilities are not clearly defined. Supervisors function as inspectors.
9 *Administrative control* is local, flexible and autonomous.	9 Administration is centralized and rigid, residing in bureaucracies.
10 *Information* is collected and used to make changes. Methods to determine at risk individuals are effective.	10 Information collection is haphazard and there is little feedback. At risk measures become ends, not means.

Source: D. Pyle, *Life After Project*, Boston, John Snow Inc., 1984.

Accountability is affected by how precisely goals are stated, how monitoring is set up and how training occurs. In most settings the structure and influence of *interest groups* favour those who are urban, educated, and established professionals.

The political analysis of programmes, in terms of the *self-sufficiency* sought for/by beneficiaries, quickly exposes the potential political threats that can accompany programmes promoting participation and involvement. Pyle suggests there is a need for more precise definition of what is meant by community participation 'so that we can distinguish real community involvement from community-based service delivery' (p. 219). He notes that an active role by the community in all phases of a project or programme, however desirable, may be idealistic and unrealistic.

> The important thing to remember is that while community participation and involvement have definite advantages and benefits for all concerned (e.g. increased control for the community and decreased economic and administrative role for the bureaucracy), it is not always required to achieve impressive impact.

An emerging blueprint for going to scale?

In the above discussion what emerges as the preferred approach to achieving scale successfully is a rather deliberate, focused, phased approach beginning with a single service, then adding on. It is an approach requiring not only political commitment and resources, but flexibility, time for learning and adjustment, teamwork, and innovative and continuous leadership capable of fitting programmes to existing environmental, organizational, and material resources. Pilot or demonstration projects linked specifically to plans for expansion are seen as potentially important, not only to work out technical details but also as a training ground for those who will follow a programme to scale and as a source of information that can help gain or sustain commitment.

Before falling into the trap of accepting a new blueprint, albeit one that emphasizes flexibility and learning, we should consider alternatives to the phased, flexible, learning-oriented approach to achieving scale described above. In the following section, three paths to achieving scale are distinguished.

ACHIEVING SCALE: THREE APPROACHES

The three approaches to be discussed are labelled expansion, explosion, and association. Scale through *expansion* begins typically with one model which is tested on a small scale, adjusted, and then extended (usually with further adjustment) to other locations until the desired coverage has been attained. Scaling up through *explosion* bypasses the pilot stage. Programme implementation starts on a large scale, usually with one model serving all parts of a nation. A process of local adjustment and filling in may occur after an initial explosion in order to make the programme more responsive to diverse social needs and to intensify coverage in some areas covered in the original burst, but in a token way. An *association* mode achieves scale by piecing together coverage obtained in several distinct (and not necessarily coordinated) projects or programmes, each responding to the needs of a distinct part of the total population served.

The conceptual distinctions made above blur in the real world. Expansion to large scale may, for instance, be programmed over such a short time after the initial model has been tried out successfully that it is, in effect, an explosion. Or, expansion might occur as several very different models are tried out and applied successively within different parts of a country. In that case the result approximates scale achieved by associating different models. Nevertheless, distinguishing the three approaches is useful because each requires different preconditions for success, related to differences in timing, organizational needs, learning potential, initial costs, and other features.

Scale by expansion

Virtually all the cases of successful programmes reviewed by the three authors summarized in the previous section would be characterized as part of a process of expansion. Ideas were developed first on a relatively small scale and expansion occurred in stages with adjustments based on learning from experience along the way. According to Korten, expansion occurs through a 'learning process approach' (see Figure 14.1) to programme development that proceeds, ideally, through three stages, each emphasizing a different learning task. In the first stage, the major concern is with *learning to be effective.* In this stage, efficiency and coverage are low, and errors may be high. Once a programme is found to be effective in responding to an identified need and achieves an acceptable level of fit among beneficiaries, the working programme model, and the capabilities of the action research team, concern shifts to *learning to be efficient* – to 'reducing the input requirements per unit of output'. Modest programme expansion during Stage 2 will increase the cadre of persons experienced in making the programme work and who are available to help build the expanded organizational capacity of Stage 3 in which emphasis is on *learning to expand* and on organizational capacity (rather than programme). Constant attention to ensuring an acceptable level of fit (among organization, programme, and beneficiaries) will mean some inevitable sacrifice in effectiveness and efficiency. The rate of expansion will be governed largely by how fast the necessary organizational capabilities can be developed to support it. Once Stage 3 has been completed, the organization may return to the solution of new problems.

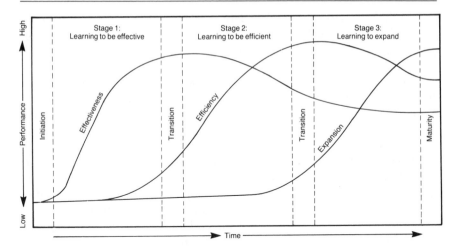

Note: It should be expected that some effectiveness will be sacrificed in the interest of efficiency and expansion. With expansion efficiency will likely suffer due to trade-offs with the requirements of expansion.

Figure 14.1 Programme learning curves
Source: Korten (1980), p. 500.

Note that going to scale along the expansionist path is seen to require a scaling up of an organization to achieve increased coverage.

Scale by explosion

A 'big bang' approach to achieving scale is usually the product of a national political decision, often motivated by a desire to gain broad political support or to build good will. Maximum coverage is sought in the shortest period possible. Typically, a major communications campaign accompanies the effort in order to mobilize demand, and political will is backed by a special appropriation of funds to reach the desired goal. In scale by explosion, programmes are centrally conceived and organized (even though community participation may be considered an important element of the programme philosophy). A blueprint approach is taken in which the same model is applied to all parts of a country or region.

Once a political decision has been taken, development organizations and implementing agencies move to take advantage of the political moment, even though they may have to compromise their usual methods of work and recognize potential problems associated with attempting to do too much too fast. Participation and the quality of the service delivered may be sacrificed in order to attain greater coverage as quickly as possible. Nevertheless, by becoming a part of the large-scale initiative, these organizations hope to secure resources not previously available and to gain a mortgage on the future, thereby turning an immediate action with short-run results into a longer-run programme with continuing benefits.

If judged from the organizational viewpoint presented in the previous pages, an explosion approach might appear undesirable. It does not embody a learning process nor allow organizational and management capabilities to adjust as a system expands. It seems guaranteed to overload the system and to open up accountability problems.

However, there are circumstances in which such an approach to scale appears to be successful. Programmes can successfully explode on the scene if they concentrate on one developmental component or idea, and are directed at a goal that is easily articulated, understood, and achieved. They can be successful if the enthusiasm and energy created as part of the explosion is not short-lived, if it becomes a base for long-term actions.

A successful explosion to scale is probably best illustrated by immunization and literacy campaigns. The Expanded Programme on Immunization has raised rates of immunization dramatically in many countries, even though it has not always achieved scale in terms of reaching an 80 per cent figure. The literacy campaigns in Cuba (1960) and Nicaragua (1980) were clearly focused national campaigns producing excellent results in a short period.

Campaigns can achieve short-term successes, which in and of themselves contribute to reductions in mortality or to advances in the welfare of living children. As suggested, however, the problem is to capitalize on that success to build the lasting programmes required to maintain the gains. No matter how successful an immunization campaign may be, for instance, it will have to be repeated frequently unless vaccination becomes a habit and unless the organizational changes are made permitting vaccination to occur on a regular basis, without mounting a new campaign. A one-time effort does not build permanent organization nor does it inculcate the habit of immunization that is necessary to ensure that the next group of children will also be immunized. A crash literacy programme does not ensure literacy unless there is opportunity to utilize the newly acquired skill.

With these observations we have introduced another dimension of scale, a time dimension. It is possible to achieve full scale or a near equivalent in the short term, but not to be able to maintain that level over time. Sustainability then becomes a main concern. That is essentially an educational and organizational task.

The Mexican 'Programme of Development for Children Ages 0 to 5 Through Parents and Community Members' (Mexico 1983) provides an example of a programme that is not a campaign but illustrates going to scale by explosion. The non-formal programme is built around a guide presenting a series of graduated activities that parents can carry out to help their children develop. Parents and other family members are trained in the use of the manual by promoters who are community members with a minimum of primary school education. Parental training is carried out over 15 days, for two hours each day, after which the promoter makes periodic home visits and calls meetings of small groups to reinforce parental actions. The promoters work with and through community committees. They are paid. A supervisor is charged with orienting and organizing the work of 16 promoters.

This parental education programme was initiated simultaneously in rural areas in all Mexican states in 1983. It did not pass through a pilot stage.[3] The programme illustrates the blueprint approach criticized by Korten and Paul. One model was used for all parts of the country and one set of materials and a manual served equally for all, even though Mexico includes more than 50 ethnic groups, many of whom must be classified among the most needy.

To serve multiple goals – nutrition, health, and early education – the Secretariat of Education, which was responsible for the programme, wisely decided not to formulate new activities in each area, but, rather, sought collaboration (networking in Paul's terms) with the Ministries of Health, Agriculture, and Culture, and with the Post-literacy Programme of the National Institute for Adult Education. As is often the case, the national programme covered a relatively small fraction of those in need. The programme was touted as a success. However, it soon ran into problems because drastic budget cuts had to be made in the government. Its sustainability was in doubt.[4]

Not all cases of scale by explosion are national programmes born of political expediency. The regional primary health care programme launched in Sine-Saloun, Senegal, with funding from USAID is a variation on the theme. In this case, health services are provided through 'health huts', each of which is to be self-supporting. Before the project began, however, there was no attempt to establish that the effective demand of the population for health care was sufficiently great to enable the huts to become self-sufficient. The model was not born of experimentation at the village level nor was it created together with communities. Nevertheless, the 'all-or-nothing' programme was directed at 880,000 rural inhabitants and launched without a test run (Gaspari, p. 19). This example, operating at a regional level, might be termed a 'small bang' rather than a 'big bang' example, about which we will have more to say later on.

Scale by association

In this third mode, scale is achieved by piecing together results of several (or many) actions, each of which is relatively small in scale, each initiated and/or carried out independently, and each approaching the problem in its own way, but with a common goal. Although a central government might set general guidelines and provide some incentives and supplementary resources, it does not dictate how coverage is to be achieved, nor impose a blueprint.

Scale by association can be visualized as the process of putting together a puzzle (perhaps contrasted with blowing up a balloon or pouring a bucket of paint over a surface in the hopes that it will cover it all, and quickly). Each piece may be a different shape and the colours will differ as well, depending on the particular place the piece occupies within the larger puzzle. When all the pieces are in place, a complete and integral picture will appear, and scale will have been achieved. The process of putting the pieces together must be a collaborative one with, perhaps, some general rules helping to guide the process and with some incentives along the way to help the picture emerge more rapidly.

It is not unusual, for instance, for several nutritional supplementation programmes to be operating in a country at one time, each linked to a separate source of food, and a separate source of financing. The programmes may be directed to the same or to different target populations. For practical reasons, a government may assign geographic areas to each programme. Taken together the different programmes may amount to large-scale national coverage and constitute a national programme, even though the type of coverage, delivery system, administration, and even type of food varies from place to place.

In nations that are themselves loose confederations of distinct cultural groups, and/or in which the natural conditions vary a great deal, or in which sheer size is a problem, achieving scale by association may be a practical and desirable approach. It allows each decentralized project to focus on a relatively homogeneous population, respond to particular needs, and make the adjustments necessary to mount an effective programme with that group. This approach does not require large start-up costs or even the introduction of a uniform technology. It could draw heavily on existing organizations and networks.

The idea of achieving scale by adding up many projects does not fit the way in which scale is usually conceived. It moves away from the idea that one model needs to be applied to all, whether through expansion and with adjustments, or as a result of an explosion. It does not require that the administration of all activity lie at the centre with one bureaucratic organization. *It allows for many parallel learning processes to go on simultaneously. It opens the possibility of real participation by communities in formulating and solving problems.*

The idea that relatively independent groups should develop and carry out their own programming (within general guidelines) has about it an air of free enterprise. That need not be the guiding philosophy, however. The example given in Chapter 7 of the parental education programme in China illustrates how a set of local education programmes can be created that add up to a large-scale effort. General guidelines for creating such programmes were applied through the All China Women's Federation at local levels, with varying results in each place. In this case, the process of adding up local initiatives to make one large programme was relatively easy because a national organization supervised the entire project.

Or, another nationally initiated and guided example is provided by the Indian National Adult Education Campaign (NAEC). The NAEC was based on a philosophy that was closer to the consciousness-raising of Paolo Freire than to a free enterprise philosophy. A programme of the Janata Party, NAEC was a politically motivated attempt to go to scale quickly with a programme that would give the party credibility and support following its defeat of Mrs Gandhi in 1977. The distinguishing feature of the unusually flexible, decentralized and varied approach to literacy was its support for the many private voluntary organizations which were already providing adult education, each in its own way, in different parts of the country and to different groups of people. A preconceived notion of how literacy and adult education should be achieved was not imposed. No one literacy method was mandated. Modest amounts of money were used to assist the various groups in small ways that made a difference. The government provided some training and guidance to existing groups. Scale was conceived as the sum of the efforts of these groups.[5]

National governments and international organizations can foster scale by association by providing funds for distinct approaches to the same problem. In the best of worlds, simultaneous funding of different approaches leads to creative competition among programmes, with broad benefits and extended coverage. In the worst cases, scarce funds are squandered and scarce human resources are destructively pulled in several directions by conflicting demands and models, reducing potential coverage and impact.

Perhaps the most crucial feature of this approach is a decentralized structure in which real power and resources are placed at the periphery rather than highly concentrated in the centre.

Combining the approaches

From the above, it seems that each path to achieving scale has advantages and disadvantages.

–   An expansionist approach to scale allows learning and adjustment and, in theory, local participation along the way. But this cautious, sensitive and technically sound model often lacks attractiveness politically and stretches out in time so that continuity and momentum can be lost.

- Scale by explosion brings with it political commitment and some momentum and often an extra bit of resources. But this model tends to be monolithic, superficial and insensitive to cultural differences and community participation.
- Scale through association facilitates the task of beginning where people are and of respecting cultural differences. But the variations that mark the strength of this model can also be a source of weakness, making it difficult for existing centralized bureaucracies to be supportive, and, perhaps, reducing potential economies of scale.

Can these approaches, which we have taken some pains to sort out, be combined, so that the advantages of each can be drawn upon? The answer is that they not only can, but should be melded together, more consciously and frequently than now occurs. Rather than think in terms of expanding one model nationally, we can think of expansion of several models simultaneously, each following the learning process described by Korten. Each model and associated learning process would expand within limits set naturally by cultural and/or administrative divisions which, taken together (our image of the puzzle), would constitute scale.

Accordingly, it is possible to contemplate supporting a series of local initiatives within a national effort that would make resources available on a decentralized basis, and would help to motivate and inform on a broad front. Such an effort could provide visibility redounding to the benefit of socially minded politicians while helping to mobilize demand. This could be done with fanfare, but also with sensitivity to the need for local variations and with an eye to strengthening local participation and organization.

It is possible also to imagine what might be termed a small explosion (or a series of small explosions) in which scale is pursued vigorously within a particular area of a country or with a particular group, with a regional or state organization taking the lead in promoting a massive effort, but again with respect for differences within the region and drawing on different models. This was the case in the Pro-Crianca project in the state of Santa Caterina in Brazil (see Myers, 1986). There, a participatory process was organized that brought together people from various groups at local, regional and state levels. A massive publicity campaign was launched by the state 'in favour of the child', that included a logo (chosen by children from among several possible logos), the distribution of information through messages placed on public mailings (including, for instance, electricity bills), and the organization of events. Each ministry at the state level was asked to indicate what they were doing to improve the welfare of young children and to present that in a report, serving as the basis for discussion and for reorientation. Several models of attention to children were developed, responding to the needs of different groups in the state – fishermen, working mothers in the capital city, rural villagers. The programme is an example of a regional explosion, with features of the association model, and with mechanisms to incorporate local participation and learning.

Beginning to think in these combined ways should help to avoid the distractions mentioned at the outset of this chapter, associated with the pursuit of numbers for numbers' sake rather than with the human condition and empowerment. Expansion within sub-regions makes easier the task of achieving scale without having to create a large new government bureaucracy, while strengthening non-governmental groups at the local and regional levels, and promoting participation along the way. It does not require a huge new infusion of resources from a national level because it begins by adding together existing resources and complementing them in ways that increase effectiveness.

In this combined view, a government can help to mobilize and communicate on a large scale, provide incentives, prepare needed information and materials, train (in direct relation to local or regional initiatives and not according to one blueprint), and promote a learning process by assisting in diagnosis, monitoring, and evaluation of the various local initiatives. It can help with networking among the various institutions involved.

CONDITIONS THAT FAVOUR SCALING UP: SECOND THOUGHTS

Organization and management

Reviews of successful cases presented at the outset of the chapter pointed to a host of organizational and management conditions that seem to favour the process of going to scale. Rather than repeat the list and try to discuss each at length, we will focus on two that are related to the programme guidelines set out in Chapter 5: the need for a multi-service, comprehensive strategy and the importance of community participation in organization and management.

Single vs. multiple services   The review by Paul suggests that successful larger-scale programmes begin with single service deliveries. He also notes that the programmes studied differed in the nature of their functional and vertical integration. Yet we have stressed a holistic view and the need to seek ways in which various services can be brought together to take advantage of their synergistic effects. We have made concrete suggestions regarding ways in which a psychosocial component might be woven into existing programmes of health and nutrition or vice versa. We have tried to bring together programmes of child care and of women-in-development. We have urged organizational convergence (rather than integration) and have stressed the need for integration in planning, and in the content of programmes.

Does this multidimensional, interactive position create an impossible barrier for going to scale? The answer is 'No'. Extending coverage by emphasizing a particular service or programme component and providing multiple services are not inconsistent. Although broad coverage may be sought first with one component or service, a phased approach can lead, over time, to the convergence of services. But some services already exist on a relatively large scale, and it is feasible to begin thinking in those cases of incorporating other elements affecting child development, and of integrating content, without the need to build another and parallel single-service delivery system. It is also possible to facilitate the convergence of several single-service systems and to assist communication among them.

The question becomes a bit more complicated if we think in terms of self-help programmes in a participatory mode rather than of service delivery. We have stressed the need to respond to the particular needs of particular communities. Because different communities will express different needs, the idea of starting with the same component everywhere and on a large scale is not appropriate. Here, the idea of going to scale in a multidimensional way can be present from the outset, but must be seen as occurring over time and in different sequences. Here, the idea of achieving scale by association is critical.

The general procedure followed may be similar in programmes designed to strengthen self-help efforts (e.g. the micro-planning procedure described in Chapter 12), even though the sequence is different and specific actions will vary. With this observation, we are led back to the question of whether or not community participation is compatible with a desire to go to scale.

Participation and scale   The three authors reviewed seem to differ with respect to the importance they assign to participation. Korten gives considerable weight to participation – as a form of learning. The participation he stresses in his discussion of the learning process is primarily participation by planners and managers in project implementation; in other writings, however, Korten is very explicit about the need for 'planning with the people' (Korten 1990). Samuel Paul notes that successful projects differ in their approach to participation, implying that the kind of deep involvement we have emphasized may not be so important. Pyle suggests that community participation may be threatening and unrealistic and is not crucial to achieving results on a large scale.

A review carried out by the American Public Health Association of 52 health projects led to the following conclusion about participation:

Although participation is important for reasons of equity, its value in improving health is not clear from the projects reviewed. Moreover, available evidence suggests most ministries of health do not have the ability (financial or organizational) to undertake the direct task of delivering health services and mobilizing communities for more than routine programme-supported activities.

(p. 17)

One way of dealing with the lack of ability observed above is to support non-governmental organizations that do have the capacity to mobilize local communities to action through involving them directly in the process. In most cases these organizations have a limited geographical range within which they are able to deliver. But if efforts of many such NGOs are added up, the results may reach scale. If governments are willing to think of scale as adding together many such initiatives, and if NGOs do actually function in a participatory mode, sometimes in conjunction with (or as a bridge to) local government, it is possible to reconcile the desire for scale with the principle of participation.

In many places, and particularly in Latin America, the growth of non-governmental networks has been extraordinary over the last decade.

The poor of Latin America are increasingly organized into dense new networks of grassroots organizations. Thickening social and political webs bind them into ever more intricate networks of social organization. While once poverty implied physical and social isolation of groups of culturally similar, equally isolated people, today the boundaries and connections have changed. A farmer, though as poor as his grandfather, is likely to belong to a village agricultural committee within a cooperative which is nested within a federation within a confederation within a movement. Each point of vertical organization, in turn, connects laterally to parallel organizations of the poor, as well as to professional organizations, universities, international NGOs, political parties, the state bureaucracy, and so forth.

(Annis 1990)

The growth of these organizations opens doors (Taller de Cooperación al Desarrollo 1989), but also makes the politics of support extraordinarily complicated. In such circumstances, it may be that community development that is tied to the healthy development of young children will provide an even wider opening than more politically charged issues such as the distribution of land. In any event, what such changes mean is that the opportunities for going to scale with programmes that have a participatory, grassroots origin have increased.

Political commitment

Both common wisdom and the reviews presented earlier in this chapter confirm that political commitment is important if a programme is to move to scale. Conversely, the lack of political will is frequently cited as a main reason for the failure of programmes.

Often, political commitment is expressed through an explosion model of going to scale. That is because political structures tend to be centralized and hold power at the centre. As suggested, one supporting condition for shifting from an explosion model of scale to either an expansion or associational model would seem to be the growth of a decentralized structure in which there is delegation of authority down to the lower levels. But, as suggested in the political analysis by Pyle, centralized bureaucracies are often reluctant to allow too much independence of action, particularly if the sub-scale programmes that would together add up to a large-scale effort are all community-based and participatory programmes. Yet it is precisely here that the major advantage of thinking about scale as the sum of projects is found. Doing so would presumably allow real community participation and empowerment and make good on the advantages that can bring.

Partial relief from this seeming dilemma appears also with the realization that it is possible to place too much emphasis on this feature of the social environment in which programmes develop. Political will can be absent but appear unexpectedly, it can be present but fickle and fleeting, or it can even be a negative force. It would be a mistake, therefore, to feel that actions cannot be taken unless a strong political will is present at a particular time. Looking beyond or around political will does not minimize the important and often determining role of politics, or the political process, in the mix of factors influencing the success of actions.

Some programme analysts would argue that social programmes building from the ground up should assume that political commitment is *not* going to support the kind of participatory programmes desired and should look for populist alternatives. They would argue that emphasis should be placed on the politics involved in creating and sustaining a civil society rather than on seeking political will from a particular government.

A comparison by Castillo[6] of three different political environments, and of varying approaches to early childhood programming, helps to provide insight into the variable place of political will in successfully going to scale. The first case, of Venezuela, is a case in which high political will is present, but is described by Castillo as a case of 'growing like a palm tree, falling like a coconut'. In a first political period, 3,000 community-based day-care centres were created, with strong support from the social democratic government, through a Foundation for the Child, headed by the First Lady. With the arrival of the subsequent Christian Democratic government, political will was again high, but the previous programme was neglected in favour of a new approach linked to a Ministry for Development of Intelligence and a massive project that relied heavily on mass media, national debate, several demonstration projects, and the education of mothers during pregnancy and at the time of birth, related to services available through maternity hospitals or other health centres. When the Social Democrats were returned to power in the next election, the massive programme of the Christian Democrats was revised and revised and revised to the point of impotence. In short, political will was high, but fickle. It did not allow learning and improvement of quality and endurance for programmes created with considerable support and fanfare.

By way of contrast, political will in Ecuador was low during a period of centre-right governments, at which time considerable emphasis was placed on technical programme development on a small scale. Three non-formal modalities were developed (day-care centres, community centres, and mobile community promoter programmes in rural areas). There was no involvement by the mass media. A learning process allowed technical adaptation and the production of manuals and evaluations pointed to the impact of the programmes in low-income areas. This case is characterized by Castillo as one in which 'the last shall be first' because, with the arrival of a new social democratic government, political will materialized and a major effort was made to go to scale, based on the good technical work done previously.

The volatile political conditions of Haiti in recent years provide yet another context for programming, one in which Castillo suggests that the best strategy for programmers was to avoid political will. Identification with a particular government in such rapidly changing circumstances can prove to be counterproductive, even if there is some evidence of political will at a particular moment. In this circumstance, rather than despair or wait for more stable times, it was thought possible to mount, with the assistance of UNICEF, a programme going directly to the people, providing information about child survival and development. One vehicle for 'sensibilizing' the public was a calendar containing information about integrated child development. The calendar was distributed through NGOs and tied both to a mass media campaign and to discussion groups. A next step was to create picture posters providing more detailed information about development, organized according to the age level of the child and lending themselves to group discussion. From this process of sensitizing and education came a move towards establishing a national child development policy and committee and a child development fund – all of which was promoted without political commitment. The case provides an example of one way to think at a national level and to work towards scale that does not fit easily into any of the going-to-scale models described above.

These examples point to the importance of considering continuity (or endurance) and quality alongside the attainment of a certain level of coverage when going to scale with programmes of early childhood care and development.

Technology

Discussions of scale must include discussion of technologies that facilitate work on a large scale. Advances in communications technologies now permit information to be disseminated rapidly to many people and often in a targeted way. Information about child survival and development can be communicated on a large scale to sensitize individuals, to help create demand for services, and to provide specific knowledge that can be applied directly by listeners to improve the condition of children. The major advances that have been made in communication technologies, and the availability of such technologies to the poor and/or their growing networks, present an extraordinary opportunity.

We have commented on the potential this technological advance brings, but also on the accompanying need for a social dimension providing opportunities for group discussion and learning. We have contrasted a social marketing approach, narrowly conceived, with a broader learning approach that draws on, but goes beyond, presenting messages through the mass media. To this, we should add the need for mastery of the technologies themselves at the local level (production of programmes for local radio stations, the use of video cameras and recorders, the mastery of personal computers) both as a means of communication among community-based organizations and as a way for communities to communicate among themselves and to express themselves to people in higher places.

Reflections on GOBI   Another kind of technology has figured prominently in the current discussion about going to scale. A set of simple health and nutrition technologies, captured in the acronym GOBI, has been at the heart of international efforts to move a programme of child survival to scale. There is a desire among some to define an equivalent technological package for early childhood development, assuming that this will facilitate the process of going to scale. Let us look closely, then, at the GOBI package.

Although grouped together, the GOBI technologies are really very different technologies, with different goals (prevention or remedy), different origins (modern science or traditional practice), and managed in different ways – by professionals or paraprofessionals or directly by family members. Examining these differences helps to uncover a source of some confusion about the process of going to scale and provides a background against which to raise questions and make proposals about going to scale with programmes of early childhood development.

The 'G', for Growth monitoring, is a diagnostic technology that has no roots in traditional culture. Because it requires measurement and recording skills and some idea of graphing, this technology has been handled, in the main, by paraprofessionals or professionals. Use by parents has been more problematic. Where it has been applied successfully, growth monitoring has not only allowed identification of children most in need of treatment, but has helped to sensitize parents and, most important of all for our purposes, has provided a relatively simple way of expressing the level of malnutrition and a way of following the progress of interventions intended to deal with malnutrition. Going to scale with this technology requires the widespread distribution of materials to weigh and measure and record. It involves convincing people that this is a useful thing to do and training them in what to do, and how to interpret the results. It implies a follow-up to deal with the cases identified as most in need. All of this requires considerable organization.

The 'O', for Oral rehydration, is a technology to be applied once a problem has been detected. Some of the rehydration methods that have been recommended originate outside local cultures, but others are based in local practices. All are fairly easy to apply and with some instruction, or sensitizing, their remedial administration can occur in the home, without recourse to a paraprofessional or professional. Going to scale with oral rehydration requires seeing that remedies are available and that their use is understood broadly in the population. Scaling up with this practice has sometimes been equated with the widespread distribution of rehydration packets or with the number of individuals who know how to prepare and use a sugar and salt solution. However, greater attention to local remedies has required a different view of what constitutes scale, less tied to a particular input, and more closely related to a widespread process of education or sensitizing of individuals to possibilities within their reach. It is closer to a view of scale by association.

The 'B', for Breastfeeding, publicizes a natural and age-old practice that hardly qualifies as a technology. It is not a scientifically invented technology. It is a preventive practice rather than a diagnostic activity or a remedy applied after the fact. It does not require a paraprofessional or professional to administer it. In this case, the drive has been to maintain a widespread practice that is fading rather than to introduce a new practice. Going to scale with a programme focused on breastfeeding requires mounting an education process. It does not require special machines or acquisition of new skills.

The 'I', for Immunization, is linked to a scientifically invented technology that is not a part of most traditional cultures. It is also a preventive rather than remedial or diagnostic technology. To administer the immunization technology, a large organizational effort is required (to distribute and preserve vaccines) and administration is handled by paraprofessionals or professionals. An educational effort may or may not accompany immunization. Typically, success in going to scale with immunization is measured by the number of individuals who have been vaccinated.

Although immunization is clearly the most demanding of the above technologies, in expense and in organization, it is the technology that has received most attention. In part that is because it is preventive. In part it is because there is a clearly established scientific relationship between immunization and the reduction of disease. In part it is because one solution can be applied to all. In part it is because it is easy to count the number of vaccines distributed and (although much less so) the number of children to whom vaccines have been administered.

As we look at technologies that might enhance early childhood care and development, the above reflection provides several lessons.

– It suggests that looking to and reinforcing existing practices may be a legitimate and useful approach to take (as in the case of breastfeeding and in the broader view of oral rehydration).
– It suggests that scale by association (as is being achieved in the oral rehydration area) can be a useful strategy.
– It suggests that, where some technologies are concerned, it is not the process of delivering the technology, but rather the process of creating social awareness and support for a healthy practice, that needs to provide the focus for action.
– It suggests that a key element in the promotion and use of all these technologies is a well-grounded belief that the result will be worth the effort.
– It suggests that being able to measure outcomes in easily understood ways is important.

GOING TO SCALE WITH PROGRAMMES OF EARLY CHILDHOOD CARE AND DEVELOPMENT

Because the period of early childhood with which we are dealing involves different ages and developmental stages of children, and a range of cultural practices and of socioeconomic contexts, a variety of different approaches to early childhood development will be necessary. Throughout the book these variations have been stressed. This characteristic of child development brings with it several implications for programming.

Look at scale with respect to different stages of development   One implication of this variation is that we should not talk about going to scale with a programme to improve care and development over the full age range from conception to schooling, but should, rather, as a first cut, look at scale with respect to specific programmes affecting different age groupings (see the programme framework on p. 84). Prenatal programmes should be distinguished from programmes for infants and toddlers and preschoolers.

For example, for the younger age groups, an approach focusing on the education and support of caregivers will dominate programming (as contrasted with seeking scale through building centres for attention to the young child). Within that approach, it is possible to consider:

- the creation of a set of materials that can serve for discussion on a large scale, allowing for local variations to be brought out while calling attention to specific areas to be considered;
- a series of regional resource centres that would be dedicated to the task of promoting these discussions and of providing and adjusting materials. These centres could have a training role for promoters as well;
- introduction of materials relating to child development through the primary school system, for instance, in the child-to-child mode which stresses active learning.

Seek scale through association. A second implication of the variation is that scale should be thought of with the puzzle image, or as scale by association, in which various programme models, applied in different locations, can add up to scale. This contrasts with a definition that attempts to expand one model of 'early childhood care and development' to cover the entire population. It implies an organizational mode that would favour local initiative and experimentation and expansion. It implies decentralization within governments and/or working with a wide range of non-governmental organizations working at the grass roots whose activities could be facilitated.

Large-scale assistance to these organizations could nevertheless be provided from the centre in the form of:

- training;
- materials providing practical descriptions of a wide range of complementary strategies and alternative models;
- travel to other areas to obtain ideas about actions that work in practice; and
- resources to help with the implementation of the particular arrangements designed by particular communities.

Seek scale in relation to children and families living in conditions that put them at risk There are a variety of ways of defining children who are at risk. We have suggested that the situations in which children may be most at risk are those in which rapid social change is occurring, including those in which people have migrated to cities. Thinking of scale with respect to these groups (or to at risk groups defined on another basis) as a first goal defines the task in a way that may not seem as overwhelming as it does when relating scale to reaching an entire population.

When the appropriate strategy seems to be to gather children together in centres and provide a direct service, this focusing is even more important, given the costs of such actions.

Seek scale by incorporating missing child development elements into existing large-scale programmes   We have suggested scale can be sought by looking to the incorporation of early childhood development components into existing large-scale programmes, of primary health care, for instance (see Chapter 9). If and when such an approach is taken, one would hope that local adjustments could be part of the process of incorporation. Other examples would include incorporation into literacy programmes or use of the existing infrastructure of the mass media.

In brief, a range of alternatives is available for going to scale with programmes of early childhood care and development. These may be programmes helping to empower and support parents and other caregivers. Or, they may be programmes in which alternative models of organized care and development are supported in different locations of a country, creating scale through association, setting in motion local and sub-regional learning processes throughout a country, but concentrating on the areas and families most in need.

We turn now to the thorny question of costs and finances.

NOTES

1   This chapter draws heavily upon and updates: Robert G. Myers, 'Going To Scale', a paper prepared for the Second Inter-Agency Meeting on Community-based Child Development, New York, October 29–31, 1984 (New York, UNICEF 1984). It also draws on comments on the paper made at that meeting, contained in a Summary Report of the meeting.

2   One case was analysed by both Korten and Paul: the Indian National Dairy Development Bank. In addition, Korten looked at the Sarvodaya Sharamadena Movement, the Bangladesh Rural Advance Committee, Thailand's community-based Family Planning Services, and the Philippine National Irrigation Administration's Communal Irrigation Programme; Paul examined the Philippine Rice Development Programme, Kenya's Smallholder Tea Development Programme, the Indonesian Population Programme, the Public Health Programme of China, and Mexico's Rural Education Programme.

3   It did, however, include preparation in terms of:

  i.   A review of pertinent social, economic and cultural studies;
  ii.   A review of literature on child development;
  iii. A survey of communities designed to corroborate the documentary research;
  iv.   Elaboration of documents, including a carefully conceived manual of operations.

4   The idea is now being given new life, but the approach is more gradual, the present effort can build on lessons of the past, and the economic circumstances are more promising than in 1983.

5   When the Janata Party fell from power, the programme did not continue. This does not, however, invalidate the principle. It does point, again, the importance of the political dimension.

6   The three examples and the basis for ideas presented in this section come from a presentation made by Carlos Castillo at the UNICEF Global Seminar on Early Childhood Development, held in Florence, Italy, from 12–30 June 1989 at the International Child Development Centre.

REFERENCES

Annis, S. 'An Information Revolution at the Grassroots: What it Means for the Poor', a paper prepared for the World Conference on Education for All, Jomtien, Thailand, March 4–8, 1990. Washington DC: the Overseas Development Council, 1990.

American Public Health Association. 'Progress and Problems, An Analysis of 52 AID-assisted Projects', Washington DC: APHA, 1982.

Cornia, G.A. 'A Cost Analysis of the Indonesian Experience with GOBI-FFF (1979–1982)', New York: UNICEF, 1983.

Gaspari, K.C. 'The Cost of Primary Health Care, A Report Prepared for USAID', Washington: USAID, December 1980.

'Going to Scale for Child Survival and Development', *Assignment Children*, 65/68 (1984), entire issue.

Korten, D. 'Community Organization and Rural Development: A Learning Process Approach', *Public Administration Review* (September/October 1980), pp. 480–511.

Korten, D. and R. Klaus (eds) *People-centred Development: Contributions toward Theory and Planning Frameworks*. W. Hartford, Conn.: Kumarian Press, 1990.

Myers, R. 'Going to Scale', a paper prepared for the Second Inter-Agency Meeting on Community-based Child Development, New York, October 29–31, 1984, UNICEF. September 1984. Mimeo.

Myers, R. 'Trip Report: Brazil, November 24–December 14, 1985', paper prepared for the Consultative Group on Early Childhood Care and Development, New York, January 1986.

Paul, S. *Managing Development Programs: The Lessons of Success*. Boulder, Colorado: Westview Press Inc., 1982.

Pyle, D. 'Life After Project (A Multi-Dimensional Analysis of Implementing Social Development Programs at the Community Level)', Boston: John Snow, Inc., 1984.

República de México, Secretaría de Educación Pública, Dirección General de Educación Inicial. 'Programa de Desarrollo del Niño de 0 a 5 Años a Traves de Padres de Familia y Miembros de la Comunidad', documento presentado al Taller Inter-Agencial sobre Evaluación y Costos de Programas del Preescolar en América Latina y el Caribe, Santiago de Chile, 17–22 de Octubre, 1983. Mimeo.

Taller de Cooperación al Desarrollo. *Una Puerta Que Se Abra. Los Organismos no Gubernamentales en la Cooperación al Desarrollo*. Santiago, Chile: Taller de Cooperación al Desarrollo, Marzo de 1989.

UNICEF. *Del Macetero al Potrero (o de lo micro a lo macro). El Aporte de la Sociedad Civil a las Political Sociales*. Santiago, Chile, 1986.

UNICEF. 'Strategies for Children in the 1990s', a UNICEF Policy Review. New York: UNICEF, May 1989.

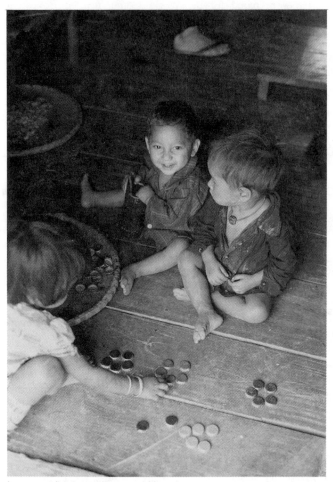
Low cost/high quality, rural Nepal

Chapter 15

Costs and resource mobilization[1]

What do ECD programmes cost?
Are there examples of cost-effective programmes?
Where will the resources come from?
Who will bear the costs?

In previous chapters we have presented a broad rationale for investing in early childhood care and development programmes, developing scientific, moral, social, and economic arguments. We have pointed to long-term benefits associated with early interventions and have shown that a variety of programmes can have measurable effects on children, families, communities and the larger society. We have shown that survival and development are fostered simultaneously through the interactions among health, nutrition and stimulation/education, making it desirable to incorporate psychosocial components into a health and nutrition programme or health and nutrition into a programme of early education. We have indicated that such programmes not only help children become more socially and economically productive adults, but also that they can free other family members, especially women and girls, to earn and learn. We have presented a range of possible approaches to helping enhance early childhood care, development and education and have provided specific programme examples, including examples of ways in which programmes can be combined.

In this chapter, we shall assume that the value of investing in early childhood has been recognized and accepted. We shall not spend a great deal of time reiterating earlier arguments about beneficial outcomes, but will focus instead on questions of costs and financing – as they relate, however, to outcomes. Costs will be approached first in this chapter by discussing orders of magnitude. Three examples of cost estimates for specific programmes will then be provided, followed by two more examples of studies illustrating cost effectiveness.

But the level of costs is only part of the issue. All programmes, whether high-cost or low-cost in concept and fact, and whether shown to be cost effective or not, require resources to begin and to continue functioning. Planners and programmers need to know where these resources will come from for programme expansion and improvement. They need to know what resources are currently being drawn upon and whether they can be extended or used more efficiently. They also need to know what resources are available but not being used, and what additional resources can be brought to the task. Above all, there is a need to examine how these resources can be organized and mobilized in the most effective and equitable way possible.

We shall argue that, in most cases, the ability to mobilize resources will be more important in determining the level of investment in programmes of early childhood care and development than the cost of a particular programme or a lack of resources. If a programme is really seen as a priority, resources will be identified and mobilized – even if that means reallocating them from another programme. Resource mobilization is as much a political process as an economic one. Decisions to seek greater programme efficiency, to allocate or reallocate funds within governmental or institutional budgets, and to seek additional revenues are linked to political concerns in most settings. Mobilizing family and community resources has its political side as well, requiring sensitivity to the real needs and burdens facing those who are asked to participate, avoiding overburdening them. Moreover, mobilization requires an ability to build partnerships.

In the following pages, several basic ideas will be elaborated:

1 Costs vary widely, depending on the programme goals and models chosen, as well as on the context and the method used to measure costs. Therefore it is not appropriate to make direct comparisons of costs across projects. Moreover, what seems to be a relatively high cost in one setting will not appear to be so high in another. Caution should be exercised when projecting orders of magnitude, even if this is done for specific programmes in specific contexts. It is probably best to make projections using several different sets of assumptions.

2 In seeking to keep costs low, it is important not to make them so low that potential effects are undermined. Indeed, the most basic point is not whether costs are low, but whether they are low in relation to desired outcomes.

3 Because early childhood development programmes usually have multiple outcomes and multiple beneficiaries, there is a general tendency to under-estimate benefits.

4 There are a number of promising ways in which the resources needed for expansion and improvement of early childhood programmes might be obtained, even within present resource constraints. These include:

   a. using existing resources more efficiently (i.e. cutting out waste from mismanagement);

b. combining the resources of existing sectoral programmes into a multifaceted programme, so as to take advantage of the synergisms among health, nutrition, education and/or other programme components;

c. coordinating disparate efforts to favour the young child within sectors (e.g. adult education and initial education, or health education with MCH);

d. changing the programme design, organization and/or technology to a less expensive one;

e. reallocating resources among or within sectors, for instance to initial education from within the education sector that will result in cost savings within the primary school level (mainly by reducing repetition), thereby offsetting the reallocation;

f. identifying dormant resources (e.g. buildings used only part-time; elderly who have time on their hands and want something meaningful to do; student time that is being employed in tasks of little social value).

5 Depending on the particular economic and political circumstances, it may be possible to increase resources through such means as payroll taxes or by legislating (or enforcing current legislation) with respect to employer responsibility for child-care programmes for employees.

6 Support and incentives can be provided by governments to the private (profit-making) sector, to non-governmental institutions operating in a non-profit way in the social sector, and to communities (e.g. funds on a matching basis, providing materials, linking programmes to the health system, etc.) to organize and run early childhood programmes for children living in conditions that put them at risk. This would help to create partnerships among governmental, non-governmental and community organizations.

7 Greater use can be made of existing channels of communication for both advocacy and education, at little or no extra cost.

8 Financing for extended and improved early childhood programmes does not need to depend on windfalls from, for instance, a 'peace dividend', or debt forgiveness. Should such funds become available, they should be pursued, but, as is evident from the listing of possible strategies above, investments in early childhood need not await them.

9 If international funds are sought, care should be exercised not to add significantly to the debt over-burden. Foreign assistance can have a role to play, but grants should be favoured over loans and the most favourable terms possible must be sought for loans. Such aid should be designed to help programmes get started and include a very strong training and capacity-building component. It needs to be selective so as to focus on children at risk, carefully phased, available over a sufficient period of time for a programme to take hold, and designed to support local initiatives (rather than imported solutions).

10 Families and communities may be called upon to contribute additional resources towards the care of their young children. However, in mobilizing these resources, which are considerable, it is important not to over-burden or exclude families that have few resources, thereby adding to an internal social debt. Equity considerations should be kept firmly in mind and the idea of partnership should not be lost.

COSTS OF EARLY CHILDHOOD PROGRAMMES: WHAT ARE THE ORDERS OF MAGNITUDE?

Answers to this question will be as varied as the programmes being carried out or considered. To seek an answer, programme goals and methods must first be specified. Because goals and methods are so different, it does not make sense to try to present one cost figure that would represent the order of magnitude for early childhood programmes generally, or that would be considered the cost of an average programme.

As we have tried to make clear throughout this book, by presenting a wide range of early childhood programme options, there are many kinds of programmes that complement each other. In Chapter 5, we suggested that, although the basic goal of any child development programme is to enhance the comprehensive development of young children, there are several possible approaches to this goal, only one of which takes as its goal direct changes in the child. Other programmes will affect the child indirectly, with their immediate focus on changing caregivers, the community, social institutions, or the broader beliefs that all affect a child's development. Even within each of these complementary approaches specific goals can differ a great deal.

Defining desired outcomes   A cost is always a cost of doing something. The desired outcome (goal) we choose for a programme can be more or less ambitious, more or less comprehensive. The choice will affect how programmes are organized and will affect the cost. It does not make sense, then, given programme differences in goals and methods, simply to compare the per person cost of one programme with the per person cost of another.

Sometimes, the early childhood development goal is defined simply in terms of *enrolment* in a programme, whether that be a programme for children or parents or community leaders or paediatricians. Or, the goal may be specified in terms of *outcomes* – what happens to the programme participant as a result of their enrolment. For the child, that might be narrowly defined in terms of a particular component of development (e.g. physical development related to change in nutritional status, or mental development as indicated by an IQ score or results on another test). Or, more comprehensive development may be the goal (as we have suggested it should be), including improvements in the physical, mental, social and emotional development. For parents, other family members, paediatricians, or traditional birth attendants, goals might be set in terms of *acquiring knowledge* or in terms of *changes in their childrearing behaviour.*

Multiple outcomes   Most of the time, the question of what we want to achieve in a programme is complicated by the fact that we have more than one goal. That is as it should be in a child development programme which starts from a holistic view of the child, which takes a multifaceted view of programming for child development, and which sees the development process as a result of interactions between the child and the surrounding environment. We want to improve the health and nutritional status of the child as well as her psychosocial well-being. We want to enhance productivity and solidarity. We want to reinforce cultural roots and foster the ability for adjustment to a changing world. And, programmes normally do have effects on more than one dimension of development.

Multiple beneficiaries   Children are seldom the only individuals who benefit from an early childhood development programme. Indeed, we have argued that the most successful programmes will be those that bring changes for both caregivers and children, and that also help to mobilize communities for continued action. Here, we are talking about effects that go beyond the ability of caregivers or others simply to help the child (or even the next child, as yet unborn). If caregivers and other community members benefit from a programme in ways that affect their lives directly (through better personal health, by improving family relationships, or by building up self-confidence, for instance), then costs should be judged also in relation to those effects. The denominator for calculating per unit costs should be greater than the number of children being reached through the programme. This is so, whether or not the programme specified desired outcomes for parents and others at the time a programme was set up.

One main implication of the above is that, because programmes have multiple outcomes and often have multiple beneficiaries, the benefits of early childhood programmes are often underestimated in relation to their costs. This will be so even if the several goals and beneficiaries have not been made explicit from the outset.

Choosing a programme option   Once programme goals have been determined, there are various ways of trying to achieve the desired outcome. To get to our destination, we can walk, purchase a bicycle or car, or take public transportation. What it will cost depends on the choice we make. At the same time, the choice we make will be affected by what we think it will cost, by what we have to spend (or can borrow or earn), by what technologies are available, and by what we think will work best under the particular conditions.

Within each of the five complementary programme approaches we have described (Chapter 5), a number of different models can be employed (examples were provided in Chapters 6 and 7). Within each model, choices can be made about the programme components to be included, the amount of time a child (or caregiver) is involved in the programme, the mix of professional and paraprofessional staff, the ratio of adults to children, the ratio of supervisors to immediate caregivers and teachers, the kind of training and the mix of in-service vs. pre-service, the choice of imported vs. locally made materials, etc.

The cost differences associated with these organizational and technological choices can be huge, even for the same early childhood model.[2] Imagine the difference, for instance, between day-care centres with the following characteristics:

	Programme A	*Programme B*
Hours per day	12	3
Days per week	6	5
Staffing	Professional	Paraprofessional
Ratio: caregiver/children	1/5	1/15
Ratio: supervisor/caregivers	1/10	1/20

Putting orders of magnitude in perspective   It is one thing to calculate actual or projected costs for a programme. It is another to judge whether these are high or low, affordable or not. To interpret cost figures, it helps to put the per unit cost figures for a programme in perspective in at least two ways: 1) in relation to indicators of the economic context in which a programme operates. This serves as a kind of proxy for ability to pay. 2) Costs should be related to the expected or actual effects of a programme.

To relate costs to the particular economic context in which they are incurred, costs are sometimes compared to: household income, the level of a minimum wage, the per capita GNP, or per capita expenditures by local, state and national governments. This comparative exercise is most useful at the extremes. If a programme cost per child is higher than a minimum salary, for instance, it will obviously not be a programme the poor can afford on their own. In such cases a judgement needs to be made about whether the benefits to individuals and to society at large make a public subsidy appropriate, without which those most at risk cannot possibly afford to participate (see the Perry Preschool project example later in this chapter). If the per capita programme cost is the same as the per capita expenditure by local state and national governments, or even the per capita expenditure in one sector (e.g. education), the programme must be regarded as too expensive to be considered seriously on a large scale (but might be considered on a very limited and targeted basis if effects were high). Conversely, if the programme cost is, let us say, one per cent of a minimum wage, it would seem to be affordable. What is not so clear is an intermediate ground. Does a ratio of 1 to 15 when comparing cost with a minimum wage indicate a high or low cost, relative to ability to pay?

A second way of putting cost figures in perspective is to relate them to measures of the effectiveness of a programme. If a per child cost of, let us say, $10.00 produces little or no effects, it is obviously not a good investment, no matter how affordable that level of expenditure might be. But if a cost of $150.00 per child produces a very large effect, it may be an excellent investment, even though it appears to be a relatively high cost. Accordingly, *the most basic question is not whether costs are high or low, but whether they are high or low in relation to outcomes.*

Against this background, and with the understanding that direct comparisons should not be made among programmes that have different goals and use different methods, we turn by way of illustration to three rough estimates of the costs of particular programmes. These examples provide some idea of orders of magnitude, but they cannot be generalized. Perhaps more important, the examples show how estimates can vary according to how they are calculated. In different ways, the three examples share a design as community-based and integrated programmes, including components of health, nutrition and education. In all three, paraprofessionals are central. However, the three also differ in specific goals, in scale, in programme organization and content, in the degree of actual community involvement, and the importance of a parental education component, as well as in their economic, political and cultural contexts.

1 India: The Integrated Child Development Service (ICDS)

The ICDS (described in Chapter 6, p. 103) is probably the largest-scale programme of integrated attention in the Third World, covering (in 1989) an estimated 11.2 million children, aged nought to six and two million pregnant and lactating women, all concentrated in rural, tribal and urban marginal groups. The programme design includes nutrition, health, and preschool education interventions for the children and education and referrals for the women. The paraprofessional who runs each local centre (Anganwadi) is trained (3 months initially, plus periodic refreshers) and is supported by a helper and a supervisor (a ratio of about 1 to 20).

One unofficial estimate of the cost to the federal and state governments of the ICDS programme, made in 1989, arrived at a figure of US$10.00 per child per year (see Hong 1989). This rough figure was made by taking the estimated total yearly cost to the national government per administrative block (US$67,670) and dividing it by the approximate number of children under age six in a block (17,000) to arrive at a figure of US$4.00 per child per year. But the national government covers only about 40 per cent of total governmental costs, the rest falling to the states. Adjusting the per child figure upwards to include the state costs gives the very rough figure of $10.00 per child per year.

Another way to arrive at a per child cost estimate for this programme is to look at the funds that were budgeted or expected from various sources in a given year and to divide them by the number of children actually enrolled in the programme. In 1989, approximately US$250,000,000 was budgeted for ICDS at national and state levels (approximately US$70,000,000 of this amount was estimated as originating with international organizations, and approximately one-half of it was for food aid). Taking the figure of 11.2 million children aged nought to six covered by the programme, we arrive at an estimate of about US$22.00 per child – more than double that reported above. The main reason for this difference is that less than 7,800 of the 17,000 children in an administrative block who are potential participants are actually enrolled in the programme; this reduced figure for coverage yields a higher per child cost. (Most of those not enrolled are children under age three.)

Not included in either of these estimates are the 'in kind' costs borne by families and communities. And, the calculation of per child costs leaves out approximately 2,000,000 women participating in the programme to whom some of the costs are directed. If they were included, the per person (rather than per child) cost estimate would be about $19.

Another estimate of costs reported for the ICDS programme makes a comparison with costs for comparable services with a nutrition monitoring and feeding programme carried out in the state of Tamil Nadu (the Tamil Nadu Integrated Nutrition Project – TINP). 'The annual per capita cost is Rs10 (or US$0.81), compared with RS18.4 (US$1.49) *for comparable services* in the ICDS' (Berg, p. x of the Author's Note, emphasis added). The problem with this comparison is that the services are not comparable. To set the two approaches against each other when they really should be viewed as complementary, and to make a cost comparison only with relation to the nutrition outcomes does not seem to be appropriate.

Suppose we accept the larger cost figure of $22 per child per year (or about $0.10 per day, assuming that the Anganwadis are operating 220 days per year) for the ICDS programme. Is this high or low for India? The daily minimum wage rate for the same period was about $1.50. Therefore, the per child cost of the programme amounts to about 1/15th of a minimum wage. Or, if we relate the $22 figure to the per capita GNP of $340 for India (1988), the Anganwadi cost is 1/15th of the per capita GNP.

In Chapters 6 and 10 we reported some positive outcomes of the ICDS programme, based on studies of nutritional status, health indicators, educational readiness and school participation and progress. In spite of its relatively low quality, the programme is effective at one level. These effects have not been converted into any kind of a monetary figure and so a cost–benefit ratio is not possible.

What may be most interesting about the ICDS case is that, among the many evaluations of the ICDS, one finds very little information about programme costs. And, although it may be that serious cost analyses and projections have been done internally of which we are not aware, it is striking that the programme has expanded to such a large size without more obvious attention to its cost effectiveness. This might suggest that the effects of the programme, as measured, have been judged to be adequate in relation to costs, so that more refined measures of cost effectiveness are not considered necessary. It might also suggest that political rather than economic forces drive the programme.

2 Peru: a non-formal programme of initial education (PRONOEI)

In 1984, an evaluation was carried out of a project designed to extend and improve a community-based non-formal preschool programme in Peru. The project covered approximately 2,000 villages and an estimated 60,000 children in four states. In the PRONOEI model, children aged three to five are gathered together in groups of about 25 to 30 for several hours four or five mornings most weeks of the year. The children participate in activities intended to improve their physical, mental and social development. The paraprofessional 'animators' who are in charge receive a short initial training of ten days to two weeks and periodic refresher training. The community is responsible for providing a place for the children to gather, for preparing the food, for selecting the 'animator', who is paid a gratuity but who is essentially serving the community, and for managing the PRONOEI.

The analysis of programme expenditures and costs carried out in 1984 produced an estimated per child per year cost of $40 (Myers *et al.* 1985). The estimate varied from $28 to $61 across the four states included in the analysis. This variation was related to the level of enrolment (apparently economies of scale were at work) and to the differential attention given in budgets to the community development component of the programme.

The $40 estimate per child included cost estimates for the value of donated resources from the community (estimated at 23 per cent of all costs). Thus, the calculation is different from that made for ICDS, where community contributions were not included. The estimate also included costs of income-generating activities in the community. If the income-earning activities are excluded, the cost of the PRONOEI programme drops to $38 per child per year. Of this figure, public sector funding covered $19, foreign assistance $11, and the community $10 (of non-monetary resources). If we focus on the monetary contributions from the government and from international sources, omitting the 'in kind' community contributions, the per child per year cost is $28.

Comparing the Peruvian cost of $28 with the prevailing minimum wage at the time of about \$2.00, the ratio of cost to minimum wage is 1 to 14. If, however, we make the comparison with the GNP per capita, the ratio is about 1 to 40.

The Peruvian evaluation found that participation in the PRONOEI project had significant effects on the development of children and their readiness for school. These effects did not, however, carry over into school in terms of lowered repetition, reflecting major problems of primary school quality, organization and management. The effects on nutritional status were found to be moderate and indirect, and to differ by project site. Community involvement and awareness was found to have increased as a result of the project.

The per child costs of the PRONOEI were found to be less than one-half the cost of a formal preschool centre. We have argued, however, that such comparisons are spurious. We do not have comparable measures of the results of participation by children in the formal centres. Moreover, the goals of the two preschool programmes were different – with the PRONOEI programme explicitly including elements of community development and taking a broader child development view than the narrower attention to preparation for school characterizing the formal programme.

3 Chile: the parents and children project (PPH)

The PPH programme, described as an example of community-based parental education in Chapter 7, is a much smaller-scale programme than the Indian or Peruvian ones, reaching only 50 communities at the time an evaluation was carried out in 1984. This cultural action programme was developed and implemented by a non-governmental research and action organization working closely with a local radio station operated by the Catholic church. The general and interrelated objectives of PPH are: 1) enhanced child development, 2) personal growth of adults, and 3) community organization.

To achieve its goals, weekly meetings are organized in participating communities at which discussions are held related to living with and bringing up children. The discussions are stimulated by pictures and questions asked by locally selected coordinators (two per village) and by radio transmissions heard by the group. The process is supported by ten general coordinators who train, visit villages and help prepare and present radio dramas, by manuals, and by worksheets that parents take home for their children. The content of discussions deals with helping children to learn to talk, read and count, with human relations in the family, alcoholism, nutrition and how to make the best of food supplies, food preservation and sex education.

The programme evaluation showed positive effects on the children, their parents and on the community at large (Richards 1985). These results are described in Chapters 7 (p. 140) and 10 (Table 10.4, p. 246). Children participating in PPH scored better on readiness tests and did better in school than those who did not participate. Changes occurred in adult attitudes and perceptions and community organization was fostered, as indicated by a long list of constructive activities.

The annual cost per child was calculated at US$77. This calculation did not include the resources, mostly time, donated by the community, under the assumption that those who donated their time were benefiting from their involvement and it was therefore inappropriate to count their time as a cost. In some cases, the time used was not taken from any productive activity and was, in a sense, unused time. Nor did the estimate include the technical assistance from the NGO (considered to be a 'sunk cost' and not part of the ongoing operation of the programme). Nor did it include an estimate for powdered milk donated by Caritas (and distributed by PPH) nor the donated air time of the radio station. Had these costs been included, the estimate would have increased considerably.

The ratio of the estimated cost of $77 per child per year to a minimum wage (using the Minimum Employment Programme figure) at the time was approximately 1 to 5. The ratio of cost to the GNP per capita was approximately 1 to 18. The cost of a high-quality kindergarten was estimated at six times the PPH cost and the cost of a low-quality day-care centre was double the PPH cost.

If the cost calculation was made on a per person basis, including adults in the community who benefited from the programme as well as children, the cost of the programme was only $19 per person per year. (In this case, however, it would probably be appropriate to include an estimate for the community costs and the figure would rise somewhat.)

In the three studies presented above, no attempt was made to establish a direct monetary comparison between costs and benefits. In each programme, outcomes were evaluated, and each programme could claim to be effective at a certain level and with respect to certain outcomes. Each programme could claim to be less expensive than a more formal preschool alternative, even though each took a broader view of child development, including nutrition and health components as well as educational components. Lacking a direct comparison or a rate of return, then, the planner or policymaker who wishes to be guided by economic criteria is left to make a personal interpretation regarding whether or not the outcomes outweigh the cost.

TWO COST–BENEFIT EXAMPLES

We now present two programme evaluations in which such a comparison of costs and benefits in monetary terms was made, one from Brazil, the other from the United States. In the Brazilian example, the calculation is fairly simple; the financial benefit lies in the cost savings (primarily in teachers' salaries) associated with the reduction of repetition during the first year of primary school. This is a calculation that is within the realm of possibility for most planners and it uses data that can be obtained fairly easily. The second example is based on a more sophisticated study tracing individual children over 15 years after leaving a preschool programme. The calculation of costs and benefits was more inclusive. This second study is probably the only study of its kind and is not easily repeated, but it provides an enlightening perspective on the relationship between costs and potential benefits of early childhood programmes over time.

4 Brazil: the preschool feeding project (PROAPE)

PROAPE, described briefly in Chapter 6, was conceived as a strategy for reducing malnutrition among Brazilian preschoolers living in marginal economic conditions in urban areas. The general goals of the project were broad, including improved nutritional status and the psychomotor, cognitive and social development of preschoolers.

In the PROAPE model, children aged four to six were brought together in centres during weekday mornings in groups of about 100 children for supervised psychomotor activities and a snack. A health component, involving immunizations, dental care, visual examinations, and hygiene was also included. Children were attended by a combination of trained personnel and participating family members, on a rotating basis. In the original model, one certified professional was assisted by six community members.

The PROAPE programme can be called community-based in the sense that paraprofessionals came from the local community, family members helped out in the programme, and the locale was often donated by the community. However, control over the programme did not lie with the community. The programme did help to converge services on a particular population of children thought to be in need, by bringing together nutrition, health and education components.

The prototype for PROAPE was a pilot programme carried out in the city of Sao Paulo. An evaluation of that programme suggested that school performance scores were better and repetition rates were lower among programme children than among those who did not participate. The programme was then taken into the north-east of Brazil where it was tried out in the state of Pernambuco. Subsequently, it was extended to 10 states. One programme evaluation showed that, 'The measured impact of PROAPE itself on physical growth was only marginal, but evaluations showed that 73.5 per cent of former PROAPE participants got passing grades in the first and second years of elementary school, compared with

59.5 per cent in a group that did not participate. And the academic performance of children with two years of exposure to PROAPE was consistently better than that of the non-participating group, ranging from 2 to 21 per cent in three variations of the model' (Berg, p. 20).

In 1980, a study was made of the cost effectiveness of the PROAPE programme, comparing 22,298 first grade PROAPE entrants with 22,298 non-PROAPE entrants to first grade, then following them to second grade. This study concluded that:

> The total cost of schooling (including preschool PROAPE services) per second-grade graduate was about (US$50.00 (or 11 per cent) less for students who had been in the PROAPE programme than for those who had not been in PROAPE.

(Berg, p. 58)

Yet another evaluation was carried out in the state of Alagoas, one of the states to which the programme was extended and where adjustments had been made. In the Alagoas variant of PROAPE, centres were run by three trained paraprofessionals who received help from parents. The paraprofessionals were paid 70 per cent of a minimum salary for their morning's work. The programme was carried out in locations donated by the community. Supplementary feeding consisted of a glass of milk, and bread with jelly and margarine. As in other programmes, health support was also provided to the programme.

Table 15.1 presents primary school data for children who participated 1) in PROAPE, 2) in an alternative form of preschool called a Casulo, or 3) formal kindergartens, and similar information for 4) children who did not participate in any preschool experience. The table shows that 73 and 76 per cent of the PROAPE and Casulo children, respectively, passed the first grade in 1982, as compared with only 63 per cent of the formal kindergarten children, and 53 per cent of those without a preschool experience. Only 9 per cent of the PROAPE children actually failed (vs. 16 per cent for the Casulo, 28 per cent for kindergarten, and 33 per cent for non-preschool children). This is so despite the fact that the PROAPE children attended for only 78 days as compared with a 180-day period for Casulo children and a 2-year programme for kindergarten children. The cost per child for the programme was estimated at US$28. (The ratio of this cost to the minimum wage at the time was approximately 1 to 2.)

Using Table 15.1, and knowing the cost per child per year for PROAPE ($28) and the cost per pupil per year for the first grade of primary school ($205), we can make an interesting calculation. Let us assume that all 27 per cent of the PROAPE children who did not complete the first grade in one year, as indicated in Table 15.1, will repeat the year and will pass on the second try. Let us make the same very conservative assumption for the 47 per cent of children without any preschool experience. Then the per

Table 15.1 A comparison of academic performance of children in the first year
of primary school, with and without preschool: the PROAPE
programme, Alagoas, Brazil*

	PROAPE		Casulo		Jardim** Infantil		Children without preschool education	
	No	%	No	%	No	%	No	%
Registered children	184	100	557	100	320	100	2,334	100
Children remaining								
until year end	150	82	517	92	291	91	2,000	86
Dropouts	34	18	40	8	29	9	334	14
Passed	134	73	426	76	201	63	1,245	53
Failed	16	9	91	16	90	28	755	33

*Source: Ministerio da Saude y Instituto Nacional de Alimentação e Nutrição, 'Analição do
PROAPE/Alagoas com enfoque na area ecônomica', Brasilia, MS/INAN, 1983. Mimeo.
(Data come from supervisors of schools with children from preschool projects in 1982.)
**Prior to their primary school, early intervention programmes attended to children for
different lengths of time: PROAPE, 78 days; Casulo, 180 days; Jardim Infantil, 540 days.

child cost to complete first grade for a PROAPE child would be $260
($205 per year × 1.27 years), and the cost for a child without preschool
experience would be $301 ($205 × 1.47). That means the average cost per
child of producing a first grade graduate is *at least* $41 less for PROAPE
children than for children without preschooling. This per child saving is
higher than the PROAPE cost figure of $28. *In these terms, the PROAPE
programme not only paid for itself but resulted in a primary school cost
saving in the first year over and above the cost of PROAPE.*

The effectiveness of the PROAPE model is confirmed by a more
detailed micro-level study of various preschool options carried out in 1983
(Ciavatta-Franco) in which the author concluded that '... PROAPE
constitutes an equalizing and efficient preschool education at low cost'
(p. 116). Apparently, PROAPE was able to achieve a combination of
modest resources and some quality control.

The point of presenting these data is not to argue for indiscriminate
replication of the PROAPE model, but rather to show that it is possible to
achieve cost savings in the primary school through an investment in a preschool programme that pays for itself and more.

The evaluation of PROAPE focused on the children and on their subsequent performance in school. Attention was not given to possible effects on
the participating parents and on the broader community. Indeed, the
programme was not conceived as part of a broader community development programme even though it can be called community-based. If poten-

tial benefits occurred at this level, the programme would be an even better investment.

In what must be more than a postscript to the above presentation, we must note that the PROAPE programme is no longer functioning, in spite of the seemingly positive results of the programme viewed as an investment in children. One explanation that has been given for the programme's demise is that it was formalized out of existence. The Ministry of Education which took a leading role in the programme did not easily incorporate a non-formal alternative into its operations and slowly adapted the non-formal community-based model to a more formal preschool, creating formal preschool classrooms of 30 children each with a trained preschool teacher. Undoubtedly there are other explanations that may have more to do with political changes than with bureaucratic perspectives. But the basic point to be made is that reasons other than favourable cost-benefit ratios proved more important in determining the continuity of the programme.

5 United States: The Perry Preschool Project

Effects of this combined preschool and home visiting project for lower-income children were reported in Chapter 10 (p. 227). We noted that children participating in the project who were followed up at age 19 were more likely than a comparison group to have graduated from high school and obtained employment, and were less likely to require remedial attention in school, be in trouble with the law, become pregnant while a teenager, or receive welfare payments (Berruta-Clement et al. 1984).

As part of the follow-up evaluation at age 19, a cost–benefit study was carried out (Barnett 1985). The study was done from the viewpoint of costs and benefits to society and a serious effort was made to estimate in monetary terms some of the benefits to society that are mentioned above. At the same time, the results are interesting because they allow a comparison of social and individual perspectives with respect to costs and benefits.

The following costs were included (see Table 15.2) in the analysis:

1 Programme costs, including instruction, administration and support staff, overhead, supplies, psychological screening, and capital costs (interest and depreciation).
2 Additional educational costs incurred as a result of increased demand for education (project children stayed in school longer).

Benefits were defined both in terms of cost savings and in terms of increased economic productivity over a lifetime. Cost savings were identified related to:

- Child-care savings;
- Reduced school costs due to less remedial education;

Table 15.2 Summary and distribution of costs and benefits, the Perry Preschool
Programme, for one year of preschool*

Type of benefit or cost	Total	Benefit or cost** (in US dollars)	
		For preschool participants	For taxpayers and citizens
Measured			
Presch. programme	−4,818	0	−4,818
Child care	290	290	0
Education, K-12	5,113	482	5,113
Welfare at age 19	642	546	161***
Crime thru age 20	1,233	0	1,233
Predicted			
College†	−704	0	−704
Earnings after 19	23,813	19,233	4,580
Welfare after 19	1,438	−14,377	15,815
Crime after 20	1,871	0	1,871
Net benefits††	28,933	5,082	23,852
Benefit-cost ratio = 7			

Source: Berruta-Clement *et al. Changed Lives, the Effects of the Perry School Program on Youths through Age 19.* Ypsilanti, Michigan: The High/Scope Press, 1984. Combined information from Tables 26 and 28, pp. 90 and 91.
*Table entries are present values in constant 1981 dollars (US), discounted at 3 per cent annually. (The use of a 3 per cent discount rate may seem low. However, it should be remembered that time 0 in this study is 1962. Had a higher discount rate been used, the fundamental conclusion of the study would not change because the same rate would be applied to both earnings and welfare savings.)
**Costs are indicated as negative amounts.
***Assume 25 per cent of estimated earnings is paid in taxes.
†Some college costs are undoubtedly borne by the participants and their families, but there is no estimate for that amount. The most conservative assumption towards increasing the relative benefits of participants was to assign all college costs to the taxpayer.
††Column figures may not sum to net benefits due to rounding.

−   Savings in welfare expenditures; and
−   Savings through reductions in crime and deliquency (and consequently in costs associated with prosecution, rehabilitation, and time in prisons).

Increased earnings – actual earnings figures were used for ages 16 to 19 (data collected in a longitudinal follow-up of children to age 19) and earnings differences were projected after age 19, using age–earnings profiles for different levels of schooling attained.
    The cost–benefit study suggests that:

1 *The benefit-to-cost ratio for a preschool programme can be high.* As indicated in Table 15.2, the ratio was 7 to 1, indicating a very high pay-off.

2 *Even a high-cost early intervention programme can be socially beneficial.* Note that the original cost of the programme alone was US$4,818 per child for one year. The ratio of this cost to per capita GNP was about 1 to 3 and was almost as high as the minimum wage at the time.

3 *The bulk of the benefits accrues to taxpayers and citizens rather than to the individual programme participants* or their families. When the amount of money that participants 'lose' by not participating in welfare is subtracted out from the extra amount they are able to earn, the difference is relatively small ($5082), just managing to offset the programme costs. The benefits to taxpayers from various forms of cost savings are, however, dramatic. This finding argues strongly for public subsidy of such programmes. The private incentive to invest is not strong and the disadvantaged economic position of poor families makes it unlikely they would make the initial investment required for participation in a programme of as high quality as the Perry project. In other words, the demand for the programme would not be very high if individuals had to pay for the programme, even though the social benefits are high.

4 The study shows that *it is useful to look at a range of possible effects of early intervention programmes* and to try to estimate the monetary benefit associated with the effect. This goes well beyond estimating productivity gains, as indexed by increases in earnings.

The cost–benefit findings from the Perry project serve as a point of departure only. As indicated in Chapter 10, generalizing these results to the Third World is not appropriate, given the major differences one might expect to find between children in a small city in Michigan and children in urban or rural areas of most parts of the Third World. Their nutritional and health status will be different, as will the educational backgrounds of their parents, the exposure to television and written materials, the quality of the primary schools and the welfare structure helping to buffer effects of poverty for some families. However, following the Perry project example, it is possible to imagine benefits or cost savings that are pertinent to particular settings in the Third World (e.g. reduced repetition or reduced health costs). And it is possible to think that estimates could be made of some of these as was done, for instance, in the Brazilian case.

Having provided some examples of cost magnitudes and cost–benefit calculations, we turn now to questions of financing. Before doing so, it is important to mention that we would like to have included examples of cost calculations for child development programmes in which an education or psychosocial component is incorporated into a nutrition or health programme (in a sense, this was the case for PROAPE which began as a nutrition programme but became an education programme). Although it is not too difficult to find studies relating the cost of health or nutritional services to health or nutritional outcomes or studies relating nutritional interventions to psychosocial outcomes (see Chapters 9 and 10), cost calculations and corresponding outcomes for health and nutritional programmes explicitly incorporating a psychosocial component were not found.

PROGRAMME FINANCING: WHO SHARES THE COST BURDEN?

Support for early childhood development programmes, as others, comes from a variety of sources. These include: 1) governments, 2) international funders, 3) non-governmental organizations (with a social bias and operating on a non-profit basis), 4) the profit-making private sector, 5) community organizations and 6) programme participants. The resources that each of these can provide are different, and different factors influence the ability of each to make the resources available. The total amount of funding and other resources that are available for programmes of care and development will be the sum of what is provided by all of these sources.

Governments

The total amount that a government can mobilize for care and development depends on the size of its budget and on the way allocations are made among and within sectors. Governmental revenues will be affected by the level of economic activity and the rates of economic growth and inflation. In many cases, these factors are determined as much by external factors (such as the world price for coffee or oil and other terms of trade, the world economic climate, war, the level of indebtedness) as they are by internal factors (such as the pricing, employment, monetary, taxation and social investment policies and the credibility or control of the government). With such an array of determinants, it is clear that no easy generalizations are possible about the ability of particular governments to provide funds at particular times.

In today's world, both debt repayment and military expenditures weigh heavily against the ability to pay for social programmes within education, health, argicultural, or others that might be considered early childhood development programmes. We do not lack dramatic analyses of the declining resources available through the public sector and the sad results that this trend has brought in the areas of health and education and of the need for 'adjustments' in expenditures that will be humane as well as economically justified (Cornia *et al.* 1987; Berstecher and Carr-Hill 1990). At the same time, there is a grand hope that debt repurchasing and a peace dividend will free up funds for social purposes, increasing markedly the ability to pay. Should that happen, and new funds become available, every effort should be made to see that part of those funds is directed towards 'the twelve who survive' and their development.

Even if funds did become available, however, a more basic question would still remain. How would the new funds be distributed? To capture these resources for early childhood development would require, in most countries, an important reorientation in thinking. *In the last analysis, the ability to pay is as much a matter of priorities that determine the distribution of funds as it is the availability of funds.* That is so for existing budgets as well as for hoped-for new resources. If a high enough priority is given to early childhood development, funds can be shifted from other programmes to cover the costs, even within the limited resources available.

Four examples will help to demonstrate that, with political will, resources can be found for programmes, even under conditions of relative resource scarcity.

–   By making ICDS one of her 'Twenty Points', Indira Gandhi gave priority to early childhood development. The result has been the large-scale programme described above, in a country where the GNP per capita is relatively low.
–   North Korea has established child-care centres and preschool pro-grammes for the majority of its children because a high priority has been given. The rationale is partly an economic one, based on the assumption that women should participate fully in the labour force and that child care is therefore needed. But the rationale is partly political, linked to a recognition, present in various socialist societies, that creating the 'new man' must begin with creating the 'new child'.
–   In Mexico, during the period from 1982 to 1988, the rate of coverage of children aged three to five in preschool programmes, most of which are government subsidized, grew at a rate of 9 per cent per year. This occurred in a country with, at the time, one of the most pressing debt problems in the world. This growth was possible in part because the base from which the growth began was low; nevertheless the increase suggests that priority was given to the area and occurred because funds were appropriated that could have been used for other purposes.
–   In Colombia, the government has committed itself to a major early childhood programme of home day care, to complement an existing programme of more formal Centers for Integrated Attention to Pre-schoolers. Although the groundwork for this initiative was set over time by technicians, the decision to move ahead on a large scale was a political decision at a presidential level. The two programmes are financed in the main by a payroll tax, recently increased to help cover costs.

Although there is a tendency to focus on the budgets of national govern-ments, state or municipal governments often play an important part in the financing of early childhood programmes. In the Indian ICDS case, for instance, state governments fund about 60 per cent of the monetary costs. In Brazil, most of the public funding for child care comes from municipal and state governments.

Because child development is integral, crossing bureaucratic lines, significant portions of programme resources for development are available through government and other programmes of health and nutrition. These programmes are not labelled as early childhood or child care or preschool or initial education. Often missing is the integration into such programmes of a mental and social development component. Recognizing that health and nutrition programmes are making a contribution to child development should not give a government an excuse for failing to broaden and to integrate its investments in the mental and social, as well as the physical, development of its children. The presence of these disparate programmes provides a base for integrated actions that can increase effectiveness for all of them and need not, therefore, add significantly to costs. It might even reduce them.

International assistance

In general, international assistance provides only a small percentage of the total resources for child-care and development programmes that include an educational or psychosocial component. However, if assistance through supplementary feeding programmes linked to some sort of early education programme is included, or if a particular project or programme is examined, the percentage can rise significantly. This was so in the Indian ICDS case (where about 28 per cent of the ICDS support was estimated to come from international sources), the Peruvian PRONOEI project (29 per cent if community contributions are included in total costs and 37 per cent if these are excluded), and the Brazilian PROAPE programme (which was originally funded through a World Bank loan). International resources are often provided to cover start-up costs such as the construction of buildings, the purchase of equipment (furniture or refrigerators or vehicles to facilitate supervision), or the training (retraining) of staff at various levels. Another form of support is technical cooperation, often in conjunction with pilot or demonstration projects.

If attention is focused on programmes that emphasize a child's mental and social and educational development or that incorporate a psychosocial component into health or nutrition programmes, the flow of international funding was barely visible in the 1980s. The largest institutions – development banks and bilateral agencies – rarely supported such programmes. Some assistance was provided through UNICEF, international non-governmental organizations (the Alliance of Save the Children, Foster Parents Plan, and others) or through private philanthropic initiatives (such as the Bernard van Leer Foundation). Although these organizations may provide a significant amount of money for early childhood each year, the funds are spread out over a large number of countries and projects and constitute a small proportion of the resources available in any one country.

A recent survey by UNESCO, including questions about sources of funding for early childhood education programmes, concluded that the main sources of assistance had been through UNICEF and 'in kind' donations of food, mostly through the World Food Organization. Further, bilateral aid was on the decline and 'the days of philanthropy seem to be over' (Fisher 1990).

When ten international funding organizations[3] were asked by the author in 1990 to provide information about their support for programmes of early childhood education and development, the clear conclusion was that such support was a minor part of overall operations (Myers 1990). Moreover, the absolute amount of support reported for 1989 was, with three exceptions, less than US$5,000,000 and in most cases it was less than US$1,000,000 for the entire year and for all the countries receiving funding. Moreover, funding was directed almost exclusively to support small experimental initiatives.

In brief, during the 1980s, international assistance for early childhood care and development with an educational and psychosocial dimension was weak and, with exceptions, focused on small-scale pilot or demonstration initiatives. There is some evidence that this is changing slowly in the 1990s, but international assistance still constitutes a relatively small percentage of the total resources available. One might argue that this ought to be the case, given the large debt burden of many countries. Still, international resources can have an important role to play to help get programmes started.

Resources from non-governmental organizations

A proper accounting has not been done of resources made available for early childhood care and development through not-for-profit, non-governmental organizations operating in the social sector. (We will treat community and grassroots organizations separately below even though they might be included under this heading and are often allied with national or international non-governmental organizations.) There is a growing impression, however, that an important source of resources lies with church-related organizations (e.g. the Sarvodaya Movement in Sri Lanka), major women's organizations (e.g. SEWA in India), national NGOs (e.g. BRAC in Bangladesh), national organizations affiliated with major international NGOs, or youth organizations such as the scouts and the girl guides. These organizations are often able to contribute time and energy and organizational capacity in addition to funds.

Given these NGO contributions, it would be a mistake to focus our analysis too narrowly on governmental or international funding when thinking about resources available for early childhood care and development programmes. We have argued that governments should seek to work in partnership with NGOs (as well as with communities and organizations in the private sector) in the task of mobilizing resources. We have also argued that this requires a vision of scale that does not focus on extending one particular programme model but, rather, envisions scale as the result of putting together the outcomes of many projects and programmes run by different organizations which may differ in their coverage and methods, but are part of a common cause of improving the early development of children.

Private industry and entrepreneurship

In many countries laws are on the books that require businesses employing over a certain number of people to provide child care for their employees. These laws are often disregarded and unenforced. Moreover, child care 'on site' is not always the best form of child care, as we indicated in Chapter 11. And child-care laws can lead to discrimination against women in hiring. Accordingly, mobilizing resources from businesses in the private sector, while potentially important, must be undertaken with careful attention to the possible negative side effects that could arise.

Mandated child care is not, however, the only way in which private resources might be mobilized. We have mentioned, for instance, the payroll tax that the Colombian government has legislated. This tax allows child care to occur in neighbourhoods instead of at the company site. It also makes child care available for families whose members work in the non-formal sector and who would not be eligible for programmes that companies provide for their employees. In a sense it serves a redistributive function.

Another set of strategies that can be used to mobilize resources from the private sector does not involve direct support for child care nor does it necessarily involve direct financial outlays. We encountered examples of companies that have been willing to allow their employees time during working hours for educational programmes (e.g. Kağitçibaşi *et al.* 1987). To the extent this strategy results in lost production, there is obviously a financial cost to the company. However, if the small amount of 'released time' results in more motivated employees who work better and on a more regular basis, they may pay for themselves.

Companies can be involved in advocacy activities as well. Match companies or large companies producing beverages, for instance, can incorporate information about particular programmes in their labelling and/or publicity. Electricity companies or others that have an extensive system of billing that reaches beyond the middle class can incorporate information into that system. These strategies have been used successfully in some locations.

Another way to mobilize private resources is to provide incentives for companies or individuals to establish philanthropic organizations providing funds for early childhood development.

Finally, child care and integrated attention to young children can itself be an entrepreneurial activity. In major cities throughout the world, private kindergartens and child-care centres abound, but these are usually run by the middle class for children of the middle class. In some countries, private nurseries, kindergartens, and day-care businesses constitute the main means of capturing resources for early childhood. Unfortunately, that means that attention is provided only to those children whose families have the ability to pay. Where this is the case, early childhood programmes reinforce social divisions and inequalities. To the extent that a government allows such enterprises to develop, without taking complementary action to help those most in need, it encourages social inequality rather than working to counteract it.

In partnership, however, it is possible to imagine similar centres that are run by and cater to families with scarce resources, as in the home day-care programme of Colombia. Governments can provide training, including training in how to organize and manage a small enterprise, and can help to subsidize those who attend, perhaps using a sliding scale related to the ability of participating families to pay.

Family and community resources

In this section, we will concentrate on family and community resources that are not channelled through the government (by paying taxes) or through payments to entrepreneurs, but are, rather, captured through direct application, either in the home or by participation in various forms in community programmes. These resources may be monetary resources, but are more likely to be donations of time and materials. The value of the time donations will be related to the levels of education, health and nutrition, and the childrearing experience (sometimes collective wisdom rather than individual experience) of the participants.

These family and community resources are substantial, and they can almost always be called upon more effectively than is done at present. A small initial investment in support and/or education of parents, for instance, may release these resources for direct use in the home in new ways, or by reinforcing waning practices. Calling on the volunteer spirit of community members can allow programmes to operate that would not otherwise function, for lack of resources. Increasingly, this is the hope of governments and other organizations which view community participation in an instrumental and cost-cutting way.

In many projects and programmes, costs are shared between the various sources described above and local resources provided by communities and families. In the PRONOEI case described above, somewhere between 20 and 50 per cent of the project costs were estimated as borne by the community, with variations from year to year. If we concentrate on recurrent costs rather than total (including capital) costs, the proportion borne by the community is even higher because most is in the form of volunteer work covering the recurrent cost of the project's human resources. This is not a budgetary cost, but it is a cost nevertheless and programmes could not operate unless this contribution of resources was made.

But this approach to, and hope of, capturing community resources for early childhood must be put in perspective. This is because community contributions may already be running at a relatively high level, but may be 'invisible' in budgetary terms. Efforts to place even more responsibility for projects through community financing or by charging user fees to recover costs can backfire. This is not an all-or-nothing comment; there are certainly communities in which some level of payment can be expected, as we suggested above in relation to entrepreneurial programmes of care and education. However, one result of this strategy may be to increase the community share in those communities that have a better economic base while making programmes inaccessible to poorer communities (or families) where the need may be greater. Thus, the community emphasis would undercut the potential redistributive role of the government. Another result may be that women are assigned greater burdens, adding to their already overburdened schedules and their ills.

What can be done?

We have looked at resource mobilization from the standpoint of potential contributors. Now let us focus on strategies. In so doing, it should be clear that, although we have taken a cautious position with respect to the appearance of windfalls from debt reduction or a peace dividend, this position should not discourage the reader. As has been suggested above in relation to different possible sources of support, a range of strategies can be pursued to mobilize resources for expanded and improved programmes of early childhood development. These include strategies for better use of existing resources, and strategies for obtaining new resources.

Using existing resources

Being more efficient

Cut out waste   If the management of existing resources is tightened, funds and resources will be released that can be used for extending or upgrading the programme. This may mean introducing better systems of accountability. It may mean making difficult political decisions regarding the basis for the selection of personnel (with a shift from political reward towards merit and motivation). It may mean seeking ways to cut down inattendance so that children receive the full benefit from the existing programme. It may mean seeing that preschool teachers or animators are present when they are supposed to be.

Focus   Being more efficient may require 'targeting' of resources. This process of focusing may reduce the total number of individuals involved so that efforts may be concentrated on those who are really in need – even if this means raising the per person cost, it is likely to result in greater benefits. Targeting may also be combined with changes in the model used to reach different groups, making the total process more efficient, not by extending one model more widely, but by displaying flexibility that is needed when faced by varying situations (e.g. concentrated vs. dispersed populations).

Combine   We have suggested throughout this book that a combined approach to programming will allow one to take advantage of synergisms among the various programme lines, leading to a better result with the same, or perhaps lower, cost. We have also indicated how difficult this is to do. Nevertheless, concrete suggestions have been offered in Chapters 9, 10, and 11, based on programme experiences in which health and nutrition have been combined with attention to psychosocial well-being, on an analysis of ways in which women-in-development programmes may be combined with child care (and child care with child development), and on suggestions for relating early interventions to primary schooling.

The combination of programmes may occur by adding components within an existing infrastructure. For instance, check-ups occurring through a primary health care centre (or through the health system in general) may provide the opportunity for screening children for mental as well as physical problems, and can provide the occasion for education of parents. In this case, the level of costs may increase and some new resources may be necessary, but by using existing infrastructure and phasing in (care must be exercised not to overburden people with too many duties at once) an additional component of child development, the cost increases can be relatively minor.

Adopting less costly programme design/technology

For some people, this strategy is really part of the process of trying to use resources more efficiently. Here, however, the emphasis is on changing the technology and organization rather than making the existing technology work more efficiently. It is the equivalent of changing from a car to a bicycle to reduce costs, as compared with tuning the motor of the car to make it run more efficiently.

Most cost-cutting (and the associated liberating of funds) is related to a change in project design, organization, and/or technology. The main cost item for most social and educational programmes, including early childhood programmes, is the cost, or value of, the time of people who make the programme function – the child minders/teachers, supervisors and managers, and, depending on the breadth of the programme, the health personnel, community organizers, nutritionists, cooks, etc. That seems to be the case, whether we think in terms of attending children in centres, of educating caregivers, or of promoting community development as the main programme approach. It is not surprising, then, that so much attention in alternative programmes has been given to the role of paraprofessionals and/or volunteers.

In any programme there will, of course, be costs of materials, equipment, and dwellings as well, but normally these will be a minor portion of total costs and an even smaller portion of recurrent costs. Even in a parental education programme using television, there will be significant, if somewhat lower, human resource costs in terms of the time spent by those who produce the programme (and the parents who listen to it).

Recognizing the central importance of human resource costs, cost-conscious planners are led to seek ways of reducing that lion's share of costs. Among the methods used are:

- Spreading out the human resource cost by changing the number of children per person (e.g. changing the ratio of children to caregiver from 6:1 to 10:1 or 15:1);
- Reducing the intensity of the programme by cutting back on the hours worked (e.g. from a 4-hour to a 3-hour morning, or from 5 to 4 days a week);
- Substituting human resources with a lower market value (e.g. paraprofessionals or untrained mothers as assistants);
- Substituting technology for people (e.g. a television in place of home visits).

As these changes of technology and organization are considered, it is important not to be carried away by the marvels of the mass media on one hand, or the romantic notion that an ordinary mother is, simply by virtue of her experience, a good person to run a neighbourhood home day-care centre in her home. These, and other options, need to be put in perspective and their effect on desired outcomes needs to be kept very much in mind. The risks of impersonalizing and of seeking low costs for their own sake must be avoided.

In the above listing we have not included the cost-cutting strategy of seeking volunteer labour. We have not done so because the time of volunteers should also be valued. This strategy, although representing a cost reduction for a government, really represents a redistribution of the cost burden from governments to local individuals. This may be feasible and is not necessarily bad. Indeed, it may build participation and solidarity. But, strictly speaking, it does not produce a reduction of social costs, unless the volunteers are either less qualified individuals whose market value is lower or are individuals with considerable leisure time as is sometimes the case with retirees. We have noted elsewhere that the use of volunteers may be successful for several years but that the motivation that originally drove individuals may be difficult to maintain. That has been shown to be the case in many non-formal programmes and can be a threat to sustainability of a programme.

Calling upon unutilized/underutilized resources

It is common for early childhood programmes to be carried out in locations that are not being used in a community, or which have a part-time use – churches, community centres, vacant rooms in a school or space in a school outside of school hours, etc. It is also possible to call on individuals whose human resources are not being utilized, or who are underutilized. There is an increasing recognition that retired individuals or grandparents may not only be capable caregivers with experience, but also benefit personally from continuing contact with young children. In China, for instance, retirement homes are now being built next to early childhood centres.

Transferring resources

Within a sector   It may be unrealistic to think that any major transfer of resources can be made among programmes within a sector. Only in unusual circumstances (Chile in the 1980s) does one find examples of a conscious and enforced decision to, for instance, transfer funds from higher education to early childhood development.

However, the current budgets for child care and initial education are so low, proportionately, to other programmes within the social sector or within education, that a small transfer has the potential of making an important difference. Indeed, the transfer might be made over time as current resources in, let us say, higher education are held steady while new resources are assigned to the early years.

Among sectors   In recent years, and within the framework of structural adjustments, there has been increasing attention to maintaining (or increasing) resources available to social sector programmes while reducing expenditures for such programmes as defence. This reallocation could also be a source of revenue. Again, vested interests make such reallocations very difficult, but they can be accomplished if political will is strong and if the political base is solid. A recent example comes from Venezuela where a large programme of subsidized feeding has been redirected and focused. The redirection includes funding for early education programmes.

Seeking new sources of funds or other resources

Mandating new revenue-collection schemes

Depending on the taxing (and collection) capacity of a government, new and earmarked taxes can be established. We have noted the Colombian case in which a payroll tax (now at 3 per cent) is collected from employers to support activities of the Institute for Family Welfare. Rather than put the tax burden on all taxpayers, which can easily be regressive, this tax appears to be progressive and redistributive towards the lower socioeconomic groups.

Some governments have turned to such schemes as lotteries to collect new funds.

Requiring government and private organizations to provide care and development programmes for their employees

This method contrasts with the payroll tax and places greater responsibilities on individual organizations. Although it may generate new resources for early childhood, the programmes are not likely to include families who are operating in the non-formal sector. And, it may lead to programmes that are underutilized because they are not near to the homes of the workers. This strategy might also be classified, where governments are concerned, under the reallocation heading.

Providing investment incentives

Matching funds, loan schemes with low interest rates, forgiveness of taxes on earnings and other incentives can be considered that are designed to mobilize private sector resources to invest in early childhood programmes. As this is done, care should be taken to see that these resources are not concentrated only in the upper income groups.

Charging for services

Another much discussed strategy is to ask users to pay for a service so that costs are recovered. This can be a useful strategy for covering part if not all of the costs of a programme. There is some evidence that the strategy is appropriate and workable with respect to essential drugs which are sold at subsidized prices. However, the same conclusion does not seem to be drawn with respect to reducing current costs of more general programmes of primary health care: '... of the 28 projects that used community financing to compensate community health workers, none has a satisfactory method for obtaining local support' (Burns Parlato and Favin 1982, p. 77). Before moving too quickly with this method of mobilizing resources, then, careful attention should be given to both the ability to pay of the target group and to the contributions that are already being made in time and materials to a particular programme. Sliding scales of payment may make this approach more equitable.

Linking financing to income-generating projects

In Chapter 7 (p. 138), a Thai programme was described in which self-funding for projects was achieved. A loan fund was established in some rural communities, using outside funds at the outset. When loans were paid back, the resources went into a capital fund to be used on a continuing basis for support of the early childhood development programme. While the fund was increasing in value, community members learned to manage the fund. After five to seven years, the fund was sufficient to let the programme continue without outside support.

Seeking international aid

In the previous section we have suggested that international sources of funds have an important role to play, particularly in providing help with capital and start-up costs. However, we have also emphasized that such a strategy needs to be pursued in such a way as not to overburden the overburdened. The above example of the Thai programme provides a novel case of a way in which foreign funds helped to develop and sustain a programme.

CONCLUDING COMMENTS

The foregoing discussion suggests that:
- Low-cost and affordable programme options are available and workable, and may even pay for themselves by introducing efficiencies in the use of resources or through cost savings.
- There is a variety of possible strategies for mobilizing resources in support of early childhood development programmes.
- We need not wait for major new windfall sources in order to move ahead with early childhood initiatives.
- Working in partnerships will be crucial, rather than expecting all resources to come from the government or the community or the private sector.

Finally, although costs and the question of where resources will come from loom large in the calculus of funders and planners, the importance of political factors and commitment must not be overlooked. In the last analysis, the use of resources involves choices about what is considered most important. Only if a government or another funder assigns a high priority to such programmes will the needed resources be found. That priority may be assigned because the arguments themselves are convincing and a real belief exists that children and future generations will benefit. Or, priority may be given because such programmes are seen as a way to mobilize a population and/or produce political satisfaction or loyalty. If this is so, the needed resources will be found, even where budgets are limited. A major task, therefore, for those who seek additional support for early childhood is to make both the technical and political case for such support.

In Part I of this book, we set out a rationale for investing in early childhood care and development programmes and analysed where we are with respect to such investments in terms of coverage and support. In Part II, we attempted to provide conceptual clarity by looking at how terms are used, by examining frameworks from various disciplines as applied to early childhood development, and by establishing and laying out a set of complementary programme approaches and criteria. Part III provided examples of various programme models related to each of the complementary approaches, while Parts IV, V and VI explored issues and actions related to the various criteria. It is now time to pull all the elements together, summarizing hopes and expectations for 'the twelve who survive', and putting forth a challenge to those who would build on that hope.

NOTES

1   I would like to express my thanks to Jim Himes, David Parker, and Richard Heyward for their reading and thoughtful comments on an earlier version of this chapter. As a result, a drastic revision has occurred – for which, however, I take full responsibility. The earlier version placed less emphasis on financing and was based much more directly on: R. Myers and R. Hertenberg, 'The Eleven Who Survive: Toward a Re-Examination of Early Childhood Development Program Options and Costs', a discussion paper prepared for the World Bank, Education and Training Department, Washington DC, March 1987.

2   The cost figures derived for a particular project or programme or projected into the future for a new programme will also depend on:
   - whether a social or institutional or individual perspective is taken (a cost to the society at large may not be a cost to a particular institution or to an individual because they do not have to bear the cost directly);
   - the scale of a programme (it is often assumed that 'economies of scale' will occur as a programme grows bigger so that per unit costs are reduced);
   - how particular contributions are treated (e.g. volunteer labour and other

non-monetary contributions; capital costs; the choice of unit adopted for per unit costs; the time dimension, etc.).
For additional attention to these issues as they affect cost calculations of early childhood programmes, see Myers and Hertenberg 1987.

3   UNESCO, UNICEF, the World Bank, the Organization of American States, the United States Agency for International Development, the International Development Research Centre (Canada), the Inter-American Foundation, the Ford Foundation, the Aga Khan Foundation, and the Bernard van Leer Foundation. These organizations had some difficulty providing information because accounting systems were not set up to separate out the relevant grants or loans. In only three organizations were there specific programmes labelled early childhood development or early education or child care. Therefore, staff were asked to look at the content of programmes in health and nutrition, community or rural development, and women-in-development programmes to see if an early childhood care and development component was included.

REFERENCES

Barnett, W.S. 'The Perry Preschool Program and Its Long-Term Effects: A Benefit-Cost Analysis', Ypsilanti, Michigan: High/Scope Educational Research Foundation, Early Childhood Policy Papers, Vol. 2, 1985.

Berg. A. *Malnutrition, What Can Be Done? Lessons from World Bank Experience.* Baltimore: Johns Hopkins University Press, 1987. Published for the World Bank.

Berruta-Clement, J.R., L.J. Schweinhart, W.S. Barnett, A.S. Epstein and D.T. Weikart. *Changed Lives, the Effects of the Perry School Program on Youths through Age 19.* Ypsilanti, Michigan: High/Scope Press, 1984.

Berstecher, D. and R. Carr-Hill. 'Primary Education and Economic Recession in the Developing World since 1980', a special study for the World Conference on Education for All (Thailand, 5–9 March, 1990), Paris: UNESCO, 1990.

Boianovsky, D. 'Primary Care for Pre-School Children Through Home Day-Care Centres', (description of a project carried out by the social services secretariat of the Government of the Federal District in Brasilia). July 1981. Mimeo.

Burns Parlato, M. and M. Favin. 'Primary Health Care: Progress and Problems, An Analysis of 52 Aid-Assisted Projects', Washington DC: American Public Health Association, August 1982.

Carbonetto, D. 'Informe Final de Evaluación de la Asisténcia de UNICEF al Gobierno del Perú durante el Periodo 1982–84' (Documento de Evaluación No. 1). Lima, CEDEP, Septiembre, 1984.

CEDEP. 'Estudio de Caso: Proyecto de Atención Integral al Niño y Su Familia en los Pueblos Jovenes de Cono Sur de Lima Metropolitana (Análisis Costo-Beneficio)'. Lima: Agosto, 1983.

Ciavatta-Franco, M.A. 'Da Assistencia Educativa a Educação Assistencializada – um estudo de caracterização e custos de atendimento a criancas carentes de 0 a 6 anos dei dade', Rio de Janeiro: UNICEF/Centro Nacional de Recursos Humanos (CNRH), 1983. Mimeo.

Colclough, C. and K. Lewin. *Educating all the Children: The Economic Challenge for the 1990s.* England: University of Sussex, Institute of Development Studies, March 1990.

Consultative Group on Early Childhood Care and Development. 'A Briefing Note Prepared for a Meeting of the International Working Group on Education (May 30–June 1, 1990)', New York: The Consultative Group, 1990. Mimeo.

Cornia, G.A. 'A Cost Analysis of the Indonesian Experiences with GOBI-FFF

(1979–1982)', New York: UNICEF, May 1983. Mimeo.

Cornia, A., R. Jolly and F. Stewart. *Adjustment with a Human Face: Protecting the Vulnerable and Promoting Growth*. New York: Oxford University Press, 1987. Press, 1987.

Fisher, E.A. 'Statistical Analysis of Questionnaires on Early Childhood Care and Education (ECCE)', Paris: UNESCO, January 1990. Draft.

Fuller, B. and M.E. Lockheed. 'Policy Choice and School Efficiency in Mexico', Washington DC: the World Bank, Education and Training Department, May 1987. Report No. EDT 78.

Grawe, Roger. 'Ability in Pre-Schoolers, Earnings, and Home-Environment', Washington: the World Bank, 1979. Working Paper No. 322.

Hong, S. 'Integrated Child Development Services – India Case Study', a paper prepared for Global Seminar on Early Childhood Development, Florence, International Child Development Centre, June 12–30, 1989. New Delhi: UNICEF, June 1989. Mimeo.

Iragorry, R., L. Apiolaza y L. Rojas. 'Determinación y Análisis de los Requirimientas de Recursos Humanos y Financieros del Programa Hogares de Cuidado Diario', Caracas, Venezuela: Fundación del Niño, 1978.

Kağitçibaşi, C., D. Sunar and S. Bekman. 'Comprehensive Preschool Education Project: Final Report', Instanbul, Turkey: Boğaziçi University, November 1987. A report prepared for the International Development Research Centre.

Latorre, Carmen Luz and S. Magendzo. *Atención a la infancia en comunidades marginales*. Santiago, Chile: UNICEF/Programa Interdisciplinario de Investigaciones en Educación', 1979.

Llanos, Martha y R. Myers. 'Evaluación de los Centros de Educación Pre-escolar No-Escolarizada (CEPNE) de Nicaragua', Managua: UNICEF, 1982. Mimeo.

Llanos, Martha. 'An Evaluation of the Ate-Vitarte Project', prepared for the Bernard van Leer Foundation, The Hague, 1985.

Ministerio da Saude y Instituto Nacional de Alimentação e Nutrição, 'Analição do PROAPE/Alagoas com enfoque na area econômica, Brasilia: MS/INAN, 1983. Mimeo.

Myers, R. 'Analyzing Costs of Community-Based Early Childhood Development Projects', a paper prepared for the Workshop on Evaluation and Costs of Early Childhood Development Programmes in Latin America and the Caribbean. Santiago, Chile. UNICEF, October 1983.

Myers, R. 'Programming for Early Childhood Education and Development', a briefing note prepared for a meeting of the International Working Group on Education, May 30–June 1, 1990. New York, the Consultative Group on Early Childhood Care and Development, May 1990. Mimeo.

Myers, R. and R. Hertenberg. 'The Eleven Who Survive: Toward a Re-Examination of Early Childhood Development Program Options and Costs', a discussion paper produced for the World Bank, Education and Training Department, Washington DC, March 1987.

Myers, R., *et al.* 'Pre-School as a Catalyst for Community Development: An Evaluation', a report prepared for United States Agency for International Development, Lima, Peru, January 1985.

Pontifica Universidad Católica de Chile, Instituto de Economia, 'Evaluación y Proyección del Programa CADEL', Santiago, Chile, UNICEF, Mayo de 1989.

Psacharopoulos, George. 'The Economics of Early Childhood Education and Day-Care', *International Review of Education*, Vol. XXVIII (1982), pp. 53–70.

República de México, Secretaria de Educación Pública, Dirección General de Educación Inicial. 'Programa de Desarrollo del Niño de 0 a 5 Años a traves de

Padres de Familia y Miembros de la Comunidad', documento presentado al Taller Inter-Agencial sobre Evaluación y Costos de Programas del Pre-escolar en América Latina y el Caribe, Santiago de Chile, 17–22 de Octubre, 1983. Mimeo.

Richards, Howard. *The Evaluation of Cultural Action.* London: Macmillan Press Ltd, 1985.

Robert R. Nathan Associates, Inc. *Assessing the Cost-Effectiveness of PVO Projects – A Guide and Discussion.* Prepared for the Bureau for Food and Private Voluntary Assistance. Washington, DC: Agency for International Development, August 1983.

Selowsky, M. 'Nutrition, Health, and Education: The Economic Significance of Complementarities at Early Age'. *Journal of Development Economics.* Vol. 9 (1981), pp. 331–46.

Selowsky, Marcelo. '¿Estamos subinvirtiendo en capital humano a edades pre-escolares?' en Fernando Galofré (ed.) *Pobreza Crítica en la Niñez: América Latina y el Caribe.* Santiago, Chile: UNICEF, 1981.

Smilansky, Moshe. 'Priorities in Education: Pre-school; Evidence and Conclusions', Washington: World Bank, 1979. Working Paper No. 323.

UNICEF/Dominican Republic. 'A Report on the Non-Formal Pre-School Education Experience in the Dominican Republic', March 1983. Mimeo.

Part VII

Conclusions

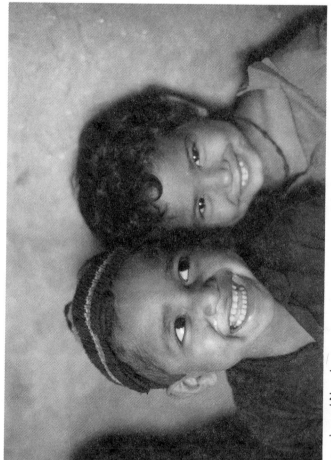

'Imps', rural Nepal

Chapter 16

Towards a fair start for 'the twelve who survive'

A straightforward and simple line of reasoning with respect to programming for early childhood development[1] emerges from the descriptive data and examples, the literature reviews and references, the discussions of terms and frameworks, and the analyses of programme characteristics presented in preceding chapters. In synoptic form, that reasoning goes as follows:

1 Millions (perhaps hundreds of millions) of children throughout the world suffer delayed, debilitated or distorted mental, social, or emotional development in their early years, affecting all of their later life.

These children are victims of social neglect in varying degrees. Deprived of the chance to develop their abilities, they are unable to cope adequately with a rapidly changing, and increasingly complex world, let alone to help in the construction of a better world. They are condemned to lethargic, dependent, unproductive and unrewarding lives. These children – and their families and communities – need help with their development if they are to have a fair start in life. Failure to do so carries a heavy moral burden and a high social cost.

2 Scientific research establishes the importance of promoting healthy development during the early years.

Evidence from physiology, nutrition, psychology, sociology and other fields continues to accumulate, indicating that the early years are critical in the development of intelligence, personality, and social behaviour. Moreover, systematic evaluations of programmes designed to foster early development show that lasting effects can occur such as improved school attendance and performance, decreased delinquency, and reduced pregnancy during the teenage years.

It is clear that children are born with extraordinary physical, social and psychological capacities allowing them to communicate, learn and develop. If these capacities are not recognized and supported, they will wither rather than develop. For normal development to occur, children need not only food, shelter, health care and protection, but also love and affection, opportunities to interact, consistence and predictability in their caregiving environment, and a chance to explore and discover.

3 Strong moral, social, political and economic and programmatic arguments exist for investing in early childhood care and development.

Children have a right to live and to develop to their full potential.

Through children humanity transmits its values. To preserve moral and social values, one must begin with children.

Society benefits economically from investing in child development, through increased economic productivity and cost savings.

By providing a fair start, it is possible to modify distressing socio-economic and gender-related inequities.

Children provide a rallying point for social and political actions that build consensus and solidarity.

The efficacy of other programmes (health, nutrition, education, women's programmes) can be improved through their being combined with programmes of child development.

In sum, whether one takes a human rights perspective or focuses on social equity, or economic productivity and social costs, or the transmission of values, or the need for better education for tomorrow's leaders and citizens, or simply the efficacy of existing programmes, attention to the development of children in the period before about age seven and entry into school turns out to be crucial. Taken together, and in combination with the scientific evidence, these reasons constitute a powerful rationale for action. (These arguments are elaborated in Chapter 1.)

4 The need and demand is increasing for programmes of early childhood care and development.

Why is that so? Changing demographic, social and economic conditions require additional attention to early development:

- Increases in the infant survival rate mean that more children are now at risk of impaired physical, mental, social and emotional development than previously.
- The rapid rate of urbanization and the dislocations of war and civil strife bring with them disruption of stable family units, the erosion of healthy traditional child-care practices, and the difficulty of adopting new practices that will be appropriate to new settings. These conspire to have a negative effect on early development.
- Revolutions in transportation, communication and education have also allowed the reach of the city into rural areas, with accompanying changes in values and practices. Confusion about what is 'right' has led prematurely to abandoning time-tested, culturally appropriate practices of child care and children are increasingly suffering the effects of this confusion.
- The dramatic increase in participation by women in the paid labour force, combined with shifts in family structures (towards nuclear families

or women-headed households) bring along an increasing need and demand for alternative forms of child care, in both urban and rural areas.
- Lingering effects of the worldwide recession of the 1980s have exacerbated problems of early development as families living at the margin in absolute poverty struggle to survive.

5 Knowledge about what to do to foster healthy and holistic child development has accumulated, providing an adequate basis for action.

Recent advances in the state of the art have been impressive. We need not wait for further research to provide additional or magical answers. Additional answers may be in the making but to wait for them would be to deprive today's child of the urgent and sound assistance to which she is entitled.

Moreover, advances in the state of the art have not been accompanied by similar advances in the state of the practice. For instance:

- We know that development occurs as children interact with their caregivers and that the child must be an active partner in the process; *but* the state of the practice continues to place greater emphasis on one-way stimulation of the child by the caregiver.
- We know that there is a synergistic (mutual interaction and effect) relationship among good health, sound nutritional status and psychosocial well-being; *but* a mono-focal approach to programming still dominates.
- We know that indigenous childrearing practices are often very healthy; *but* emphasis is placed on imported solutions.
- We know development begins prenatally; *but* programme emphasis is placed on children aged three to six.

In short, we know more than we think we know, we have not applied all we know and we have an adequate knowledge base for action.

6 Programme experience has accumulated, providing a range of potentially effective and financially feasible models.

Wide experimentation during the previous two decades, and particularly in the last five to ten years, has provided us with many examples of ways to enhance early childhood care and development in a variety of settings (see Chapters 6 and 7). These include programmes of centre-based care and education (creches, home day care, formal and non-formal preschools, play groups, kindergartens, child-care centres in the workplace, etc.), programmes of home-based support and education for parents and other caregivers (home visiting, adult education, mass media presentations, child-to-child), and broader programmes of community development built around integrated attention to the child.

7 In some countries attention to early childhood education and development has grown dramatically, well beyond a demonstration stage.

Examples of such growth (see Chapters 2, 6, and 7) include the expansion of the Integrated Child Development Service in India, the non-formal, community-based preschools for children in Kenya, the home day-care programme in Colombia, parental education in China, the incorporation of a child's right to care into the Brazilian constitution and the inclusion of child development content into the primary school curriculum of Jamaica. These examples suggest that moving from pilot projects towards major policies and larger-scale programmes is possible.

8 Cost and affordability are not the main deterrents to expanded attention.

Low-cost, effective programme options exist. In many cases, a child development component can be folded into an existing structure at marginal cost. Focusing efforts can keep costs within reason. Cost savings can moderate or even offset the investment costs in early childhood development (see Chapter 15). A variety of innovative financing schemes and cost-sharing arrangements between governments and communities are possible.

Moreover, it is possible to point to several examples of countries with low per capita incomes in which child care and development has been given sufficient priority to allow sizeable programmes to develop. These facts suggest that if a country believes the investment is a good one and there is political will, the relatively modest amounts needed can be found to give a major impulse to programmes of early childhood care and development.

In summary

- Millions of children suffer delayed or debilitated development, affecting all of later life, carrying high personal and social costs.
- Scientific research supports early intervention and shows that faltering development can be avoided or overcome.
- The moral, social, economic, political, and programmatic reasons for investment in early development are compelling.
- Need and demand has grown, affected by sociodemographic change.
- Our knowledge and experiential base for action is sound.
- Examples of how to foster early development abound.
- Cost is not the main deterrent to expanded programming.

What has been the response?

In general, despite the growth and examples, and despite what seems to be more than adequate reason to invest heavily in the intellectual, social and emotional components of early development, the response can be characterized as timid, slow and selective (with some notable exceptions). In general:

- coverage remains relatively low in most countries.
- many initiatives continue to be small pilot activities that are innovative, effective and feasible to replicate, but have not been extended in a significant way.
- the distribution of existing programmes is biased against those most in need.
- quality is often poor, undercutting results.
- reaching children before the age of three continues to be a challenge – particularly for children between the ages of one and three (as weaning occurs, talking begins, and walking allows greater possibilities for exploration).
- programmes of support and education for parents are weak in most places.
- most programmes do not provide integrated attention; i.e. education, nutrition, and health are not included together.
- day care that takes into account both the needs of children and of their working mothers remains at a very low level, both in extension and in quality.
- national policies for children are rarely found.
- international assistance for programmes of early childhood continues to be focused on survival; the importance of broader attention to child development is only beginning to be appreciated.

WHY HAS THE OPPORTUNITY NOT BEEN SEIZED?

A fairly long list of hypotheses can be offered for the failure of governments and international organizations to take on the problems of child development in a significant, large-scale, and intensive way, in spite of the seemingly persuasive arguments for doing so.

1 *It takes time.* The demographic, social, and economic changes referred to above that are increasing need and demand have really only begun to be apparent in the last two decades. It takes time for such changes to be recognized, let alone to respond to them. Typically, governments and assistance agencies react to emergencies rather than to slowly eroding conditions. Delayed or debilitated intellectual, social and emotional development is not as dramatic as death or third-degree malnutrition and the effect of deteriorating conditions on development is not as obvious. Accordingly, the child development part of the 'silent emergency' is only just beginning to be documented and realized and acted upon.

2 *Child development is seen as a by-product.* The idea that economic development does not automatically bring with it improvements in social welfare has been slow to die. Similarly, the idea that intellectual, social and emotional development will take care of itself if problems of nutrition and health are solved holds over from the 'basic needs' approach of the 1970s.

It takes time to digest the fact that these facets of child development should now be treated explicitly, because they do not necessarily improve as a result of other actions.

3 *Children are not an organized political force.* Children aged nought to six are a special category politically. They are dependent. They do not vote. They cannot go out on strike. If adults do not act on their behalf they are helpless. And low-income and marginal families in which developmental problems are often the most acute lack the political power necessary to move governments on this issue as well as on others.

4 *Specialization deters action.* A mark of our time is institutional special-ization. Our academic and bureaucratic institutions are increasingly fractured and piecemeal. But children are not made in pieces corres-ponding to nutrition, health, education, and social welfare. Because child development is best approached in a holistic way and requires the attention of all these sectors, it is at once everyone's concern and no one's concern. Putting the pieces back together and assigning responsibility for action has not been an easy task (see Chapters 8–11).

5 *A family responsibility.* The idea that the problems of children should be solved by individual families is deeply ingrained. The idea that there is a broader social responsibility for governments to support families in their efforts has been slow to take hold. Too conveniently, public concerns with child care and child development have been looked upon as interference.

6 *Cultural variations* in goals and practices have made child development and growth faltering more difficult to deal with than some other areas. For example, measles is measles, wherever found, and the causes of measles are relatively uniform. Prevention and treatment can also be uniform (at least at the level of a vaccination). Such uniformity does not exist in the causes of delayed or debilitated development. Programmes must therefore be adjusted to the particular circumstances.

7 *Misconceptions.* Many misconceptions about child development or about programming for child development deter initiatives that could be taken. Consider the following misconceptions:

- Child survival and child development are perceived as sequential processes (rather than simultaneous ones) and, therefore, program-ming to save lives comes first, programming for child development later (see Chapters 3 and 4).
- Health and nutrition are known to influence psychosocial well-being, but the reverse is seldom recognized as true. This one-way view favours programmes concentrating on health and nutrition, with psychosocial development seen as a by-product (see Chapter 9).
- The myth that mothers are the sole and best caretakers of their children in the early years is associated with the idea that programmes of care outside the home or with other people must be detrimental (see Chapter 11).

- The naive notion that real learning and education begin at school seems to have grown stronger as the system of schooling has expanded. Therefore, education ministries do not see the earliest months and years of life as falling within their charge, despite strong evidence indicating that, even at birth, children are learning. Educational investment continues to go first to educational institutions from primary school onward (see Chapter 10).
- Related to the previous point is the misconception that investments in early childhood care and education represent a direct trade-off against investments in primary school. Because this is incorrectly seen as a 'zero-sum game' a choice seems necessary, and because learning begins in primary school, that should come first (see Chapter 15).
- There is a tendency to think that all so-called traditional childrearing practices and beliefs are outmoded and need to be corrected or replaced with more modern practices. This biases early childhood programmes towards a compensatory model rather than a supportive and constructive one, working with the strengths of families and communities (see Chapter 13).
- There is a misconception that non-professionals are unfit to be teachers of young children. This misconception can keep excellent people from participating in early childhood programmes.

WHAT NEEDS TO BE DONE?

Create awareness/demystify/inform

The previous discussion suggests that a great deal of energy must be put into raising awareness about what the process of child development is, about the deteriorating conditions affecting early childhood development and about the long-term effects of developmental faltering on individuals and societies. An effort is needed to demystify child development and to overcome misconceptions. Available alternatives must be made evident.

These actions must involve a range of individuals and groups approaching child development at different levels and in different ways. The means used to reach and involve each group will vary and the content of the exercise must be appropriate to each:

- *Politicians* need to understand the problem, potential solutions and the broader social, economic and political implications of action or inaction. Awareness of technical details is not so important for this group.
- *Planners* require a greater technical understanding, must have a feel for the specific options open to them and need to know about costs. They must be shown that intellectual, social and emotional develop-

ment of young children is not simply a by-product of other programmes. They need examples of integrated attention.

- *Professionals* may need to be helped to redirect their thinking towards more supervisory roles and towards actions that draw upon experience as well as on their academic preparation. Curricula will need to be reviewed and revised so that medical doctors in training learn about psychosocial health and teachers learn about child health and nutrition.
- *Programme implementors* (in governments, NGOs, communities) need to be versed in the art of the possible, in thinking holistically, and in the various ways in which real participation can be incorporated into programmes.
- *Families and other caregivers* need concrete information about actions they can take in the home. They need to know they are the child's first teachers. They need to be supported with knowledge about what they do that is right as well as about what they should do that they do not.
- *National and international funders* need examples that help to debunk myths about costs and that show outcomes. They need also to made aware of the interdependence of survival and development.

Mass media can play an important role in helping to raise awareness, correct misconceptions, and provide basic information about child development. But more than dissemination of information is required for changes in awareness and attitude to occur. An active strategy is needed creating opportunities for discussion, dialogue, experiencing of alternatives, and participation in all phases of programming for child development. Such a strategy must build on both academic knowledge and experience.

Establish a comprehensive strategy

In Chapter 5, a framework was presented that provides the basis for establishing a comprehensive strategy. The framework, summarized below, describes five complementary approaches, suggests a set of programme guidelines, and distinguishes several age groups of young children requiring different treatment.

Five complementary approaches

Strengthening awareness and demand   This approach, which concentrates on the production and distribution of *knowledge* and *information*, has a degree of urgency that has led us to emphasize it above as our first point under 'What must be done?' Unless political understanding and will is present, unless programme planners and implementors have a broad vision backed by solid knowledge and experience, and unless the population at large is aware of options, actions will continue to be deterred, biased, or ineffective.

Strengthening institutional resources and capacities   Efforts to strengthen governmental and non-governmental *institutions* working to improve early childhood care and development may involve setting proper legal bases (including constitutional and legal reforms) as well as strengthening the financial, material and human resources available to plan, organize, implement and evaluate programmes. New forms of organization may be necessary to tie together various institutional efforts. Training will be a key activity, both to provide the kind of awareness and knowledge stressed above and to strengthen specific capacities.

Promoting community development through an emphasis on early childhood development   This approach stresses *community* initiative, organization, and participation in a range of interrelated activities to improve the physical environment, the knowledge and practices of community members, and the organizational base, allowing common action and improving the base for political and social negotiations. These activities, although centred around the healthy development of the young child, will be of benefit also to the community more broadly.

Supporting and educating caregivers   This approach focuses on *family* members and is intended to educate and empower them in ways that improve their care and interaction with the child and enrich the immediate environment in which child development is occurring, rather than substitute for it. Education and support for parents and other caregivers may be provided through home visits, in adult education courses, through the mass media or in child-to-child programmes.

Attending to children in centres   This direct approach, focusing on the *child*, seeks to provide conditions for healthy development of the child outside the home, compensating for or enriching what occurs in the home. These programmes can take such diverse forms as a creche, home day care, formal and informal preschools, play groups, kindergartens and child-care centres in the workplace.

Each of these approaches is directed towards improvements in a different level of the environment influencing development of the child, each at a different distance from the child. Each approach is directed towards a different audience or group of participants although all share the overarching goal of improved child care and development. The balance among these complementary approaches will differ according to particular situations, but some attention to each one is probably warranted in all settings.

Programme guidelines

A comprehensive strategy requires a set of guidelines to be followed as programmes are formulated and implemented. We have suggested the following:

- Focus on children and families whose living conditions put them most at risk for delayed or debilitated mental, social and emotional development.
- Take a multifaceted view of child development, seeking integration (or convergence) of programmes in order to take advantage of the synergisms among health, nutrition and early education.
- Seek community participation that goes beyond superficial or one-time donations to real involvement in the planning, management, and evaluation of programmes.
- Be flexible enough to respect and adjust to different sociocultural contexts, reinforcing local ways to cope effectively with problems of child care and development, even while introducing new ideas.
- Adopt approaches and models that are financially feasible and cost-effective, taking advantage of appropriate technologies that have proven to be effective.
- Try to reach the largest possible number of childen who are at risk.

Different ages and stages require different treatments

A comprehensive strategy must take into account the major differences that are related to the child development process itself. These can be defined roughly as the prenatal, infancy, toddler and post-toddler, pre-school, and early primary school periods. Different kinds of programmes will have to be fashioned for these different periods.

Work towards partnership

The responsibility for the healthy development of young children is not a sole responsibility of families or governments or communities or non-governmental organizations constituting a 'civil society'. In order to make the best use of resources and to cumulate efforts, there is a need for mechanisms that will facilitate working together by these very different institutions and groups. At a national level this may mean, to use the term favoured by UNICEF, creating a 'grand alliance' that mobilizes many groups to work together in common cause.

   In the long run, working towards partnership requires something less glorious and more difficult than mobilization of many people and organizations in common cause at a national level. (See Chapter 12 for a more complete discussion of the following abbreviated points.) It means creating lasting forms of cooperation in the field, at the level of the village or neigh-bourhood. For that to happen, important shifts need to occur that take one beyond simply working together. It means establishing conditions favouring dialogue and mutual learning (as contrasted with the imposition of ideas). It means joint participation at all points in a project or programme, beginning with diagnosis and planning, and carrying through to imple-mentation and evaluation. It means recognizing that both academic knowl-edge and experiential knowledge have validity. It means strengthening local organization. It means selecting and training professional and tech-nical personnel who believe in and know how to work in a participatory way with community and other grassroots groups. Unless these shifts in the form of work occur, the empowerment of local groups necessary to work in true partnership will be slow to appear and quick to disappear and we shall be left with yet another slogan.

CHALLENGES

Embedded in the above suggestions are several special challenges.

Moving from a compensatory to a constructive programme view   A negative approach to programming has dominated in the past, based on identifying what is missing or harmful and trying to compensate by filling in the holes. A challenge for the future is to take a positive view, beginning with the strengths in a given environment and working with people to reinforce those strengths, even while adding new dimensions.

Thinking in a holistic way and translating that thinking into combined actions   One of the greatest challenges to be faced is that of recovering the holistic, and integral, way of thinking that has been so eroded by our world of specialization. In approaching child development, a broad and integrative view is essential, not only in concept, but also in various ways in the operation of programmes.

In trying to respect the unity of the child when operationalizing activities, it may be necessary to admit that we shall not easily integrate bureaucratic structures, each established for a specific purpose such as health delivery or education. We might, instead, stress cooperation among existing programmes of health, nutrition and education and their conver-gence on those areas and people where the need is greatest. Organizational devices such as placing coordination outside specialized agencies, creating inter-organizational activities, and building networks will help to provide integration.

But in the last analysis, integration will occur in the actions of family members and others who are responsible for child care. That integrative process can be helped along by making planning a collaborative process crossing bureaucratic lines and involving grassroots organizations which have an integrated view. Thus, programmes of parental education, with integrated content, and within a context of participatory community development, offer promise for affecting early development.

Drawing on academic and experientially derived knowledge   One reason why working towards partnership is difficult is because those who provide resources or who are charged with implementing programmes bring with them knowledge (or a technology) that they feel is superior because it has a scientific base. But knowledge that is based in time-tested accumulation of experience can be of equal or higher value in specific situations. For there to be a fruitful dialogue that draws from the best of both these traditions, it is necessary to recognize that both are valid.

Being flexible: avoiding blueprints and magic solutions   Another challenge facing us is overcoming the natural desire to discover and apply one specific solution or technology to all children. Programming to enhance the mental, social and emotional development of young children cannot be built around the hope of discovering a child development vaccine. Children are different. Contexts are different. But, fortunately, a range of available technologies exists that can be called upon, some more appropriate to one context, some to another.

In approaching this challenge, it is obvious that a decentralized organization will have an advantage over a centralized one. It is also clear that the greater the involvement of individual families and local communities in establishing and implementing programmes to foster integrated child development, the more likely these are to be adjusted to local realities.

Reconciling a desire for scale with the need for flexibility and the importance of local participation   The challenge of flexibility does not mean that programmes must be small in their conception or in the number of participants. It does mean, however, that such large-scale, centralized meaures as information campaigns must contain within them devices allowing content to be adjusted locally. It does mean that providing information to people on a large scale cannot be regarded as *the* solution – equivalent to an inoculation. Such campaigns need to be part of a process that allows and fosters face-to-face discussion and strengthens social ties.

Scale by association – There is a tendency to equate scale with centralized programming and with single approaches to a problem, but, as has been elaborated in Chapter 14, that need not be the case. In contrast to a centrally run immunization or literacy campaign reaching large numbers of individuals, we might think of scale as the sum of a great many local or regional programmes, each distinct, and each directed towards the same end: improvements in child survival and development. In this jigsaw puzzle view of scale, it is possible to envision programme effects for large numbers while incorporating the ideas of flexibility and local participation. Expansion of particular approaches can be encouraged within cultural or geographic limits, with the sum of the various efforts constituting scale.

The role of governments or other centralized organizations in such programmes would be to provide general guidelines, to motivate, to assist with additional resources when they are needed, to provide ideas, and to help with the monitoring and evaluation. This view of going to scale allows for expansion of local programmes over time, within districts and regions, but does not require expansion to a national level in order for a project to be considered successful beyond its original demonstration or pilot phase.

Monitoring and evaluating   We have suggested (Chapter 10) the need for the creation of a Child Readiness Profile incorporating indicators, at age five, of a child's health and nutritional status, of pre-literacy and numeracy skills, of self-esteem, and of parental expectations. This profile, which would need to be adjusted to particular settings, could be applied periodically, using a sampling frame, to monitor and evaluate the well-being of young children about to move from the confines of the home into the larger world, including the world of schools. Such a profile, or another instrument, is needed for monitoring, evaluation and advocacy.

SOME PRIORITIES

With the above considerations and suggestions in mind, what deserves special attention in programming for early childhood care and development?

1 **The younger ages**   Among the several age groupings that can be distinguished roughly as a child experiences developmental changes between the time of conception and age eight, priority should be given to the period before about the second birthday. Development and learning during this period occurs extraordinarily fast and the results form the basis for most of later learning. Not only is this the period when connections in the brain will take shape, but it is a period that encompasses weaning and walking and the beginnings of spoken language.

Viewed from a standpoint of intellectual, social and emotional development, this earliest period in life has been neglected. However, the fact that development is so closely tied to health and nutrition in these early months and years, and the fact that considerable attention is being given to these dimensions, opens innumerable opportunities for incorporating a psychosocial dimension into ongoing health and nutrition programmes.

2 **Support and education of parents and other family members**
Because the family, in all its varieties, provides the primary environment

for child development during the early years, the first focus of programmes should be on helping families in their task. In Chapter 7, advantages and cautions of this programme approach were listed and several examples given of different ways in which support and education might be operationalized. These include home visiting programmes as well as programmes incorporating education into adult education (for instance, nutrition and health education) and literacy programmes. They also include working with prospective parents through child-to-child programmes.

3 The articulation of home and school environments   Schools often differ dramatically from homes, not only in the physical setting and the people with whom a child will interact, but also in activities, expectations and rules of conduct, and in ways of learning. There are differences also between organizations and agencies responsible for schools and those that work with the child and the family in the home and community during the preschool years. This artificial division emphasizes rather than moderates differences and leads to uncoordinated programming that is not in the best interests of children who are expected to cope with school. Nor is it in the best interests of schools.

Even within the educational sector, a division is made between preschool and primary school, when it would make more sense to treat the two together (at least the first one or two years of primary school). This organizational arrangement merits some rethinking. At a minimum, a semi-autonomous unit within the Ministry of Education might be created that would be charged with the responsibility for programmes covering the ages three to eight (or even one to eight). This unit could be a multidisciplinary unit, including individuals with health, nutrition, adult education, and community development backgrounds. The non-education people might be loaned from other ministries, with the understanding that they would serve as a liaison to programmes in the health, nutrition and other areas from which they came. This group could be overseen by an inter-ministerial committee.

There is a tendency to think that a child should be adjusted to the particular school he or she will enter. But schools should have an equal, or greater, obligation to adjust themselves to the kinds of children they receive. Thus, the relationship between home and school should be viewed as the interaction of a child's readiness for school, and a school's readiness for the child (which might be measured by a School Readiness Profile including indicators of accessibility, quality, adjustment to local realities, and teacher attitudes and expectations). The preschool/primary school unit described above could help to work on this interaction from both sides. In Chapter 10, several concrete ideas are offered of how the adjustments between home and school could be assisted.

4 Children and families in circumstances of rapid social change or of social displacement   Among those children who are most at risk of delayed or debilitated development are those being cared for in unfamiliar environments in which not only are the conditions precarious, but familiar patterns of childrearing do not function well. Among the groups that fall in this category are migrants from rural to marginal urban areas, refugee children, and children in conditions of war. In addition, special attention should be given to care and development where major modernization projects are being carried out (e.g. building a new dam), where new technologies are being introduced, or where there is a shift to a cash crop economy.

5 **Child care and development for children of working mothers in low-income and single-parent conditions** Special attention to children in these conditions is becoming more and more important. To some degree, this priority overlaps with the previous one. There is a pressing need to bring together programmes that are often separated from each other bureaucratically: programmes promoting women's income-earning capacity, and programmes to enhance early childhood development in preschools and child-care centres.

A CALL TO ACTION

In this final decade of the twentieth century, we are in a much better position to make a major and sustained advance in our programming for improved early care and development than we were in 1979 during the International Year of the Child. We have sounder knowledge and experience and technologies to draw upon. Consciousness of the importance of care and development has grown, evident in a new willingness to look beyond survival. That consciousness is indicated by the recent expansion of early childhood programmes, even in a time of economic retrenchment and adjustment. There is indeed hope that 'the twelve who survive' will have an opportunity for healthy mental, social and emotional development.

In spite of these advances, the level of investment by many national and international organizations in early childhood is still low, and their stance is lukewarm at best. If actions are not taken to change that position, an important moment will have passed us by.

If a new and conscious and broad-based initiative fails to materialize, we shall continue to drift, slowly, towards greater, but not necessarily improved, attention to the needs of young children. Meanwhile, the measured and dilatory pace of that drifting will deprive several generations of at risk children of a fair start in life.

But more, failure to act could easily prejudice future generations as well by allowing an outmoded, monolithic, socially biased, bureaucratic, centralized, formal and uncreative model of early childhood care and development to expand, taking its cue from a problem-riddled primary school. This trend must be arrested. Action must be taken to place much greater emphasis on the earliest years, on social as well as mental development, on family and community involvement, and on constructive rather than compensatory programming. These shifts in focus and organization will not happen by themselves. And, if they do not begin to occur now, we shall soon have passed the time when we are early enough in the process to be able to make a real difference in the organizational outcome.

This, then, is a call to national governments and to the international community to open themselves to new and worthy ventures and to proceed with all due haste towards an enlightened programme of child survival *and development.* It is a call also to communities and non-governmental organizations to make the child a central part of their grassroots efforts as they take advantage of the present opening towards civil initiatives and the growing movement towards a civil society.

The challenge we face in building strong programmes of child survival, care and development is at once immediate and long-term. In the remaining years of this century, many pages will be written about preparation for the twenty-first century. Many assessments will be made, accompanied by dreams for a better future. In all of this it would be well to remember that the primary school graduates of the year 2000 have already been born and are being prepared for their future lives. They have already, for the most part, passed the critical period from age nought to six. We are, then, already thinking well into the twenty-first century as we talk about the newborns who will be the dreamers, builders and leaders of tomorrow. They will be responsible for seeking economic and social justice, for halting the devastation of our environment, and for building a world in which neighbours and nations can live together in peace.

What seems so far away is being influenced now. It is time to act if we wish to bolster development of tomorrow's citizenry, with a vision of a more equitable, humane, productive and peaceful world. It is time to act not only with money, but with personal commitment to seeking a fair start for 'the twelve who survive'.

And it is with urgency, then, that this call to action is made.

NOTE

1   As a reminder: human development involves more than growing bigger. Simply stated, human (and child) development refers to the process of change in which people (children) become able to handle ever more complex activities. Development includes a physical dimension (the ability to move and coordinate); an intellectual dimension (the ability to think and reason); a social dimension (the ability to relate to others); and an emotional dimension (self-confidence and the ability to feel). Development begins prenatally. For a child to develop in a healthy and normal way, it is necessary not only to meet the basic needs of protection, food, and health care, but also to meet basic needs for affection, interaction and stimulation, security (associated with consistency and predict-

ability), and learning through exploration and discovery. Programmes to enhance child development promote conditions of care, socialization and education – in the home and community, formally and informally – that are required to meet these needs.

Afterword

The re-edition of this book in paperback provides an opportunity to identify and comment on changes that have occurred since the initial writing as well as to up-date thoughts on what needs to be done. It also provides me with a welcome opportunity to re-examine ideas presented in the first edition of the book – to present a kind of personal review, with the benefit of five years' hindsight. What holds up? What would I modify? I will begin this Afterword with that re-examination and review, then close with comments on recent changes and their implications.

A REVIEW OF "THE TWELVE WHO SURVIVE"
by the Author

The basic arguments

Does the general line of argumentation for supporting investment in programmes of early childhood care and development (ECCD) presented in the first edition of "The Twelve Who Survive" (see Chapter 1) hold up over time? In my opinion, the general line of argument has, if anything, been strengthened during the past few years. To wit:

- The number of children at risk of delayed or debilitated development continues to be very high and may even have increased.
- We have an even stronger scientific base from which to argue the importance of the early childhood years in the development of intelligence, personality and social behaviour.
- The moral, social, political, economic and pragmatic programming arguments for investment have been increasingly accepted.
- Programme experience has continued to accumulate, providing us with examples, lessons learned, new starting points and insights; our knowledge and experiential base for action is sound.
- Cost is not proving to be the major deterrent to expanded programming – will, imagination, organisation and training are major deterrents.

– Moreover, trends in conditions that create new needs and demands for alternative forms of promoting the integral development of young children continue apace. The move of women into the paid labor force continues to occur. Disruptive migration to cities has accelerated in many countries, with a new push from neo-liberal economic policies. The infant (and child) mortality rate continues to decline in most countries. If this book were to be written today, it would be titled "The Fourteen Who Survive," because 14 of 15 children born worldwide now live until at least their first birthday. These surviving children continue to live in conditions that previously put them at risk to die and now put them at risk of delayed and debilitated development. Even more than before, the question, "Survival for What?" takes on significance.

Key concepts and frameworks: reaffirmations and some changes

The book presents a set of concepts that are intended to provide a basis for policy, planning, programming and implementation of ECCD programmes. I will briefly revisit several of the major concepts, reaffirming their treatment or suggesting modifications.

Survival, growth, development and care   I would not change the conceptualisations of survival, growth, development and care used in the book (see Chapter 3). The emphasis on each of these as a process rather than a state is increasingly accepted. The idea that survival and development are simultaneous, not sequential, processes, although seemingly obvious, is only now beginning to be accepted by policy-makers and programmers. If anything, I would put even greater emphasis on the synergistic character of child development, and particularly on the idea that the psycho-social condition of children affects their health and nutrition status, not just the reverse (see Chapter 9). Evidence mounts that human interaction and love affect growth and health, acting through reductions of stress, the functioning of the immune system, and the effect on growth hormones. Slowly, the health sector is bringing this viewpoint back into its way of thinking, but there is a long road ahead for this conceptualisation to be accepted as it should be if mental health and attention to psycho-social development are to become part of everyday practice in programmes of health and nutrition.

Integration   My experiences with programmes since the first edition confirm the value of treating the concept of "integration" and integrated programming on several levels, as presented in Chapter 8, substituting "convergence" for integration in the delivery of services, and with emphasis on integrating plans and programme content as well as on the ability of communities to bring different services at local levels. If re-writing, I would place even more emphasis on trying to see that services converge on the same population and also more emphasis on the importance of helping these populations integrate those services locally.

Community participation The concept of "community participation" set out in Chapter 12, although continuing to be difficult in practice, holds as an ideal. Participation must go well beyond the notion of using services or donating resources or even administering programmes to include active involvement in setting goals and priorities, helping shape content, implementing and evaluating programmes. The related concepts of "empowerment" and of "partnership" need to be reinforced.

Scale The concept of "scale" based on the image of a jigsaw puzzle, in which various project and programme models are put together to achieve scale in coverage, has proven particularly useful (Chapter 14). This contrasts with "scale" as the extension of one model to all children. The jigsaw or mosaic view of scale provides room for local participation and the adjustment of local differences even while trying to reach many children with actions that will improve their chances of survival and development. It avoids the rigidities that are bound to occur when scale is conceived as extending one model to all.

In the discussion of scale, however, I would, if rewriting, place greater emphasis on the process of setting the borders that frame the larger picture puzzle. Seeking agreement on the general guidelines for programmes is important.

Preparation for school/life, and "transition" The idea of joint attention to "the preparation of the child for school" and "the preparation of schools for the children" has been well received as part of a growing concern about the so-called "transition" of children from home to school (see Chapter 10). Joint attention to child and school helps us to avoid thinking that we should (or can) simply change the child to fit a fixed setting called the school. Schools must also change.

In Chapter 10, these twin concepts are set within a broad framework relating early childhood development to schooling and later achievements. This broader model takes as key points in time the important life changes for a child defined by birth, entrance into school and exit from school.

Given the emphasis of the book on early childhood development, and given the increase in organized programs of child care and pre-school education, I would now include in the model the point of entrance by children into programmes of care or education that occur outside the family during the pre-school years. I would also incorporate "family" much more directly and continuously into the model. True, the family in most cases has primary responsibility for development and learning during the preschool years. But, a child does not leave the family to enter into the school. Rather, at the time a child moves into school (or into a pre-school or another center-based program), the child moves into another learning environment. The child now functions in multiple learning environments. (The concept of multiple learning environments is at odds with the concept of a "transition" from home to school.)

Constructive vs compensatory programming I reaffirm the conceptual emphasis placed on "constructive" rather than on "compensatory" programming. This conceptualisation carries with it the idea that a great deal of knowledge is discovered. Therefore, active and participatory learning is important (for communities and for government planners and technocrats as they go about their tasks, as well as for children). Therefore the discoveries of traditional knowledge (constructed over time and through experience) must be recognised, with attention given to building upon positive elements in a given setting rather than on simply identifying and correcting errors.

Complementary programming approaches The programming framework presented in Chapter 5 defines five complementary approaches to be considered at each of several stages of a child's development. Each strategy focusses on a different audience or group of participants: immediate caregivers in the family; alternative caregivers working in centers, communities, social institutions; and the population at large.

In its work, UNICEF has found it useful to make explicit two additional strategies (which were hidden within the broad category of strengthening institutions), one directed toward developing supportive legal frameworks and the other toward establishing national child care and family policies. In general, greater emphasis should be given to the institution-building strategy, seen in all of its dimensions, and particularly with respect to training and re-training.

In writing about the first two of the five complementary strategies – creating centers and the education of parents – I would now put more emphasis on not only enhancing the knowledge that caregivers bring to the task but also, and perhaps more importantly, enhancing the development and the self-esteem of the adults involved directly in interaction with children. The idea is too narrow that adults can work well with children if they simply have knowledge about how a child develops and are taught some activities to be carried out with the child. Caregivers need to feel good about themselves if they are to be good caregivers. They also need to develop.

With some slight shifts of emphasis, then, and an occasional addition, the concepts and frameworks provided at the time of original writing seem as appropriate today as they were five years ago.

Programme examples and data

Inevitably, some of the specific information provided in this book is now dated. The figures given for programme coverage in Chapter 2 and in other parts of the book come from the mid or late 1980s. As examples, the figure of 650,000 given for Kenyan children in non-formal community pre-schools has grown to at least 900,000 (Kipkorir and Njenga, 1993). Coverage in the Integrated Child Development Service of India has increased from 35 percent to at least 40 percent of all blocks.

Moreover, some of the programmes described have changed character, sometimes considerably. As an example, the home day care in Venezuela that is described in Chapter 6 maintained a moderate coverage of approximately 10,000 children up to the year 1989 when it was selected by the government to be part of a massive extension of social programmes. During the period from 1989 to 1993, the programme grew in coverage to approximately 236,000 children. Moreover, the original model was modified in order to reduce costs per child. Day care mothers are now responsible for 8 children rather than 5. Supervisors cover 25 rather than 20 homes. A new model was created called a "multihogar," taking in up to 30 children. The population to be served was redefined to include not only the children of working mothers but also the children of families living in poverty. With this redefinition came a necessity to create a category of day care homes called "exonerated homes" for families that cannot contribute toward the costs of the care received by their children. Finally, in the expansion non-governmental organisations were asked to function as partners. (Ministerio de la Familia y Fundación del Niño, 1993)

In some cases, the cited programme no longer exists but has usually been replaced by another. That is the case for the example of home day care cited for Ecuador; despite its success, it disappeared and was replaced by another model. In these cases, it seems that the changes are more often related to political decisions than to an objective reading of evaluation results.

Although numbers have changed, the general conclusions in Chapter 2 about coverage still hold. Growth continues to be both significant and uneven. The greatest advances have been made in Latin America and Asia.

We continue, also, to lack good accounting systems that will let us know what the current coverage of early childhood programmes is. For the reader who is interested in data about ECCD projects and programmes in a particular country, perhaps the most accessible source of information is that provided in the various "Situation Analyses" that have been carried out as part of the process that UNICEF and national governments have developed to help determine where to put assistance priorities for the next period of time. These documents are in the public domain. and should be available from UNICEF offices. Another source of recent information is the set of periodic reports prepared by countries that are signatories to the Convention on the

Rights of the Child. In some cases governments have not made these public, but the information contained in them is supposed to be available to all. Information about "pre-primary education" can be found in the World Report on Education issued by UNESCO every two years.

Some omissions that should be corrected

Inevitably, also, omissions become obvious with the passage of time. For instance, were I to begin writing now, I would make an effort to include discussions of the following topics:

– child abuse
– disability
– children living in conditions of war or internal conflict

The programming principles espoused in the book are, in general, equally applicable to these topics, which represent special circumstances of child care and development. Looking back, it seems to me that my choice not to deal directly with them was influenced in part by a desire to counter the tendency in all of us to look first, and sometimes exclusively, at the extreme cases and to build programmes around them, i.e, to look at the one who dies but forget about the 12 who survive. But this bias should be modified, and the topics should be dealt with more forthrightly than I have done in this first edition or will do in this re-edition. In approaching these difficult topics, all of which have gained additional prominence over the last five years, I would insist on a combination of preventive and curative approaches.

Having revisited the conceptual bases for writing, having alerted the reader to the lag in specific information about ECCD programmes in particular countries, and having noted several omissions from the original writing, I now turn to a discussion of 1) some broad changes in the environment for ECCD programming, 2) some possible reasons for changes, and 3) some disturbing implications for future programming.

RECENT CHANGES AND THEIR IMPLICATIONS

An upsurge in attention

The concluding chapter of this book (Chapter 16) was written approximately five years ago, at a time when early childhood development had not yet captured the attention of the international community. It seemed appropriate at that time to dedicate part of the chapter to considering why the opportunity had not been seized to invest in ECCD when the arguments for doing so seemed to be so strong. I went on to suggest some things that could be done to help overcome the apparently tepid response from governments and international organisations, noted some special challenges and some priorities, and ended with an urgent call for action.

To some extent times have changed. During the last five years, there has been a selective upsurge in willingness of governments and international organisations to consider and mount programmes providing attention to children of pre-school age. This upsurge includes programmes that attend to the psycho-social as well as to the physical dimensions of early development. It includes programmes located variously within the education and health sectors, within social welfare organisations, and occasionally within other programmes dealing, for instance, with women or rural or urban development.

Part of this upsurge can be attributed to the growth of formal pre-school programs directed to children just before entering primary school, at ages 5 or 6. Indeed, "pre-school" may be the fastest growing sector within the field of education. Several countries of Latin America, for instance, now enroll more than 70 percent of their 5-year-olds in official pre-schools (Argentina, Chile, Mexico, and Venezuela). In a number of Third World countries, education for 5-year-olds has been (or is in the process of being) included as a compulsory grade within the formal education system. When the year immediately prior to primary schooling becomes universal, that part of the upper/middle class and urban bias associated with limited access to pre-schools is eliminated. In most cases, however, differences in the quality of pre-school education persist, related to social class and to urban or rural location, which have a social sorting effect similar to that previously associated with access. This makes attention to quality in preschool important for social as well as educational reasons.

Another part of the recent growth in ECCD comes from the expansion of so-called non-formal programmes. ("Non-formal" programmes are often very formal in the methodologies that they apply, but they are characterized as non-formal because in some sense they lie outside the formal, public system. The main distinguishing characteristic of most of these programmes is that locally hired caretakers are not paid for through the formal system.) Although it might be logical to assume that this non-formal growth is primarily a product of the continuing expansion and growing influence of non-governmental organisations managing innovative ECCD programmes, most such programmes run by NGOs continue to be small in scale. Indeed, although it may seem contradictory, the bulk of the expansion of non-formal programmes is financed by, and usually managed by, governments which apparently see a non-formal approach as a relatively inexpensive way of meeting needs and demands on a larger scale. That is the case, for instance, with the introduction and expansion of systems of home day care, particularly in Latin America.

In a very few cases, significant programmes of parental education are being created. However, attention to children in their earliest months and years in ECCD programmes through such programmes remains on the horizon in most countries or is still very limited.

One indicator of a change in attitude toward investment in ECCD is the level of availability of international funding. Five years ago international financing for ECCD programmes (which go beyond survival and growth considerations to include psycho-social development) was virtually restricted to remnants of UNICEF's Child Survival and Development funding and to some support from smaller international Foundations (such as the Bernard van Leer) or from international NGOs. In 1995, the World Bank, the Interamerican Development Bank, the Asian Development Bank and to a certain extent international bi-lateral organisations such as USAID and Canadian CIDA find themselves considering requests for loan or grant support of ECCD programmes. During this five-year period, the World Bank, for instance, has provided funds for ECCD programmes of various types in Nigeria, Mexico, Colombia, Bolivia, Chile, Argentina, Brazil, Venezuela, El Salvador, and India. ECCD programme discussions are being held between the Bank and governments of the Philippines, Malaysia, South Africa and Kenya.

Ironically, support for ECCD within UNICEF's Headquarters seems to have declined during this period, despite the fact that at least 70 field offices include support for ECCD in their programmes. To the continuing priority given to child survival, UNICEF has now added a primary school priority, with ECCD defined as a "supporting strategy".

In brief, there have been selective but significant changes in ECCD coverage and in the attitude toward investment in ECCD during the 1990–95 period.

Why the apparent change?

One possible explanation for the recent increases in attention to young children might be that the accumulation of knowledge and experience and the compelling arguments for investing in ECCD are now being recognised and acted upon. Although the accumulation of knowledge and experience and its presentation may have contributed in a minor way, this is clearly a minor force driving change.

Another possible explanation is that the changing objective circumstances and the pressing developmental needs of millions of children have finally been recognised, leading to action. This seems a more plausible hypothesis. We have noted continuing demographic, social and economic changes and their potentially debilitating effects on children (migration and concentration in cities, reduced mortality rates, increased labour force participation of women, the 1980s recession affecting most of the world).

These have created new developmental challenges and a need for alternative forms of child care. But the idea that these growing needs have been fully recognised or that their recognition automatically generates programmes is näive and is at best a partial explanation.

Although each of the above may have had some part in making ECCD programmes more prominent in 1995 than in 1990, several changing circumstances must be taken into consideration in explaining the change. These circumstances have little to do with knowledge or basic need and have more to do with general economic and political pressures experienced by countries. For instance:

1 *In response to economic problems of the 1980s, many governments adopted a neo-liberal economic strategy that, at least in the short run, has exacerbated economic inequalities and increased poverty levels.* Often, social programmes were cut as a part of economic adjustments. This not only has had a debilitating effect on the condition of children from poor families but also has produced a reaction expressed through increased pressure on governments to support compensatory social programmes, among which we find programmes to improve the survival and development of young children. This reappearance of social programmes may be seen either as an act of social conscience or as a means of avoiding conflicts leading to more fundamental change in society. The strategy has been supported of late by the World Bank and other international organizations through adjustments in their loan policies.

2 *The growing strength of NGOs and of a "civil society" has added to the political pressure on governments to democratize, decentralize and respond to disfavoured sectors of society in many parts of the Third World.* This has also helped to favour a rebirth and growth of social programmes that were cut back as economic adjustments were made, including attention to ECCD.

3 *Also in play are growing concerns centered on the preparation of children for school, related in turn to concerns about the efficiency and effectiveness of primary schools.* On one hand, there has been a growing pressure for affordable and effective preschooling from parents who want their children to do well in school. On the other hand, as primary school coverage has increased, a concern with efficiency and quality has grown. This shift in emphasis has led some governments to mount programmes that take advantage of the apparent causal connection between the preparation of children for school and repetition or dropout in the early years of primary school.

4 *To the above must be added effects of international organisation and lobbying activities in favour of children occurring over the past five years.* A great deal of this influence has resulted from activities originating in new attention to children's rights. The Convention of the Rights of the Child was approved by the General Assembly of the United Nations in 1989. A

Summit on Children (September 1990) and related follow-up efforts have led to the signing of the Convention by over 170 countries. A mechanism has been established whereby governments that are signatories to the Convention must report periodically on their efforts to conform to provisions of the Convention. Further, within the framework of the Convention, UNICEF offices throughout the world have worked closely and insistently with governments to create National Plans of Action to improve, among other things, the rights of children to integral development.

To these must be added the more modest influence resulting from the World Conference on Education for All that incorporated early childhood development into basic education. The International Year of the Family also helped focus attention on children.

These events and actions have helped to put children and ECCD "on the agenda," to shift attitudes, and to loosen at least some purse strings.

What have these changes produced?

To those who have dedicated their lives to furthering the cause of improved early childhood care and development, the above increase in attention may seem to be an extremely positive development. And it may be. However, both an analysis of the possible reasons for the recent upsurge in ECCD and a look at the way in which new programmes are being planned and executed gives one cause for caution if not concern.

1 *The "compensatory" undercurrent associated with many new programmes, for instance, runs counter to the "constructivist," participatory position that we have placed at the center in this book.* In most cases, compensatory programmes are handout programmes that begin with a centrally determined idea of what needs to be compensated. Such programmes do not do a good job of helping people to solve their own problems or of listening to them in order to identify their solutions, or of involving them in planning or management or evaluation.

2 *The overtly political origins and purposes of some ECCD programmes, while potentially positive, can lead to unfortunate consequences.* The desire of politicians to demonstrate that they are having a broad and significant effect on a problem in order to stay in power often leads to rapid, superficial and disorganized growth of programmes in which the principal preoccupation is with numbers and coverage; quality is often sacrificed. Programmes are not allowed to grow, learn and adjust along the way. They spring full-blown. Considerable pressure is placed on bureaucracies to standardize curricula and materials, so the logistics of rapid expansion can be handled more easily. This does not allow for cultural and regional differences. As a result, the programmes may be hard-pressed to show effects and

are open to criticism, sometimes leading to their undoing. In addition, the pressures to "go to scale" quickly place an unmanageable short-run burden on budgets, which in turn leads to a search for cheap alternatives, which in turn often results in second-rate programmes for those who are most in need—poor programmes for poor people.

The political origins of programmes can also bring with them adherence to a timetable set by the length of time of a period in office rather than by the length of time necessary to consult and construct. And, with changes of political regimes come discontinuities in programming that are destructive, undoing the positive accomplishments of the previous regime rather than building upon them and making needed adjustments. In addition, technical criteria for hiring, managing and locating are sometimes subordinated to political criteria. These time, hiring and continuity constraints make it difficult to strengthen institutions and to develop the cadre of human resources needed to carry out sustainable and effective programmes.

3 *Unfortunately, international pressures on governments and NGOs can reinforce the tendency to think in terms of the number of children "covered" in a programme rather than in terms of the children most in need and/or in terms of the quality of programmes.* International accounting and reporting systems still tend to be quantitative rather than qualitative. And national responses tend to be superficial to the extent that governments are responding to international pressures rather than responding because they are themselves convinced that ECCD is a good investment.

4 *The emphasis placed on formal pre-schools and on preparation for school has biased ECCD methods and content, leading to the extension downward of formal primary school methods in many places.* This extension helps to undercut the essence of many well-intentioned early childhood development programmes when placed together with an understandable desire by parents to be sure that their children know how to read and write, and with the growth of selection systems for entrance into primary schools in some places. Skills are taught pre-maturely and mechanically. Children are not allowed to learn in an active and creative manner through discovery and play. Emphasis is placed on cognitive development at the expense of social development.

The concerns listed above are legitimate concerns expressed by ECCD advocates and practitioners. We do not want cheap solutions for poor people. We would like to see effective programmes of good quality, not hastily conceived programmes focussing on children as *ciphers* rather than as *persons*. We do not want top-down, monolithic, culturally insensitive programmes. We do not want compensatory programmes that provide handouts, leave out the opinions and participation of the people being "served," and do little or nothing to change the conditions that cause debilitated or delayed development.

A SECOND CALL TO ACTION

Against this set of concerns, the "Call to Action" offered in Chapter 16 needs to be modified. Five years ago the call focussed on obtaining commitment to move beyond programmes emphasizing survival in order to give early childhood care and development the concerted attention it merits. The challenge seemed to be to put ECCD firmly on the agenda, to engage, to respond to opportunity, and to act aggressively so as to counteract a slow drifting toward greater but not necessarily improved attention to the needs of young children.

But against the description of changes and concerns described above, the problem today seems to be less one of urgently stirring people to action, although this is obviously still necessary in some places. Rather, our emphasis is on *assuring the effectiveness and quality of actions that are taken.* There is now reason to worry that rather than drifting into programmes that are "outmoded, monolithic, socially biased, bureaucratic, centralized, formal and uncreative," the field is moving consciously in that direction faster than is justified or prudent, propelled by political and bureaucratic interests rather than by a combination of social/humanitarian interests and technical knowledge and experience.

To meet the still unmet developmental needs of millions of children throughout the world, we again call upon communities, non-governmental organisations, governments and the international community to open themselves to new and worthy ventures and to move aggressively toward an enlightened programme of early childhood care and development. In this process we caution against allowing urgency and/or a quantitative view to replace need, knowledge, experience, quality and participation as prime programme criteria. We must be able to show much more for our efforts than that a large number of children are involved in some kind of ECCD programme. We must avoid creating second-rate programmes for the poor. We must insist on an active, constructive, culturally attuned approach to programming. Moreover, we must keep a human dimension at the center of all that we do. Our approach must stimulate and support local initiatives that will establish enduring processes and allow continuous learning from experience. And, while keeping attention firmly on the child, our call is also to seek, within early childhood programmes, opportunities for personal and collective development by adults and community members.

These must be our central challenges if we are to provide a genuine "fair start" for the (now) Fourteen Who Survive. Let us act accordingly, and with all due haste.

Robert G. Myers
January 1995
Mexico City

REFERENCES

Kipkorir, L.I., and A.W. Njenga. "A Case Study of Early Childhood Care and Education in Kenya," a paper prepared for the EFA Forum 1993, Nairobi, Kenya Institute of Education, September, 1993. (Mimeo.)

Ministerio de la Familia y Fundación del Niño. "Programa Hogares de Cuidado Diario. Plan de Extension Masiva: Venezuela, A Case Study," a paper prepared for the EFA Forum 1993, Caracas, Ministerio de la Familia, September 1993.

Name index

Subject index